Makeup for Asian Women

Makeup for Asian Women

Edited by
Erika De Smet

Larsen & Keller
www.larsen-keller.com

Makeup for Asian Women
Edited by Erika De Smet
ISBN: 978-1-63549-749-6 (Hardback)

Larsen & Keller
Published by Larsen and Keller Education,
5 Penn Plaza,
19th Floor,
New York, NY 10001, USA

Cataloging-in-Publication Data

Makeup for Asian women / edited by Erika De Smet.
p. cm.
Includes bibliographical references and index.
ISBN 978-1-63549-749-6
1. Beauty, Personal--Asia. 2. Cosmetics--Asia. 3. Beauty culture--Asia.
4. Women--Health and hygiene--Asia. I. De Smet, Erika.
GT499 .M35 2018
391.6--dc23

Table of Contents

Preface

Cosmetics and makeup are important aspects of beauty and fashion. Cosmetology has become an important industry in the care and styling of a person's appearance. Cosmetologists need to be familiar with makeup theory as well as be familiar with different effects of makeup. A number of modern professional makeup techniques have been elaborated in this text. Constant effort has been made to make the understanding of the difficult concepts of makeup as easy and informative as possible for the readers. This book attempts to assist those with a goal of delving into this field.

A detailed account of the significant topics covered in this book is provided below:

Chapter 1- The products that are used to improve an individual's appearance are known as cosmetics. Makeup that is commonly used comprises of skin cleansers, foundation, mascara, eyeliner, lipstick, mousse, etc. These products are mainly made up of mixtures of chemicals and natural products such as rose water and coconut oil. This chapter introduces the readers to the concept and application of makeup.

Chapter 2- There can be different ways of choosing makeup, as there are different tools for makeup. Companies can have different products for the same purpose. Some of the tools used by Asian women are rouge, eyelash curler, glitter, lotion, kohl and eyelash extensions. Those interested in the field of makeup will be greatly benefited from this section.

Chapter 3- Face base is mainly applied on the face and the neck area to hide scars and pimples and to create a uniform skin tone. It is mainly classified in different shades, such as warm, cool or neutral. Foundation can be applied by using either one's fingers or sponges and brushes. The topics discussed in this section focus on the methods and techniques used by Asian women for applying foundations and face powder.

Chapter 4- Lipsticks are applied on the lips to color them and to protect them from drying. Lipsticks have different shades, ranging from dark red to a nude shade. Matte, shimmery and normal lipsticks are distinctive types of lipsticks that are worn by women as per their taste. The following chapter explains to the readers the various kinds of lip makeup and how to apply it.

Chapter 5- This chapter focuses on the cosmetics used for eye makeup. Some of the products used for eye make up are false eyelashes, curlers, mascara, kohl and eye shadows. In order to completely understand the application of makeup on the eye, it is important to understand the manner in which make up tools are used. The section below elaborates the modern techniques and looks created with a range of eye makeup products.

I would like to make a special mention of my publisher who considered me worthy of this opportunity and also supported me throughout the process. I would also like to thank the editing team at the back-end who extended their help whenever required.

Editor

Chapter 1

Introduction to Makeup

The products that are used to improve an individual's appearance are known as cosmetics. Make-up that is commonly used comprises of skin cleansers, foundation, mascara, eyeliner, lipstick, mousse, etc. These products are mainly made up of mixtures of chemicals and natural products such as rose water and coconut oil. This chapter introduces the readers to the concept and application of makeup.

Cosmetics

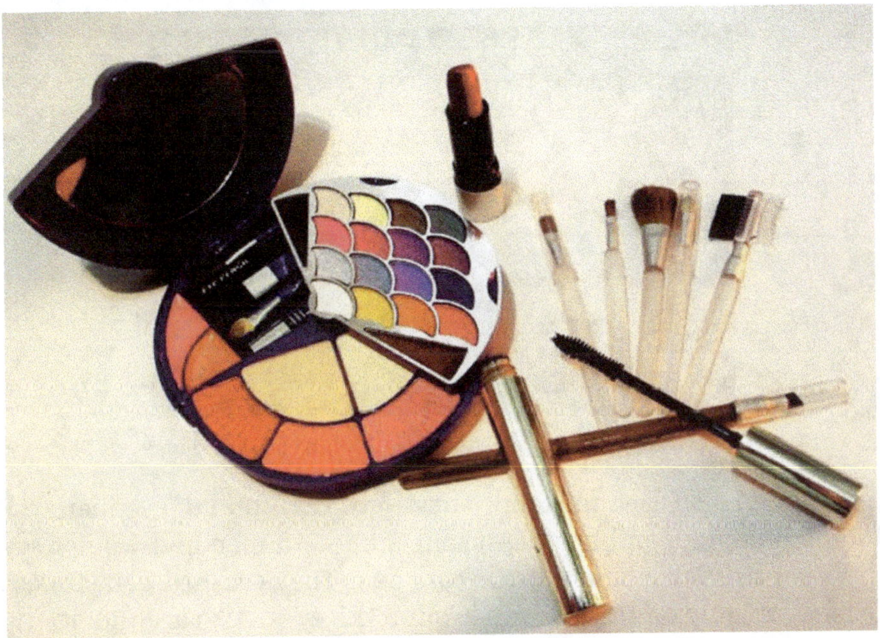

Assorted cosmetics and tools

Cosmetics, also known as make-up, are substances or products used to enhance or alter the appearance or fragrance of the body. Many cosmetics are designed for use of applying to the face and hair. They are generally mixtures of chemical compounds; some being derived from natural sources (such as coconut oil), and some being synthetics. Common cosmetics include lipstick, mascara, eye shadow, foundation, rouge, skin cleansers and skin lotions, shampoo, hairstyling products (gel, hair spray, etc.), perfume and cologne.

In the U.S., the Food and Drug Administration (FDA), which regulates cosmetics, defines cosmetics as "intended to be applied to the human body for cleansing, beautifying, promoting attractiveness, or altering the appearance without affecting the body's structure or functions". This broad definition includes any material intended for use as a component of a cosmetic product. The FDA specifically excludes soap from this category.

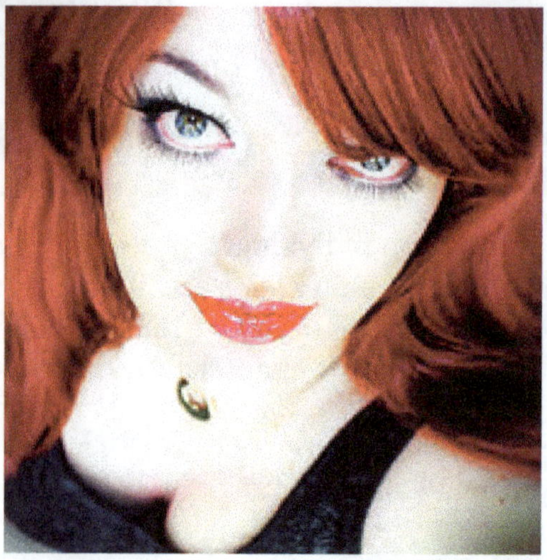

Woman wearing several forms of cosmetics, including lipstick, eye liner, eye shadow, and hair color

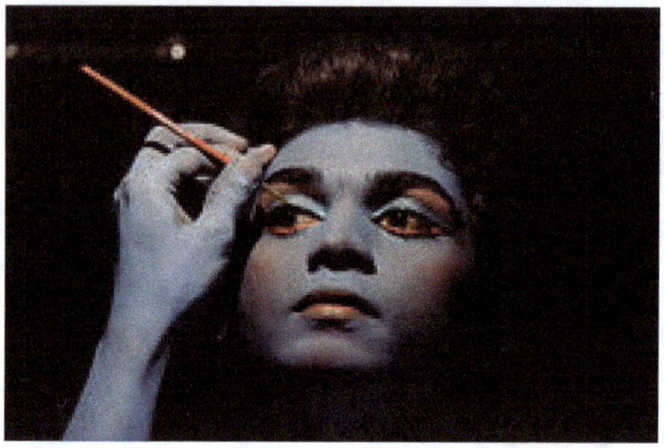

An artist applying make-up for an Indian classical dance

Egyptian women and men also used makeup. They were very fond of eyeliner and eyeshadows in dark colors including blue, red, and black. Ancient Sumerian men and women were possibly the first to invent and wear lipstick, about 5,000 years ago. They crushed gemstones and used them to decorate their faces, mainly on the lips and around the eyes. Also around 3000 BC to 1500 BC, women in the ancient Indus Valley Civilization applied red tinted lipstick to their lips for face decoration. Ancient Egyptians extracted red dye from fucus-algin, 0.01% iodine, and some bromine mannite, but this dye resulted in serious illness. Lipsticks with shimmering effects were initially made using a pearlescent substance found in fish scales. Six thousand year old relics of the hollowed out tombs of the Ancient Egyptian pharaohs are discovered. According to one source, early major developments include:

- Kohl used by ancient Egypt as a protective of the eye kohl
- Castor oil used by ancient Egypt as a protective balm.
- Skin creams made of beeswax, olive oil, and rose water, described by Romans.
- Vaseline and lanolin in the nineteenth century.

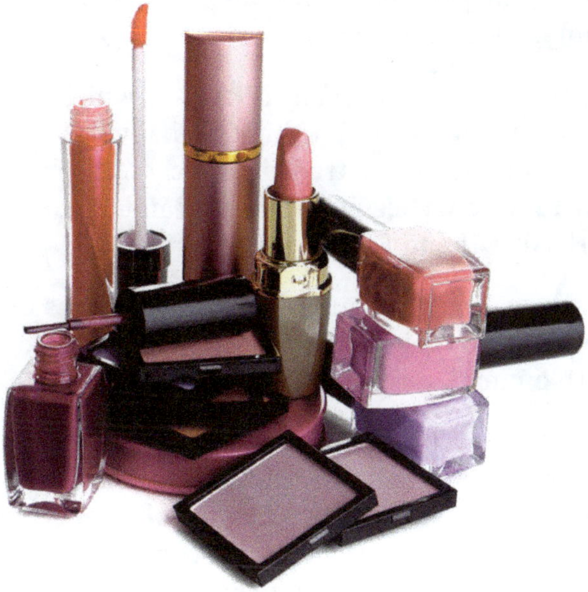

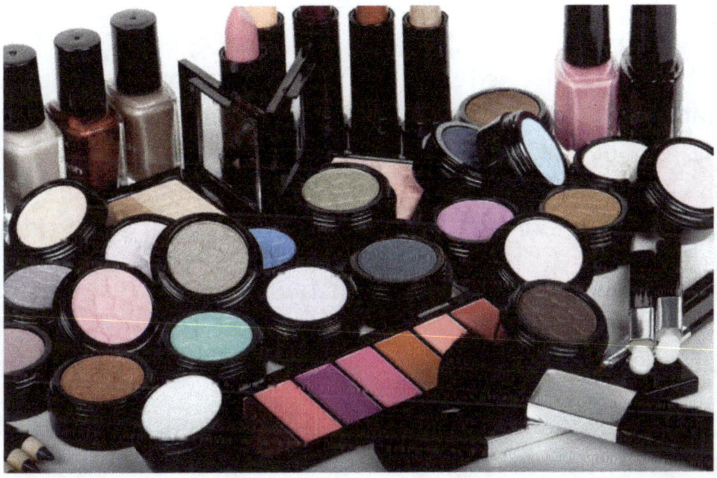

The Ancient Greeks also used cosmetics as the Ancient Romans did. Cosmetics are mentioned in the Old Testament, such as in 2 Kings 9:30, where Jezebel painted her eyelids—approximately 840 BC—and in the book of Esther, where beauty treatments are described.

One of the most popular traditional Chinese medicines is the fungus Tremella fuciformis, used as a beauty product by women in China and Japan. The fungus reportedly increases moisture retention in the skin and prevents senile degradation of micro-blood vessels in the skin, reducing wrinkles and smoothing fine lines. Other anti-ageing effects come from increasing the presence of superoxide dismutase in the brain and liver; it is an enzyme that acts as a potent antioxidant throughout the body, particularly in the skin.

Cosmetic use was frowned upon at many points in Western history. For example, in the 19th century, Queen Victoria publicly declared make-up improper, vulgar, and acceptable only for use by actors.

During the sixteenth century, the personal attributes of the women who used make-up created a demand for the product among the upper class.

As of 2016, the world's largest cosmetics company is L'Oréal, which was founded by Eugène Schueller in 1909 as the French Harmless Hair Colouring Company (now owned by Liliane Bettencourt 26% and Nestlé 28%; the remaining 46% is traded publicly). The market was developed in the US during the 1910s by Elizabeth Arden, Helena Rubinstein, and Max Factor. These firms were joined by Revlon just before World War II and Estée Lauder just after.

During the 18th century, there was a high number of incidences of lead-poisoning because of the fashion for red and white lead makeup and powder. This led to swelling and inflammation of the eyes, attacked tooth enamel, and caused skin to blacken. Heavy use was known to lead to death.

Although modern make-up has been traditionally used mainly by women, an increasing number of men are using cosmetics usually associated to women to enhance or cover their own facial features such as blemishes, dark circles, and so on. Concealer is commonly used by men. Cosmetics brands release products especially tailored for men, and men are increasingly using them.

Types

Cosmetics are intended to be applied externally. They include but are not limited to products that can be applied to the face: skin-care creams, lipsticks, eye and facial makeup, towelettes, and colored contact lenses; to the body: deodorants, lotions, powders, perfumes, baby products, bath oils, bubble baths, bath salts, and body butters; to the hands/nails: fingernail and toe nail polish, and hand sanitizer; to the hair: permanent chemicals, hair colors, hair sprays, and gels.

A subset of cosmetics is called "make-up", refers primarily to products containing color pigments that are intended to alter the user's appearance. Manufacturers may distinguish between "decorative" and "care" cosmetics.

Cosmetics that are meant to be used on the face and eye area are usually applied with a brush, a makeup sponge, or the fingertips.

Most cosmetics are distinguished by the area of the body intended for application.

- Primer comes in formulas to suit individual skin conditions. Most are meant to reduce the appearance of pore size, prolong the wear of makeup, and allow for a smoother application of makeup. Primers are applied before foundation or eyeshadows depending on where the primer is to be applied.
- Lipstick, lip gloss, lip liner, lip plumper, lip balm, lip stain, lip conditioner, lip primer, lip boosters, and lip butters: Lipsticks are intended to add color and texture to the lips and often come in a wide range of colors, as well as finishes such as matte, satin, and lustre. Lip stains have a water or gel base and may contain alcohol to help the product stay on leaving a matte look. They temporarily saturate the lips with a dye. Usually designed to be waterproof, the product may come with an applicator brush, rollerball, or could be applied with a finger. Lip glosses are intended to add shine to the lips and may add a tint of color, as well

as being scented or flavored for a pop of fun. Lip balms are most often used to moisturize, tint, and protect the lips. Some brands contain sunscreen.

- Concealer makeup covers imperfections of the skin. Concealer is often used for any extra coverage needed to cover blemishes, undereye circles, and other imperfections. Concealer is often thicker and more solid than foundation, and provides longer lasting, more detailed coverage as well as creating a fresh clean base for all the rest of the makeup.

Some formulations are intended only for the eye or only for the face. This product can also be used for contouring the face like ones nose, cheekbones, and jaw line to add a more defined look to the total face.

- Foundation is used to smooth out the face and cover spots, acne, blemishes, or uneven skin coloration. These are sold in a liquid, cream, or powder, or most recently a mousse. Foundation provides coverage from sheer to matt to dewey or full. Foundation primer can be applied before or after foundation to obtain a smoother finish. Some primers come in powder or liquid form to be applied before foundation as a base, while other primers come as a spray to be applied after the foundation to set the make-up and help it last longer throughout the day.
- Face powder sets the foundation, giving it a matte finish, and to conceal small flaws or blemishes. It can also be used to bake the foundation, so that it stays on longer. Tinted face powders may be worn alone as a light foundation so that the full face does not look as caked-up as it could.
- Rouge, blush, or blusher is cheek coloring to bring out the color in the cheeks and make the cheekbones appear more defined. Rouge comes in powder, cream, and liquid forms. Different blush colors are used to compliment different skin tones.
- Contour powders and creams are used to define the face. They can give the illusion of a slimmer face or to modify a face shape in other desired ways. Usually a few shades darker than the skin tone and matte in finish, contour products create the illusion of depth. A darker-toned foundation/concealer can be used instead of contour products for the same purpose.

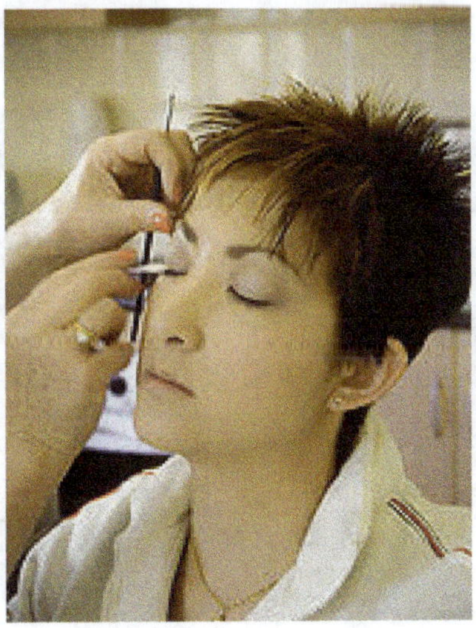

Eye shadow being applied

- Highlight, used to draw attention to the high points of the face as well as to add glow, comes in liquid, cream, and powder forms. It often contains a substance to provide shimmer. Alternatively, a lighter-toned foundation/concealer can be used.
- Bronzer gives skin a bit of color by adding a golden or bronze glow and highlighting the cheekbones, as well as being used for contouring. Bronzer is considered to be more of a natural look and can be used for an everyday wear. Bronzer enhances the color of the face while adding more of a shimmery look. It comes in either matte, semi matte/satin, or shimmer finishes.

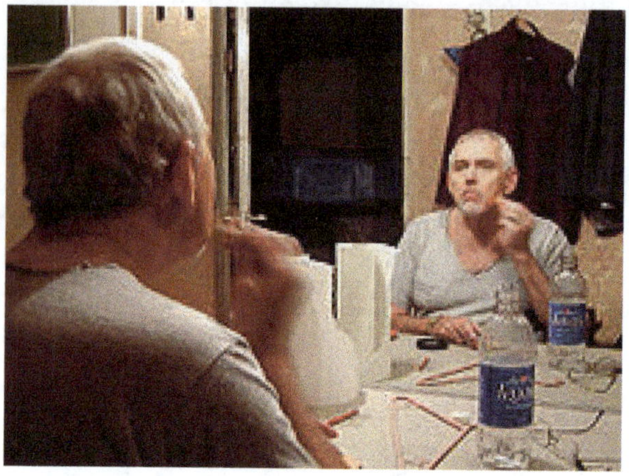

Broadway actor Jim Brochu applies make-up before the opening night of a play.

- Mascara is used to darken, lengthen, thicken, or draw attention to the eyelashes. It is available in various colors. Some mascaras include glitter flecks. There are many formulas, including waterproof versions for those prone to allergies or sudden tears. It is often used after an eyelash curler and mascara primer. Many mascaras have components to help lashes appear longer and thicker.
- Eye shadow is a pigmented powder/cream or substance used to accentuate the eye area, traditionally on above and under the eyelids. Many colours may be used at once and blended together to create different effects. This is conventionally applied with a range of eyeshadow brushes though it isn't uncommon for alternative methods of application to be used.

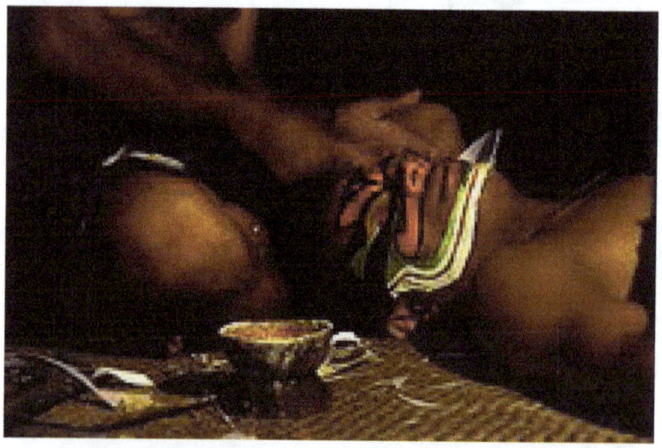

The chin mask known as *chutti* for Kathakali

- Eye liner is used to enhance and elongate the apparent size or depth of the eye. For example, white eyeliner on the waterline and inner corners of the eye makes the eyes look bigger and more awake. It can come in the form of a pencil, a gel, or a liquid and can be found in almost any color.
- Eyebrow pencils, creams, waxes, gels, and powders are used to color, fill in, and define the brows.
- Nail polish is used to color the fingernails and toenails. Transparent, colorless versions may strengthen nails or as a top or base coat to protect the nail or polish.
- Setting spray is used as the last step in the process of applying makeup. It keeps applied makeup intact for long periods. An alternative to setting spray is setting powder, which may be either pigmented or translucent. Both of these products are claimed to keep make-up from absorbing into the skin or melting off.
- False eyelashes are used when exaggerated eyelashes are desired. Their basic design usually consists of human hair or synthetic materials attached to a thin cloth-like band, which is applied with glue to the lashline. Designs vary in length and color. Rhinestones, gems, and even feathers and lace occur on some false eyelash designs.
- Contouring is designed to give shape to an area of the face. The aim is to enhance the natural shading on your face to give the illusion of a more defined facial structure which can be altered to preference. Brighter skin coloured makeup products are used to 'highlight' areas which we want to draw attention to or to be caught in the light. Whereas darker shades are used to create a shadow. These light and dark tones are blended on the skin to create the illusion of a more definite face shape. It can be achieved using a "contour palette" - which can be either cream or powder.

Cosmetics can be also described by the physical composition of the product. Cosmetics can be liquid or cream emulsions; powders, both pressed and loose; dispersions; and anhydrous creams or sticks.

Makeup remover is a product used to remove the makeup products applied on the skin. It cleans the skin before other procedures, like applying bedtime lotion.

Products

Cleansing is a standard step in skin care routines. Skin cleaning include some or all of these steps or cosmetics:

- Toners are used after cleansing the skin to freshen it up, boost the appearance of one's complexion, and remove any traces of cleanser, mask, or makeup, as well to help restore the skin's natural pH. They are usually applied to a cotton pad and wiped over the skin, but can be sprayed onto the skin from a spray bottle. Toners typically contain alcohol, water, and herbal extracts or other chemicals depending on skin type whether oily, dry, or combination. Toners containing alcohol are quite astringent, and usually targeted at oily skins. Dry or normal skin should be treated with alcohol-free toners. Witch hazel solution is a popular toner for all skin types, but many other products are available. Many toners contain salicylic acid and/or benzoyl peroxide. These types of toners are targeted at oily skin types, as well as acne-prone skin.

- Facial masks are treatments applied to the skin and then removed. Typically, they are applied to a dry, cleansed face, avoiding the eyes and lips.
    - Clay-based masks use kaolin clay or fuller's earth to transport essential oils and chemicals to the skin, and are typically left on until completely dry. As the clay dries, it absorbs excess oil and dirt from the surface of the skin and may help to clear blocked pores or draw comedones to the surface. Because of its drying actions, clay-based masks should only be used on oily skins.
    - Peel masks are typically gel-like in consistency, and contain acids or exfoliating agents to help exfoliate the skin, along with other ingredients to hydrate, discourage wrinkles, or treat uneven skin tone. They are left on to dry and then gently peeled off. They should be avoided by people with dry skin, as they tend to be very drying.
    - Sheet masks are a relatively new product that are becoming extremely popular in Asia. Sheet masks consist of a thin cotton or fiber sheet with holes cut out for the eyes and lips and cut to fit the contours of the face, onto which serums and skin treatments are brushed in a thin layer; the sheets may be soaked in the treatment. Masks are available to suit almost all skin types and skin complaints. Sheet masks are quicker, less messy, and require no specialized knowledge or equipment for their use compared to other types of face masks, but they may be difficult to find and purchase outside Asia.
- Exfoliants are products that help slough off dry, dead skin cells to improve the skin's appearance. This is achieved either by using mild acids or other chemicals to loosen old skin cells, or abrasive substances to physically scrub them off. Exfoliation can even out patches of rough skin, improve circulation to the skin, clear blocked pores to discourage acne and improve the appearance and healing of scars.
    - Chemical exfoliants may include citric acid (from citrus fruits), acetic acid (from vinegar), malic acid (from fruit), glycolic acid, lactic acid, or salicylic acid. They may be liquids or gels, and may or may not contain an abrasive to remove old skin cells afterwards.
    - Abrasive exfoliants include gels, creams or lotions, as well as physical objects. Loofahs, microfiber cloths, natural sponges, or brushes may be used to exfoliate skin, simply by rubbing them over the face in a circular motion. Gels, creams, or lotions may contain an acid to encourage dead skin cells to loosen, and an abrasive such as microbeads, sea salt, sugar, ground nut shells, rice bran, or ground apricot kernels to scrub the dead cells off the skin. Salt and sugar scrubs tend to be the harshest, while scrubs containing beads or rice bran are typically very gentle.

- Moisturizers are creams or lotions that hydrate the skin and help it to retain moisture; they may contain essential oils, herbal extracts, or chemicals to assist with oil control or reducing irritation. Night creams are typically more hydrating than day creams, but may be too thick or heavy to wear during the day, hence their name. Tinted moisturizers contain a small amount of foundation, which can provide light coverage for minor blemishes or to even out skin tones. They are usually applied with the fingertips or a cotton pad to the entire face, avoiding the lips and area around the eyes. Eyes require a different kind of moisturizer compared with the rest of the face. The skin around the eyes is extremely thin and sensitive, and is often the first area to show signs of aging. Eye creams are typically very light lotions or gels, and are usually very gentle; some may contain ingredients such as caffeine or Vitamin K to reduce puffiness and dark circles under the eyes. Eye creams or gels should be applied over the entire eye area with a finger, using a patting motion.

Other Products

There are two categories of personal care products. The Federal Food, Drug, and Cosmetic Act defines cosmetics as products intended to cleanse or beautify (for instance, shampoos and lipstick). A separate category exists for medications, which are intended to diagnose, cure, mitigate, treat, or prevent disease, or to affect the structure or function of the body (for instance, sunscreens and acne creams). Some products, such as moisturizing sunscreens and anti-dandruff shampoos, are regulated within both categories. There are also many types of tools used such as makeup brushes or face sponges.

Ingredients

A variety of organic compounds and inorganic compounds comprise typical cosmetics. Typical organic compounds are modified natural oils and fats as well as a variety of petrochemically derived agents. Inorganic compounds are processed minerals such as iron oxides, talc, and zinc oxide. The oxides of zinc and iron are classified as pigments, i.e. colorants that have no solubility in solvents.

Natural

Handmade and certified organic products are becoming more mainstream, due to the fact that certain chemicals in some skincare products may be harmful if absorbed through the skin. Products claimed to be organic should, in the U.S., be certified "USDA Organic".

Mineral

The term "mineral makeup" applies to a category of face makeup, including foundation, eye shadow, blush, and bronzer, made with loose, dry mineral powders. These powders are often mixed with oil-water emulsions. Lipsticks, liquid foundations, and other liquid cosmetics, as well as compressed makeups such as eye shadow and blush in compacts, are often called mineral makeup if they have the same primary ingredients as dry mineral makeups. However, liquid makeups must contain preservatives and compressed makeups must contain binders, which dry mineral makeups do not. Mineral makeup usually does not contain synthetic fragrances, preservatives, parabens, mineral oil, and chemical dyes. For this reason, dermatologists may consider mineral makeup to be gentler to the skin than makeup that contains those ingredients. Some minerals are nacreous or pearlescent, giving the skin a shining or sparking appearance. One example is bismuth oxychloride. There are various mineral-based makeup brands, including: Bare Minerals, Tarte, Bobbi Brown, and Stila.

Benefits of Mineral-based Makeup

Although some ingredients in cosmetics may cause concerns, some are widely seen as beneficial. Titanium dioxide, found in sunscreens, and zinc oxide have anti-inflammatory properties.

Mineral makeup is noncomedogenic (as long as it does not contain talc) and offers a mild amount of sun protection (because of the titanium dioxide and zinc oxide).

Because they do not contain liquid ingredients, mineral makeups have long shelf-lives.

Careers

An account executive is responsible for visiting department and specialty stores with counter sales of cosmetics. They explain new products and "gifts with purchase" arrangements (free items given out upon purchase of cosmetics items costing over some set amount).

A beauty adviser provides product advice based on the client's skin care and makeup requirements. Beauty advisers can be certified by an Anti-Aging Beauty Institute.

A cosmetician is a professional who provides facial and body treatments for clients. The term cosmetologist is sometimes used interchangeably with this term, but the former most commonly refers to a certified professional. A freelance make-up artist provides clients with beauty advice and cosmetics assistance. They are usually paid by the hour by a cosmetic company; however, they sometimes work independently.

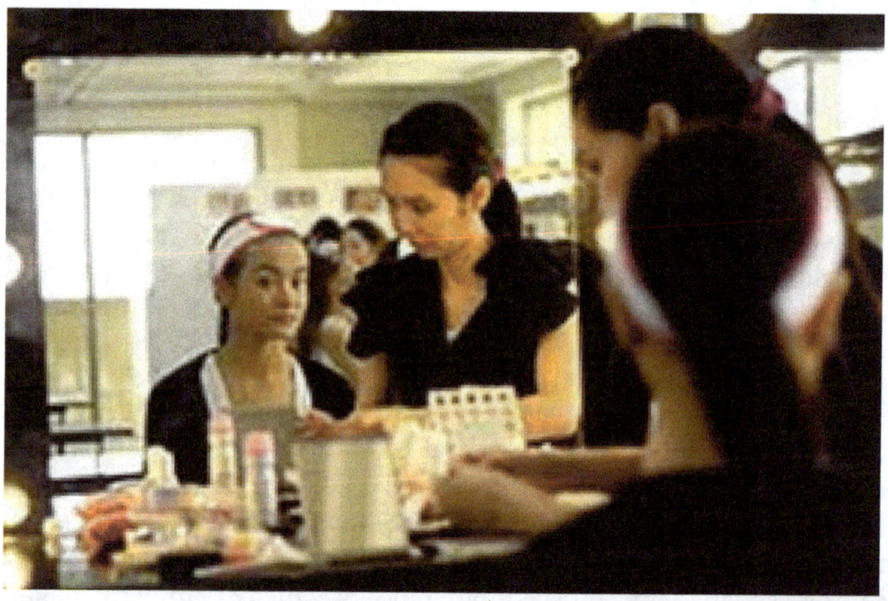

A professional make-up artist servicing a client

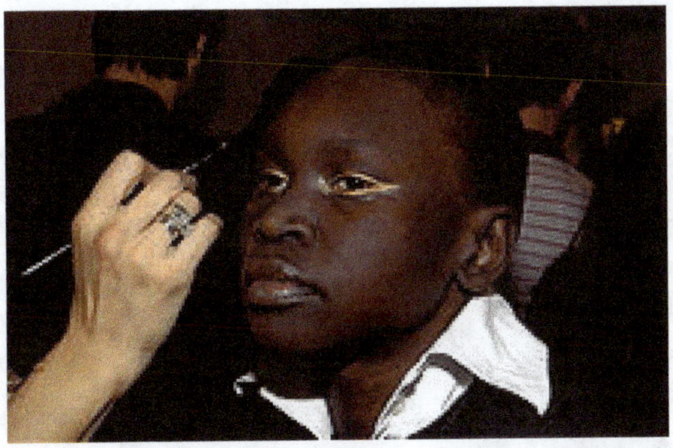

Model Alek Wek receiving make-up from a professional.

Professionals in cosmetics marketing careers manage research focus groups, promote the desired brand image, and provide other marketing services (sales forecasting, allocation to retailers, etc.).

Many involved within the cosmetics industry often specialize in a certain area of cosmetics such as special effects makeup or makeup techniques specific to the film, media, and fashion sectors.

How to Apply Makeup

Prep your face with moisturizer and primer, then apply foundation. Apply some concealer, if needed, and blend it in. Follow up with your choice of blush, lipstick, eyeshadow, eyeliner, and mascara. Once you get the hang of it, you can step things up with contouring to help emphasize your facial features.

Makeup Application Chart

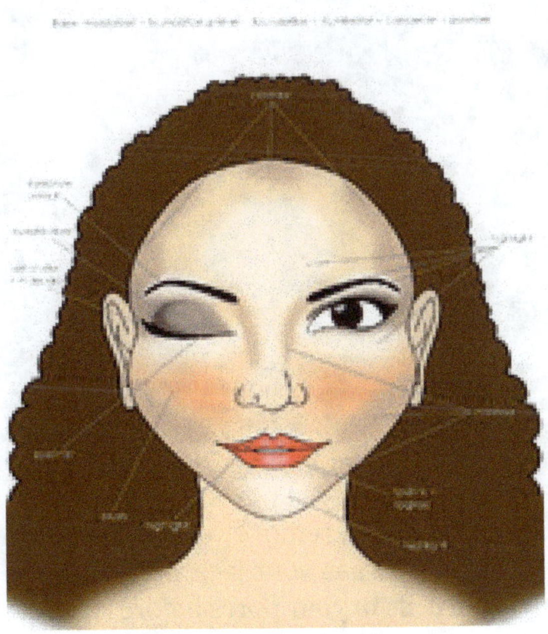

Makeup Application Chart

Part 1

Preparing Your Face

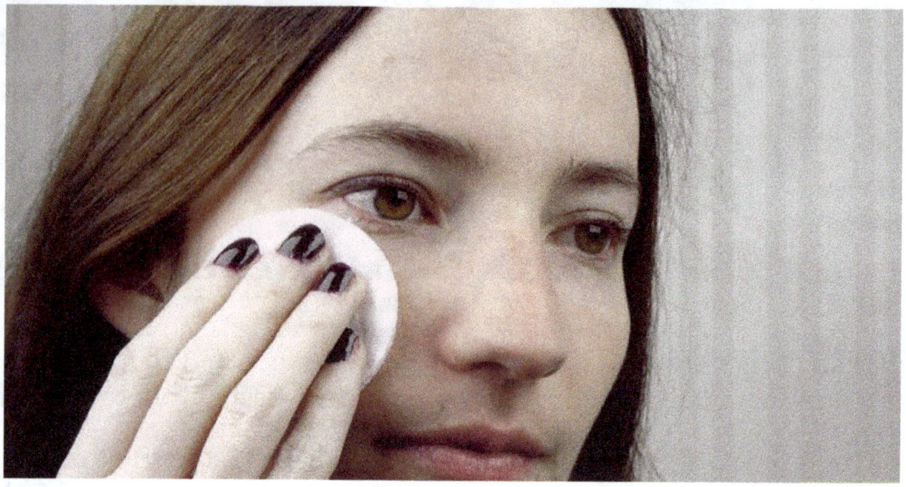

1. Remove any old makeup. When you're applying makeup, it is necessary to start with a clean palette. Remove any makeup that you might have slept in, and wash off makeup from earlier on in the day. If you try to apply more makeup over the top of old makeup (not including touch ups), your end look will appear caked on and more unnatural than makeup put on a fresh face. You also need to cleanse any makeup residue to keep your skin from getting clogged and irritated. You can use a good makeup remover or a mild baby oil to get rid of all makeup residues.

- Keep in mind that you should always remove your makeup at the end of the day; sleeping with your makeup on can clog your pores and cause blemishes and wrinkles.

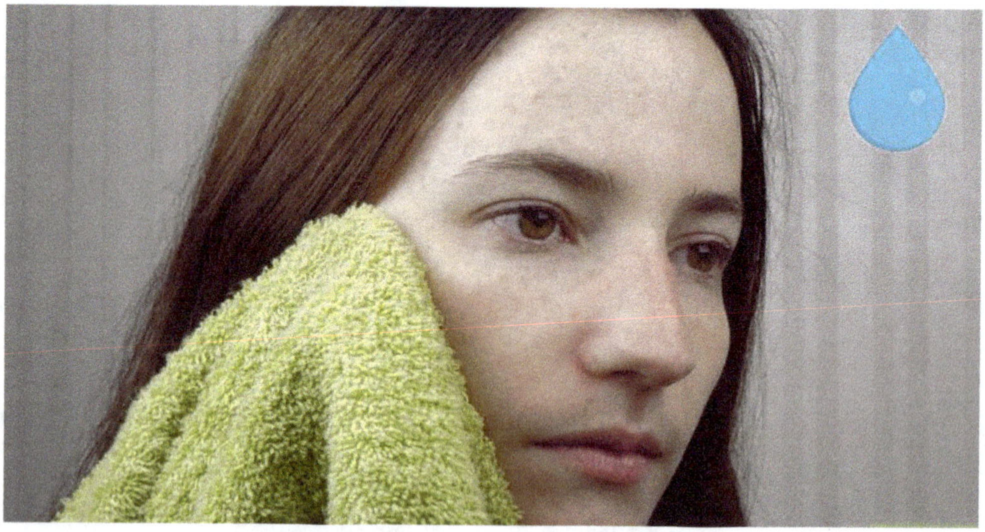

2. Wash your face. For the same reason you remove your old makeup, you should also wash your face. Use a mild facial cleanser to gently wash your face, spending about one minute of massaging to remove all bacteria and dead skin cells in your pores before rinsing with cool water. Finish up by applying a facial moisturizer, regardless of your skin type.

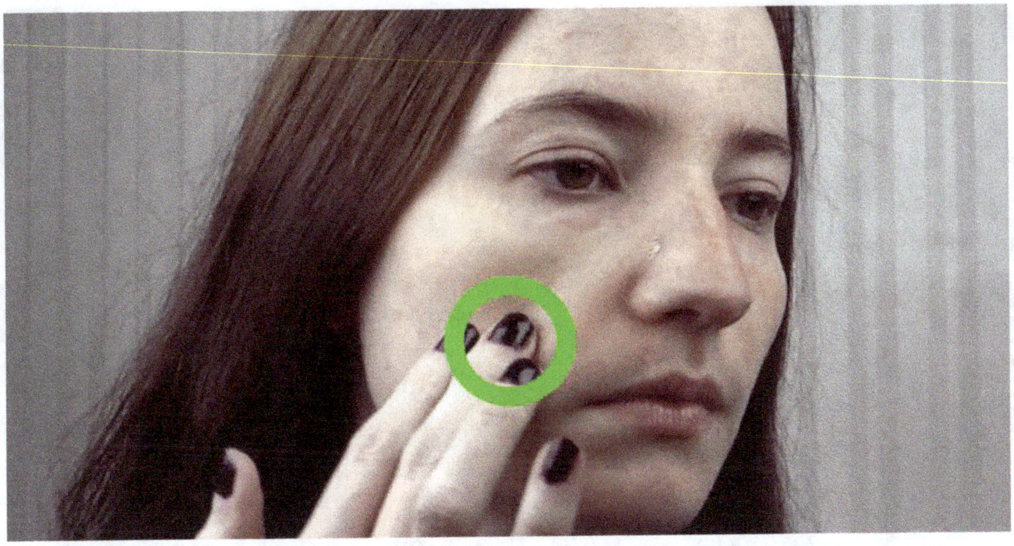

3. Prime your face. Before you add any makeup you need to prime your face. The purpose of a face primer is to enhance the appearance of makeup and increase the longevity. You can apply the primer with your fingers, covering your whole face with a small amount.

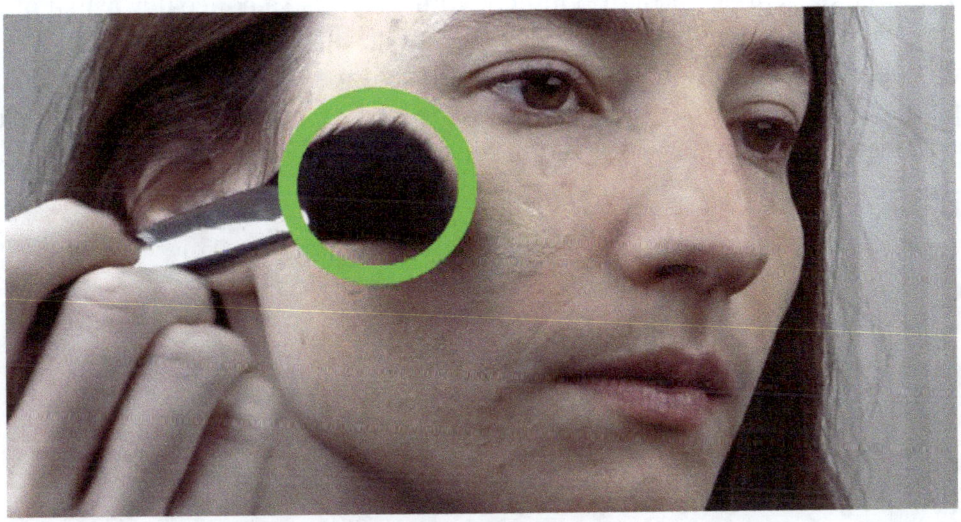

4. Put on a coat of foundation. There are several types of foundation, but they are generally applied the same way. Liquid, cream, and powder foundations all act to create a more even complexion, working to create a even base for your other makeup. Use a foundation brush or damp beauty sponge to apply foundation to your face, blending into your neck and earlobes if necessary. Keep in mind that your foundation should be the same color as your natural skin tone, not much darker or lighter. It helps to match your foundation to your chest and neck so your face isn't a different color then the rest of your body.

- You can use a concealer brush to add a little extra foundation to cover up stubborn blemishes.
- Liquid foundation can be applied with your fingertips, although this is more likely to introduce bacteria to your skin and cause future breakouts.

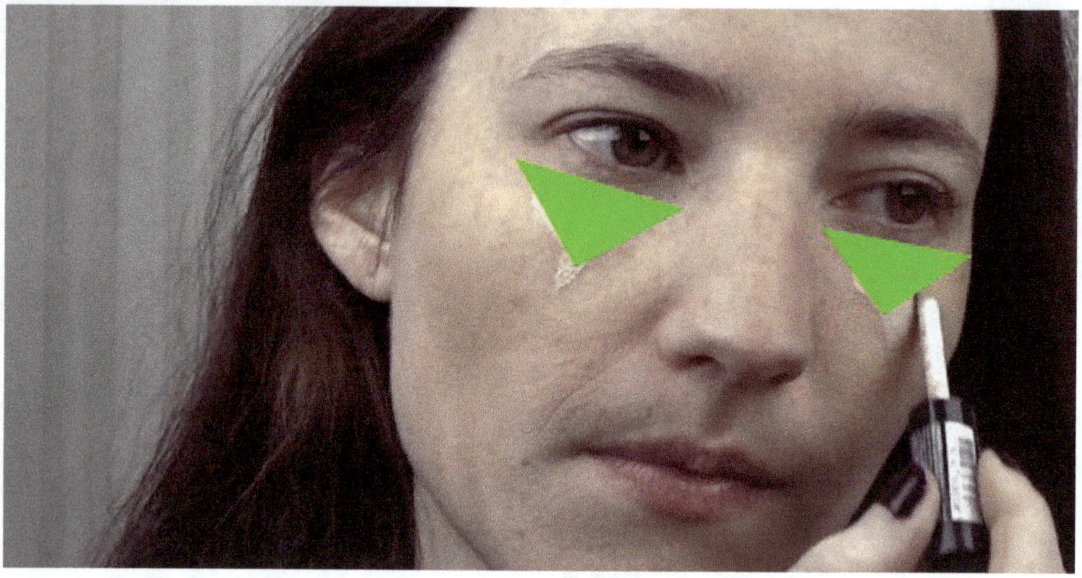

5. Apply your concealer. The purpose of concealer is to even out uneven skin tone as a result of blemishes or dark under-eye circles. You can also use a concealer in a shade slightly lighter in your skin tone to brighten dark areas or high points of your face. Use a concealer brush or your (clean) fingertips to blend concealer on your undereye area in an upside down triangle shape, down the bridge of your nose, chin, center of forehead, and above upper lip. You can use a shade matching your skin tone to cover any red areas or over any acne or dark spots. Blend the edges of your concealer so it seamlessly blends in to your foundation.

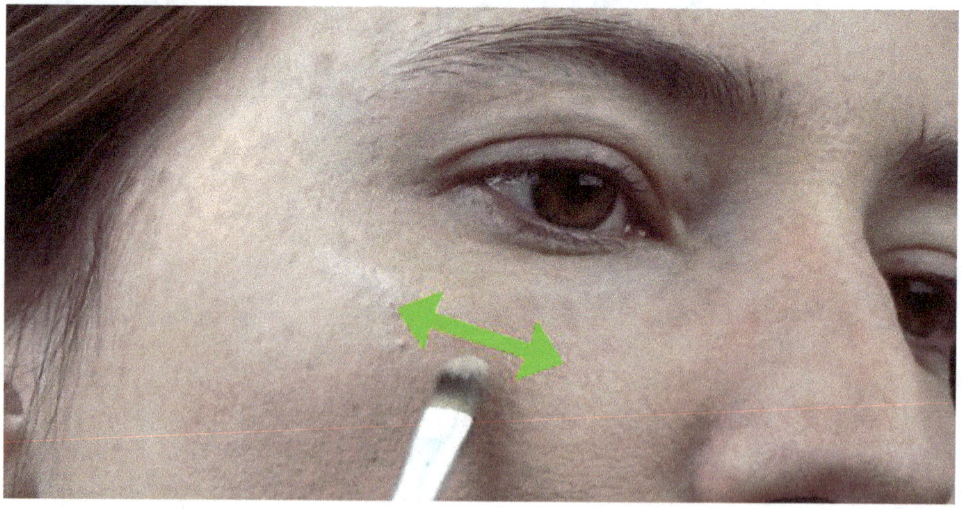

6. Set your foundation and concealer. This step is optional, but if you're looking for long-lasting, crease free makeup you should use a setting powder to hold your foundation and concealer in place. Use a damp beauty sponge to pick up loose powder and press into the under eye area, then gently sweep off any excess with a brush. Use a large, fluffy brush to cover your whole face in a translucent or matching setting powder. This step is particularly useful if you're using liquid foundation, as it will help to set the foundation and remove any shine or tackiness.

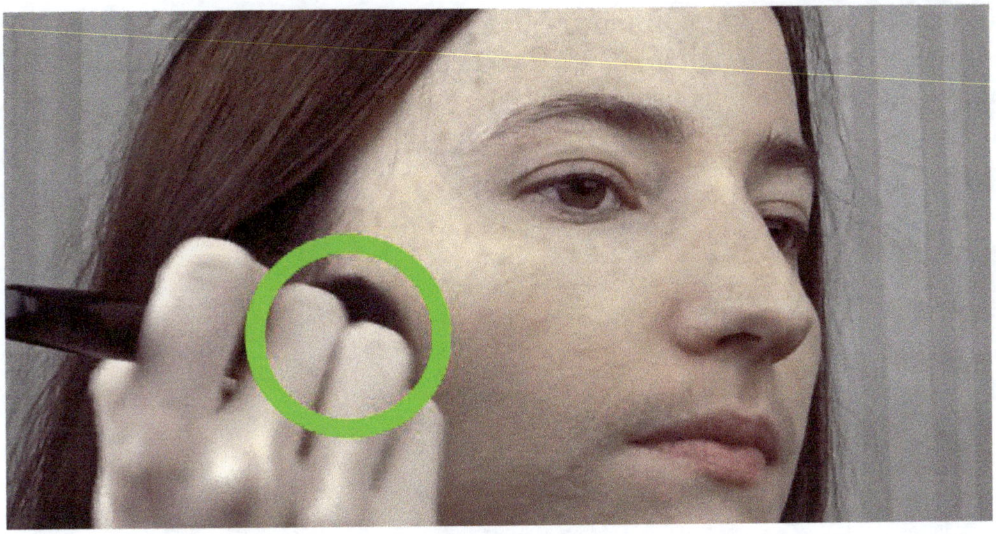

7. Apply a highlighter. With your foundation completed, it is likely that your face now looks contour-less and flat because of the uniform color. In order to provide some depth, you'll need to create the illusion of highlights and shadows. You can use a cream (apply before you set your face) or powder highlighter to brighten up the deepest areas of your face: the inside corners of your eyes, underneath your eyebrows, in the center of your cupid's bow, and on the tops/sides of your cheekbones. This will make your face look more bright and awake than it would otherwise.

- Create a '3' shape on your cheekbones, into your eyebrows, and up to your forehead for the perfect highlight.
- You can use your fingers or a small highlighter brush to apply the highlighter.

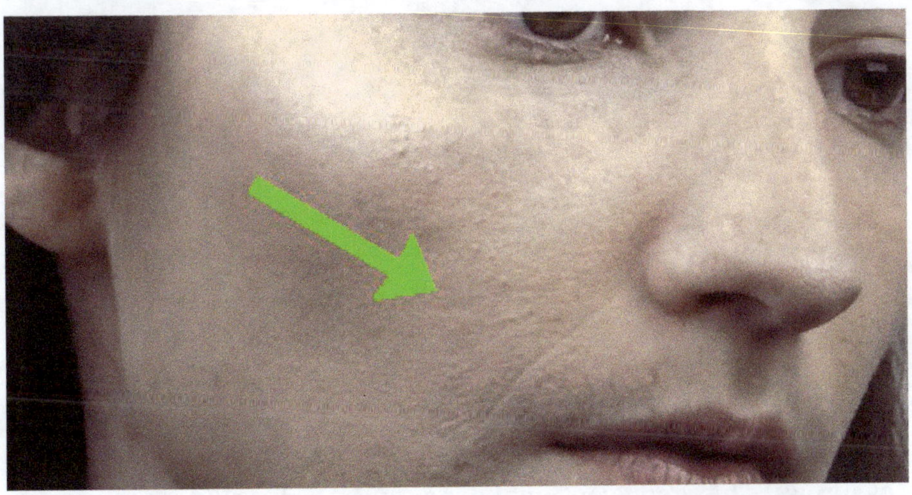

8. Add depth with contouring. The opposite of bringing out the highlights on your face, contouring involves adding a powder that is a few shades darker than your actual skin tone (different than a bronzer) to the areas you want to look minimized or further away. Typically, you should contour under your cheekbones in the hollows of your cheeks, on the sides of your nose, and under your jawline. You can also make a large forehead appear smaller by applying contour near your hair-

line. This will make your face look thinner and longer in appearance, and provide the shadows that naturally occur without foundation. After you contour your face, you can go in with bronzer to add color to your face. Use a big bronzing brush and buff out your bronzer right over where you contoured.

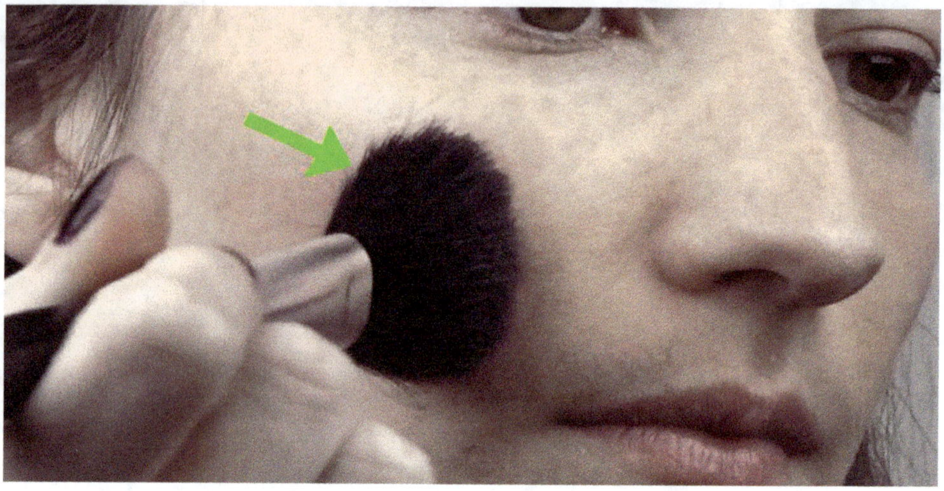

9. Apply a little blush. The final step in prepping your face is to add blush to your cheeks. Everyone's cheeks have a bit of color, but this color varies for every person. Apply your blush with large brush on the apples of your cheeks (the round part that forms when you smile). Don't go too heavy with your blush, just add enough to replenish the color that would form naturally.

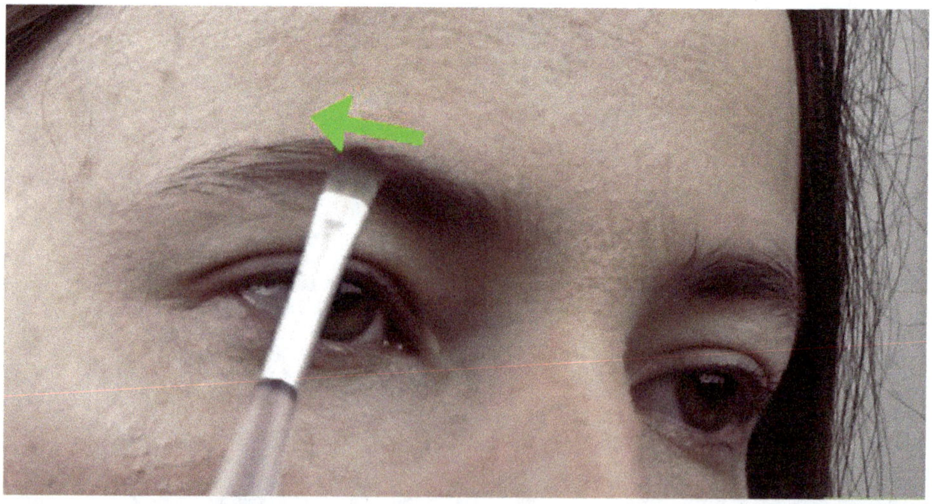

10. Fill in your eyebrows. This step is optional depending on the fullness of your eyebrows, but is generally recommended for those who have thin or sparse eyebrows. Select a color of brow pencil, powder, or pomade that is close to your natural hair color. Start by outlining the edges of your eyebrows with small dashing motions to mimic hair, and then fill in the center using the same small strokes. Go in the same direction of your hair growth, and set with a clear or tinted brow gel to make them stay all day.

Part 2

Adding Your Eye Makeup

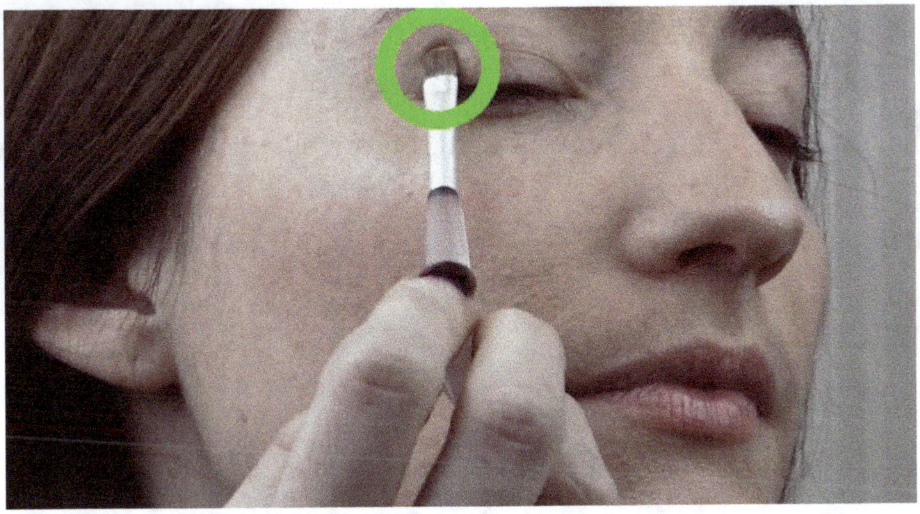

1. Apply an eyeshadow primer. This is another optional product, but applying an eyeshadow primer will help your eyeshadow to stay on for much longer. If you've gone without it, you may have noticed that your eyeshadow fades or becomes oily and collects in the creases of your eyelids after several hours. Use your fingertip to dab on your eyeshadow primer, blending it from the roots of your lashes to the top of your crease. Set with a powder to make a perfect base for blending your eyeshadow.

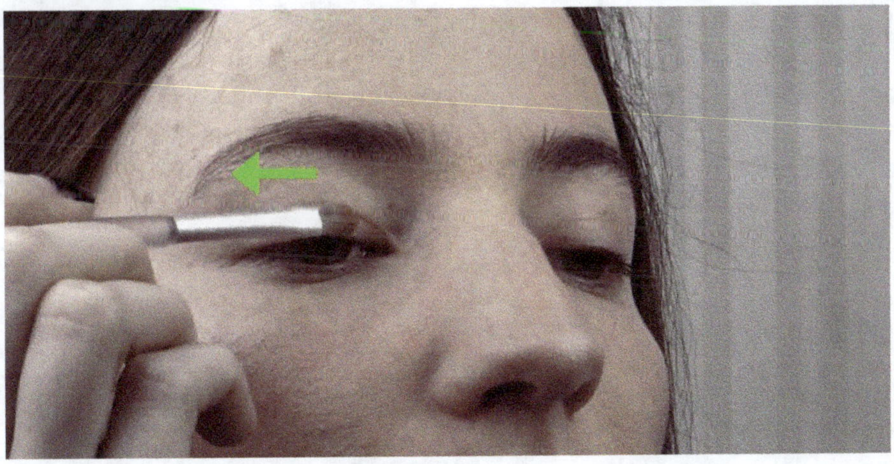

2. Put on your eyeshadow. There are many ways to apply eyeshadow, although the most basic and classic look is to apply a single color over the entirety of your eyelid. Use an eyeshadow brush to apply your eyeshadow to your eyelid, starting in the center near your lash line and blending outwards. Fade your eyeshadow into your natural skin tone near your crease and the inside and outside corners of your eyes, to prevent any harsh lines from forming. If you want a bit more dramatic look, apply a second darker matte color of eyeshadow in a 'C' shape from the outside corner of your lash line up to the top, outer ⅓ of your eyelid crease. Finish by sweeping a lighter shimmer color starting from the inner corner and ending in the middle, blending with the rest.

- Your main color of eyeshadow should never go all the way to your eyebrow, and should not extend further off your lid than the end of your eyebrow (unless you're going for a very dramatic look).
- You may, however, highlight your browbone (the area under your eyebrow but above your crease) by applying a lighter shade of eyeshadow. Be sure to use natural colors such as cream, sand, or white, if your skin is pale. Alternatively, try a nude shade slightly lighter than your skintone. The color doesn't have to be matte, but any sparkle it does have should be subtle.
- You can blend your eyeshadow onto your lower lid, sweeping the shadow along the lower lash line starting from the outside corner. Blend well so you don't have a harsh line.
- If you use multiple colors of eyeshadow, always be sure to blend them together.

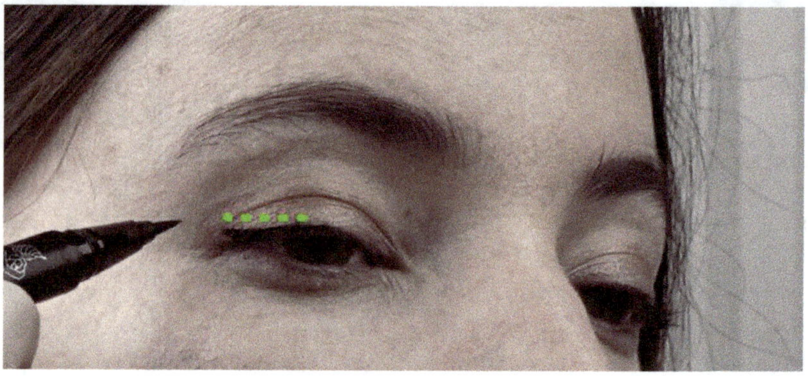

3. Apply your eyeliner. The purpose of eyeliner is to provide the illusion of a fuller lash line; therefore, choose a color that is similar to your natural hair color (or brown if you have blond hair) to go along your lashes. For a smudgy look, use an eyeliner pencil, or create a sleek and smooth look by using cream or liquid eyeliner. Create a dashed or dotted line across your lash line, and then connect the dots to create a full, continuous line. You can choose to wing the end up and outwards a bit if you want, otherwise you simply need to follow your lash line from the inside corner to the outside corner.

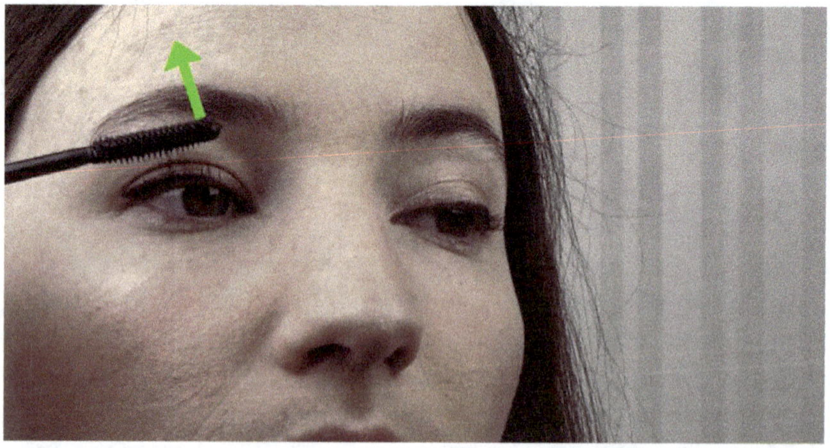

- Adding eyeliner to your bottom lash line should be done sparingly, as it will create a much darker/bolder look and appear a bit more unnatural than eyeliner on your top lash line only.

- If you feel comfortable, try tight-lining your eyes by using your eyeliner on the waterline of your eyelid.

4. Finish off with mascara. To complete your eye makeup, you'll need to top off your eyes with a bit of mascara. There are several mascaras to choose from depending on the look you want; if you have short lashes, use a mascara that will add length, or if you have thin lashes, use a volumizing mascara. Dip the brush in the mascara once and lightly wipe off the excess onto the edge of the container or a paper towel. Looking straight forward, apply it to the top lash with upward strokes. Start with the inner part of your eye and work your way outward. Do both eyes with two coats, then let dry. You can also apply mascara to your bottom lashes if you like.

- Wiggle the brush as you apply it, as this will help to coat between lashes instead of just the under layer.
- Never pump your mascara brush in and out of the mascara, as this causes air pockets.
- Avoid applying more than two coats of mascara, as this will take away the natural darkening look and give a cake-y thick look that is much less natural.
- A good trick for making your lashes look fuller is to apply a coat of baby powder between coats of mascara; this will add a bit of length and volume to your lashes.

Part 3

Adding Color to Your Lips

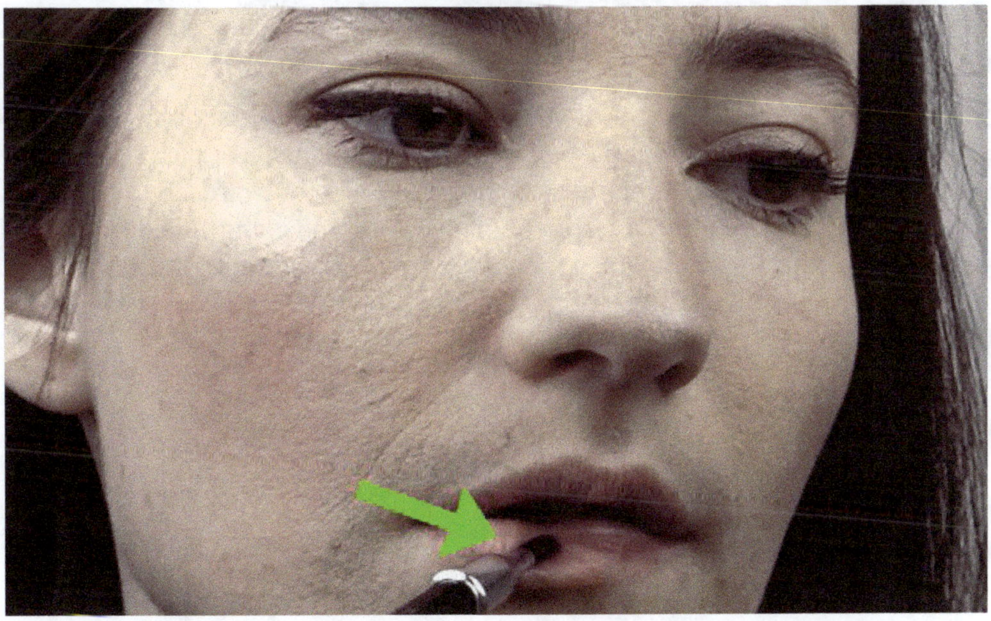

1. Smooth out your lips. Apply lip balm, primer, or sealer. This will help make all lip products applied last longer and much more vibrant. Additionally, who doesn't prefer soft lips? Adding a good balm or salve will prevent your lips from flaking later in the day.

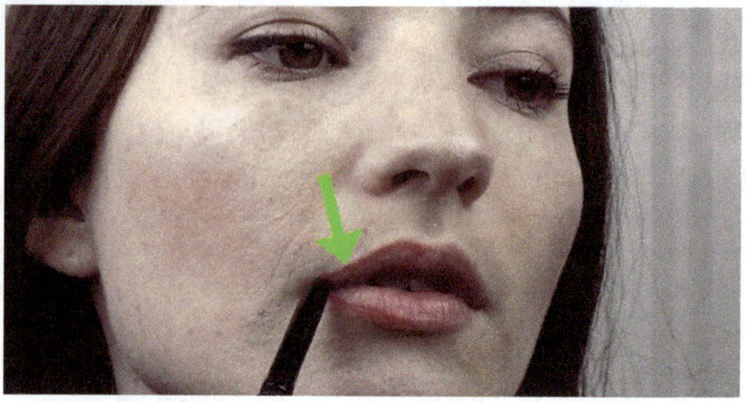

2. Apply lip liner. Line your lips with a liner that matches your lip color or the color you are going to apply. Sharpen your lip liner, and line around the natural line of your lips. With your lips outlined, use the pencil to continue filling in your lips. This works to even out the color and texture of your lips, making it easier to apply a gloss or lipstick later.

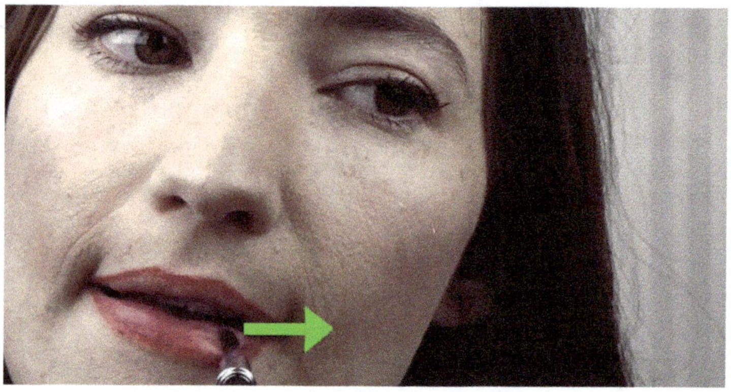

3. Apply lipstick or lip gloss with a brush or straight from the tube. Select a lipstick or gloss of your choice to go over your lipliner; for a natural look stick with a nude shade, or pick a bright hue for a more bold appearance. Start in the center of your lip, and blend the color outwards. Be sure to apply the color as close to the edges of your lips as you can without overdoing it and going outside your lip line. To prevent any lipstick from getting on your teeth, stick your index finger straight into your mouth and pull it out quickly; any excess color will stick to your finger and avoid being transferred to your teeth later on.

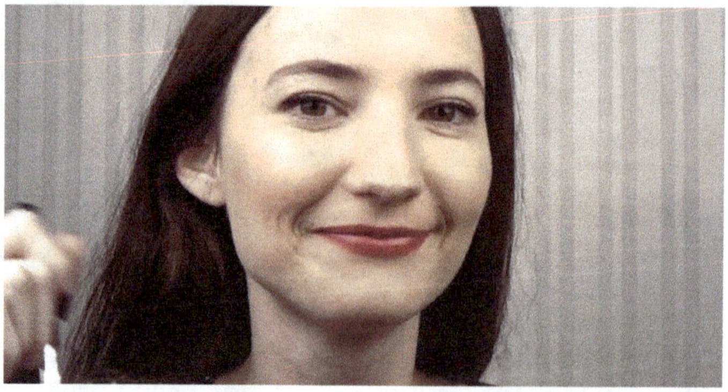

4. Finish off your look. With the completion of your lips makeup, your look is finished! Give your-

self a once-over to make sure there aren't any smudges or loose eyeshadow that needs to be removed with a fluffy brush. If you do have any mistakes, use a q-tip dipped in makeup remover to rectify them.

- After you have applied all of the makeup you desire, you should set your face with a setting spray. Simply hold the bottle 8–12 inches (20.3–30.5 cm) away from your face and spray 4-5 times on your whole face. Now your makeup will stay on longer than ever!

How to Apply Base Makeup

An important part of applying makeup is to first create the base. Base makeup doesn't have to look caked on. If you apply it correctly, it can give your face a smooth and flawless appearance.

Part 1

Applying the Base Makeup

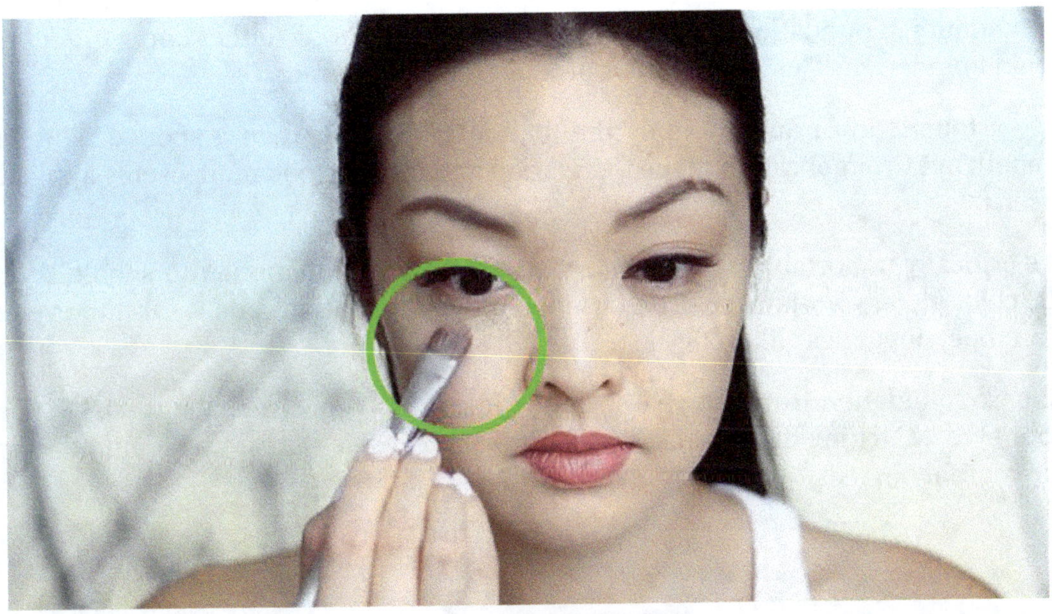

1. Use concealer. You will wreck your look if you've got dark circles under your eyes or have blemishes throughout your face. Don't feel badly about such circles or blemishes, though. They happen to almost everyone.

- Use concealer to cover up blemishes and under eye circles. You generally want concealer that matches your skin. Make sure also that your concealer matches your foundation tone. Apply the concealer in an upside-down pyramid shape.
- Use your ring finger when you apply the concealer across your skin (or a makeup brush). The ring finger is good to use for applying makeup because it will provide a softer touch to the skin.

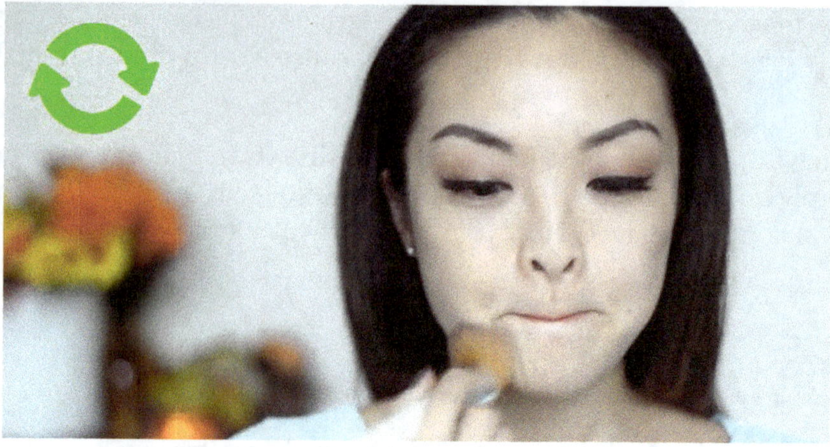

- Don't choose concealer that is several shades lighter than your skin or you will look like you have raccoon eyes. It's a myth that you should choose concealer that is lighter than your skin tone. When trying to match your concealer to your skin tone, don't test it on your arm or hand as those areas are often darker than your face.

2. Apply foundation. Foundation will complete the base. You should either apply tinted moisturizer or a liquid foundation. This is a different product than the primer.

- Use a foundation brush to apply the foundation, rather than a sponge. The brush will smooth out the application of the foundation and make it look more evenly applied on your face.
- It's critically important that you find the right color foundation. You should try to match the color along your jawline. Don't use too much foundation. You want it to even out your skin tone, not appear like a mask.
- Choose foundation from the yellow family if you are concerned about dark circles under your eyes. Matching the foundation color to your chest is a good way to find the right color for your face.

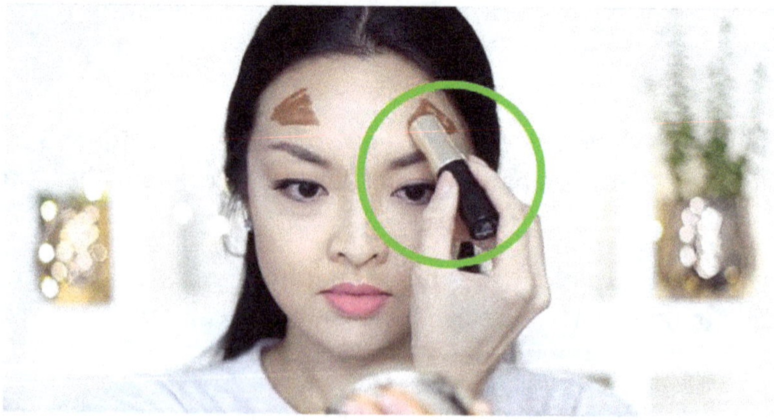

3. Try a foundation stick. Don't want to put foundation all over your face because you prefer a more natural look? You could try using a foundation stick.

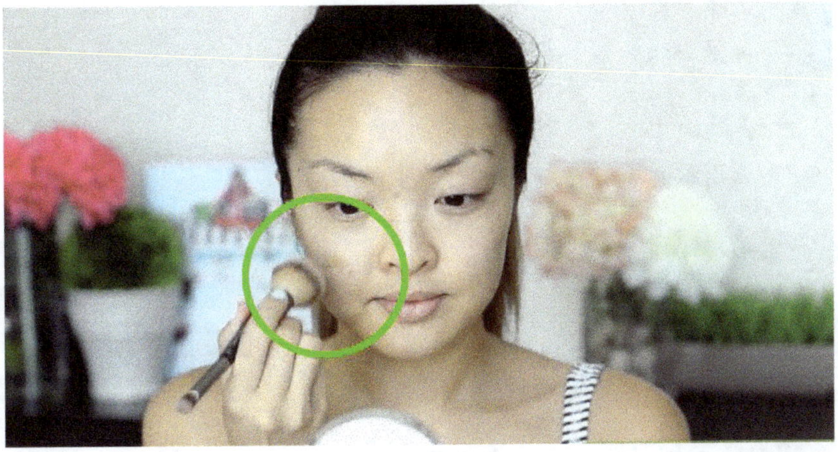

- This is also a less time-consuming way to apply base makeup. Use the stick as if it's a giant marker. Draw thick lines down your cheekbones, on the sides of your nose, and above your eyebrows, and then blend it in.
- If you want to look bronzed, you could use a stick that's a little darker, and put it in the same places over the lighter foundation. Blend both together.

4. Apply powder or compact foundation. You can also use powder or compact foundation that is not in liquid form.

- To apply this type of foundation, you will want to use a small makeup brush. Sometimes these brushes come with the makeup, and sometimes you have to apply them separately.
- Hold the brush horizontally. Brush it across the powder with short strokes. Press the brush to your face in slightly rolling motions. Then, dust the powder over your face.

Part 2

Completing the Base Makeup

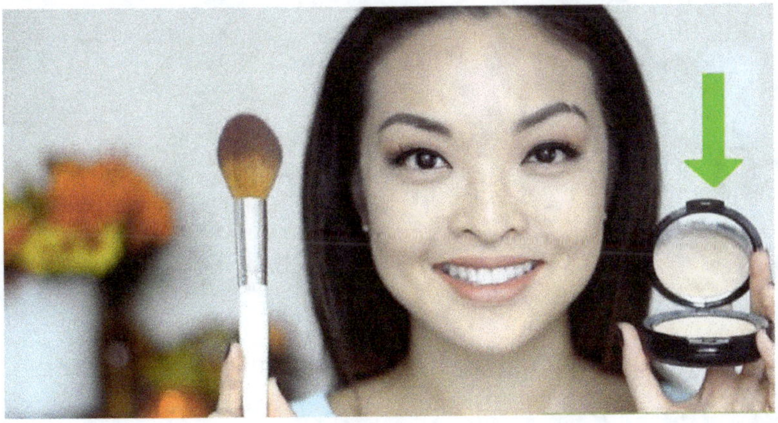

1. Finish the look with powder. Powder is an important step when completing base makeup because it will set the foundation and finish off the look.

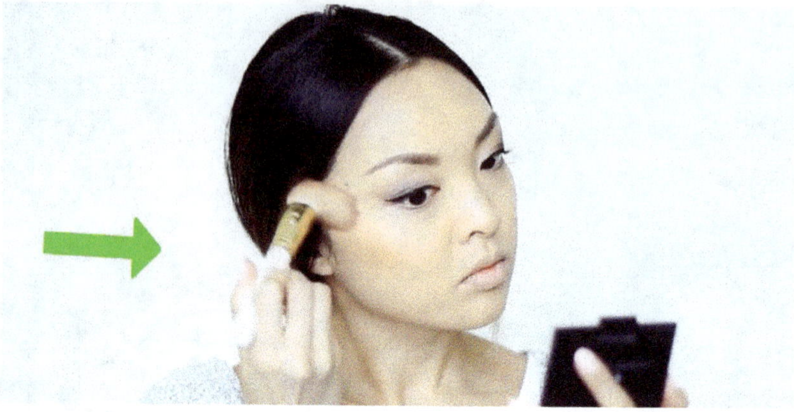

- Set the foundation with loose powder. Buy a large powder brush to apply it. Foundation will last longer if you use powder on top of it. Use translucent powder. It will control shine and provide a matte finish to your face. It's not designed to add color, but rather to set your makeup.
- Make sure you dust areas of your face that get very oily. Do this first, especially in the T-zone. Then, dust the powder throughout the rest of your face.

2. Apply bronzer or blush. Now that you've got the base makeup down, you should apply blush or bronzer in order to highlight your cheekbones.

- Put bronzer on your face, your neck, and your chest. This will even out the tone of your skin. Make sure to use a brush, and make sure the bronzer is blended.
- Smile before applying blusher. Then start by applying the blush on the apple of your cheek. Blend it back towards the top of your ear, and then brush it down toward your jawline. Blend it in so it doesn't look too stark.

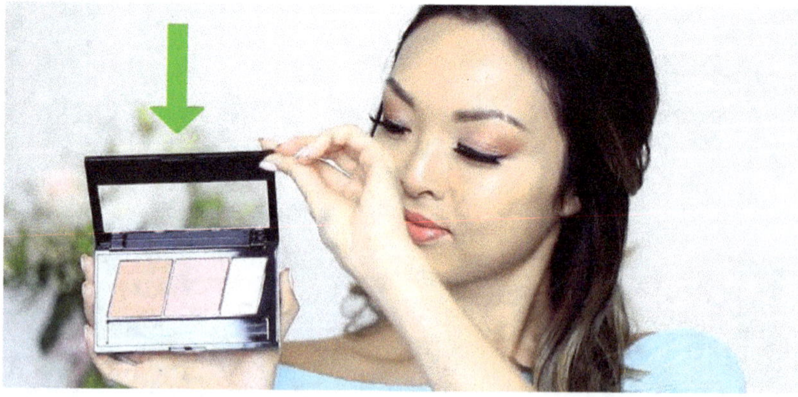

3. Try contouring. Contouring is a makeup trick used by many movie stars in order to alter the shape of their faces. The first step to contouring is to create a sound base using the steps above.

- Then, suck your cheeks in, and sweep bronzing powder on the hollows of your cheekbones. Now, take cream highlighter. Apply it above the bronzer.

- Make sure that you blend the cream in. Use stick foundations. With a darker one, trace your temples and carry it up to your hairline. To make your cheekbones stand out, place the pigment right above the cheekbones. For the nose, you can apply the stick on either side, either narrower at the top or carry it to the brow.
- Take a sponge and blend the contouring makeup into your base makeup. Now take the lighter stick, and apply it underneath your eyes. You could put some in the center of your forehead, on your chin, and on the bridge of your nose too. Dust the face with lose powder.

Part 3

Starting to Apply the Base Makeup

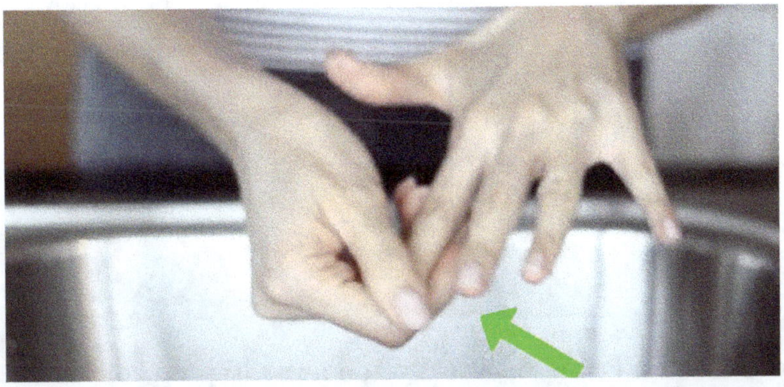

1. Clean your face and hands. This is really important. Before you apply base makeup, you will want to start with a fresh palette.

- Don't forget to clean your hands, though, in addition to your face. Use a cleanser so you aren't treating your face to harsh chemicals or soaps. Makeup remover or wipes can do a great job.
- After you clean your face and hands, apply moisturizer to your face, and make sure that it contains SPF! Wearing daily SPF is the best way to make sure your skin is protected and looks good.

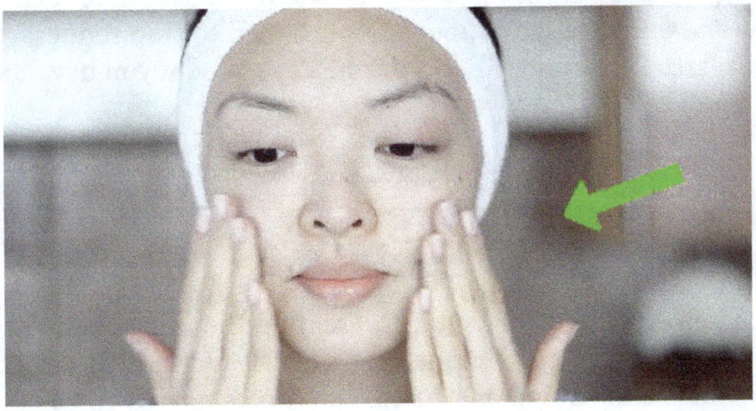

2. Exfoliate your face to prep it. By exfoliating your face, you remove dry skin from it. This evens

out your skin tone, and it makes your skin look healthier and glowing.

- After you've cleaned your face with your regular cleanser, you are ready to exfoliate it. You should do this process about twice a week.
- Mix three tablespoons of white sugar with a tablespoon of water for a homemade technique (you can also buy exfoliating scrubs at the store). Put some of the paste on a washcloth, and gently rub it all over your face in small circular motions. Then, rinse it off.

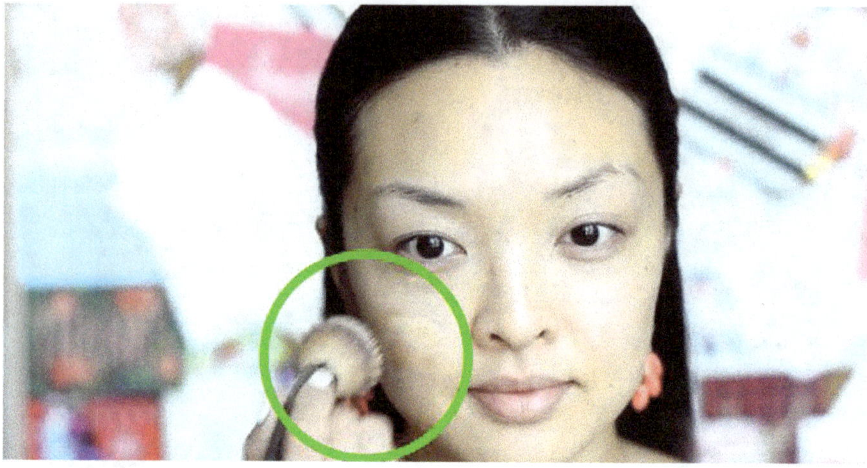

3. Apply a primer to your face. Primer is a really good way to prep your skin and to make it look smoother and more flawless. You can get it at many department store makeup counters.

- Think of primer as a much lighter foundation. You shouldn't be able to tell it's there. It provides the foundation for the rest of your makeup, and will make it last longer and be less likely to smudge.
- Make sure that you apply it evenly throughout your face, including underneath your eyes. Don't choose primer that's dramatically darker than your skin. You can buy primer for different skin types, including oily, dry and combination skin.
- When choosing the color of your primer, understand that different colors correct different issues. Yellow and green-based primers are designed to stop redness. Pink-based primers add life to dull skin. Peach and salmon primers are good if you have darker patches or circles under your eyes.

How to Apply Contour Makeup

Contouring your face helps define your features, creating the appearance of higher cheekbones and a slimmer nose and chin. It's a technique that was popularized by celebrity makeup artists, but with the right products and equipment it's easy to do on your own. Once you've applied your contouring makeup, remember to blend well for a flawless, natural look.

Contour Makeup Cheat Sheet

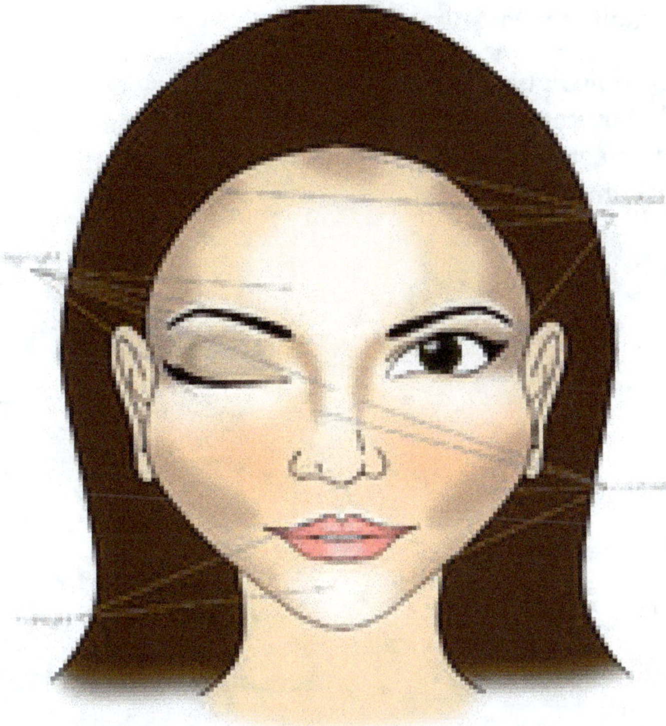

Contouring Makeup Chart

Part 1

Getting the Right Products

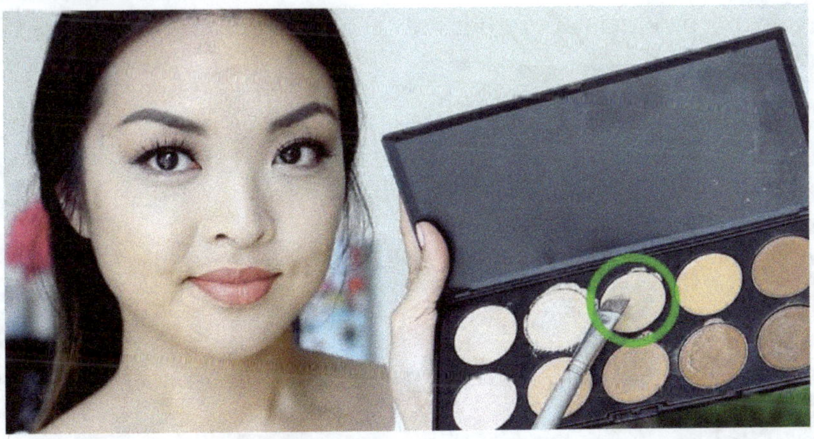

1. Start with foundation the color of your skin. Using a foundation the same (or close) color as your skin evens your skin tone and provides a base you can build upon when you contour using lightest and darkest shades. Contouring your face without first applying foundation is much more difficult, since skin tends to be uneven in color. Your face could end up looking patchy instead of smooth and contoured.

- Use a foundation composed of the same material as the other products you'll be using; for example, use all cream products or all powder products, rather than mixing the two. Mixing textures can result in a caked-on look.
- If you're having trouble figuring out what color to get, try matching your foundation to the skin on your neck. Your neck skin tends to be a bit paler than your face, and matching your foundation to your neck will ensure your face doesn't end up looking darker when you're finished doing your makeup.

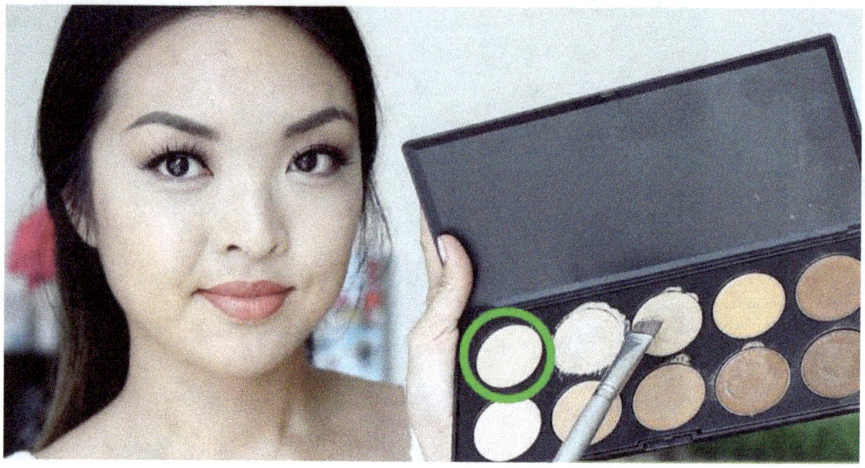

2. Get foundation a few shades lighter than your skin. Facial contouring consists of highlighting places you want to stand out, and shading places you want to recede. For your highlighting product, you need foundation that's about two shades paler than your base foundation.

- Don't go much lighter than two shades, or your makeup won't look natural.
- You can use a lighter concealer or eye shadow in place of foundation. Just remember to make sure all your products are either cream or powder; don't mix the two.

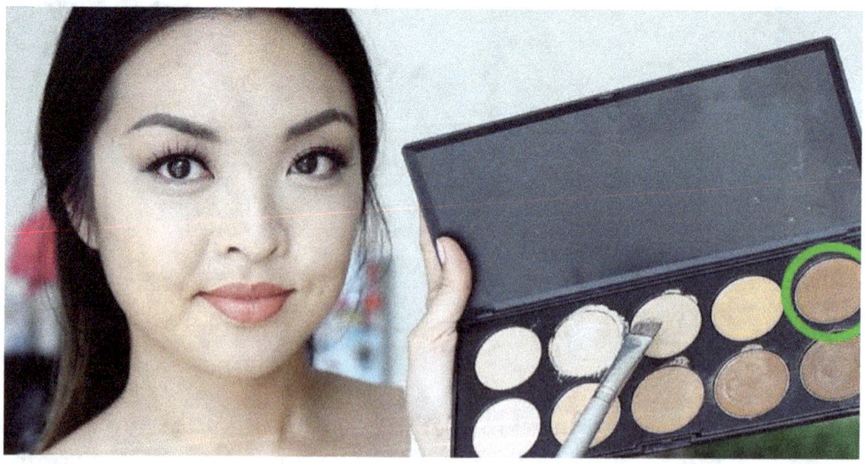

3. Choose a foundation a few shades darker than your skin. The darker tone will be used to shade the parts of your face that you want to draw attention *away* from. You'll be creating strategic shadows that make your cheekbones appear sharper and your chin more narrow.

- Don't go darker than two shades below your normal skin tone, or your makeup won't look natural.
- Bronzer, darker eye shadow or darker concealer work as well as foundation. Just remember to make sure all your products are either cream or powder; don't mix the two.

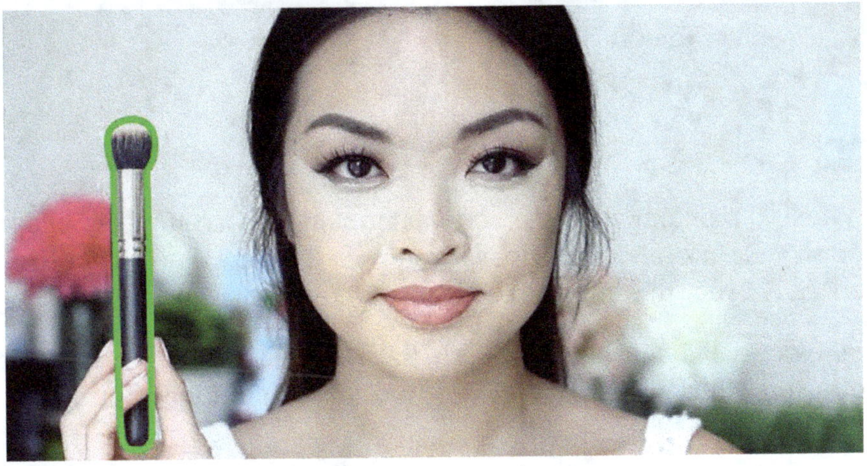

4. Get a good blending brush. Since your face will be wearing several different shades, it's important to get a good blending brush. If the different colors aren't well-blended your makeup will look unnatural. You want a big, bushy foundation brush or blending brush, rather than a smaller brush. Go for one with natural bristles to leave the softest-looking finish.

- If you don't have a brush, the next best tool to use is your fingers. The warmth from your fingers will help the makeup blend smoothly. This is especially useful when you're working with cream foundation.

Part 2

Contouring Your Face

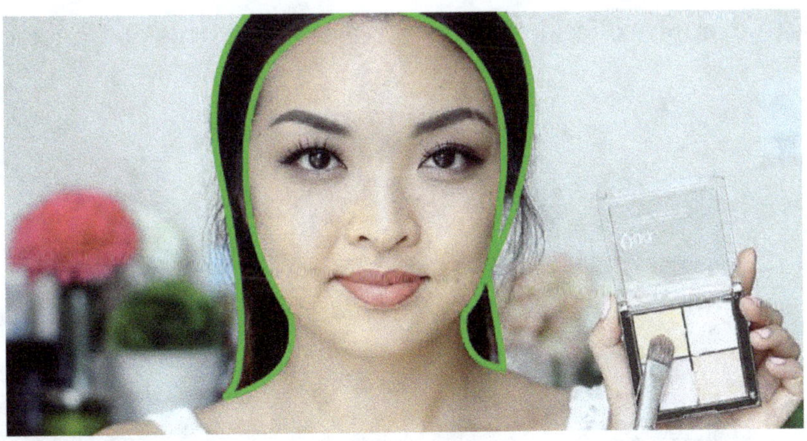

1. It is better to pull your hair away from your face. Contouring makeup reaches up to your hairline at the top of your forehead, past your temples and down the sides of your face. Pull your hair away from your face so you'll be able to see what you're doing without it getting in the way.

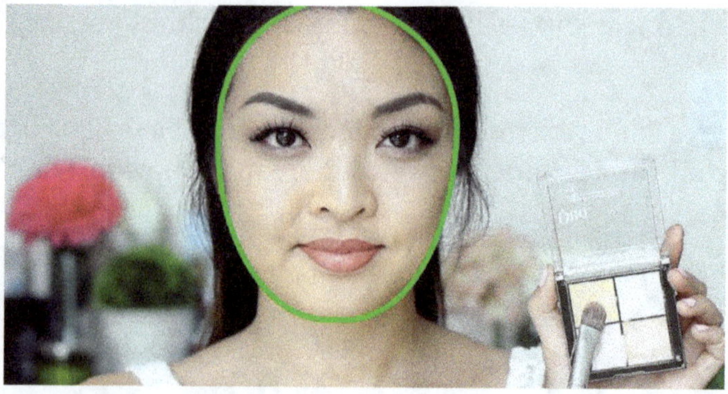

2. Prep your face. When you contour your face, you want to start with a completely blank canvas. Remove all your makeup, wash your face, and pat it dry with a towel. Exfoliate if necessary to remove dead skin, then apply moisturizer. Let your moisturizer soak in for several minutes before you apply your makeup.

- Prepping is essential if you want a smooth, flawless finish. You don't want to go to the trouble of contouring your face, only to have your makeup smudge or look dirty.

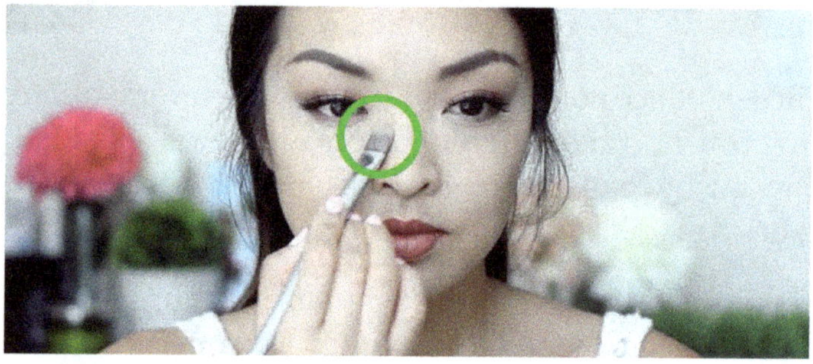

3. Apply foundation in your regular skin tone. Use your fingers or a foundation brush to apply a light layer of your normal foundation all over your face, stretching all the way to the top of your forehead and below your chin. Use a blending brush or your fingers to blend your foundation under your chin and around your neck so there won't be a line separating your face from your neck.

- You may want to apply concealer at this stage as well. Focus on under-eye circles and any blemishes.

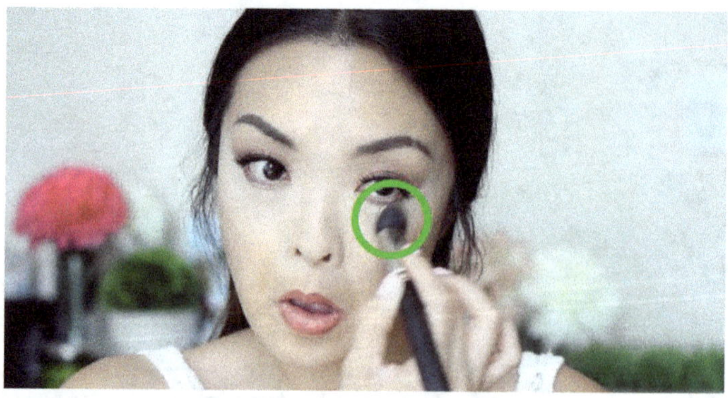

4. Apply the light foundation. Take the foundation that's a few shades lighter than your normal skin tone. Use your finger or a clean foundation brush to apply a 1/2 inch to 1 inch stroke of foun-

dation to the places on your face where the sun would naturally hit. To help you figure out where the sun would hit, stand in a well-lit room with overhead lighting and look at where it hits your face. Here's where you want to apply light foundation:

- In the center of your forehead.
- Along the top of your brow lines.
- Along the bridge of your nose.
- On the apples of your cheeks (to find them, smile).
- On your cupid's bow (the section between the tip of your nose and the top of your lip).
- In the center of your chin.

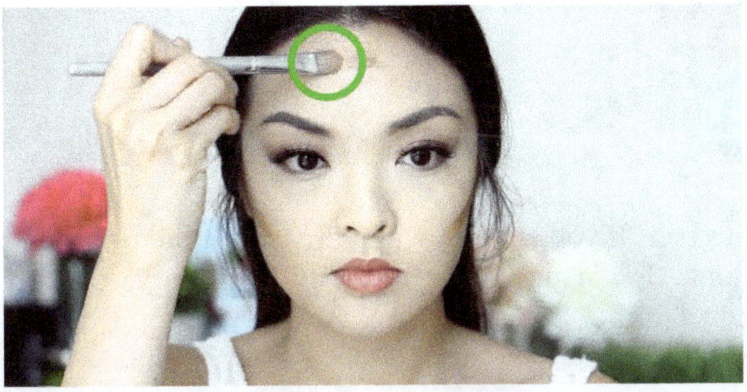

5. Apply the dark foundation. Use your finger or a clean foundation brush to apply stroke of the darker foundation in the places where your face would naturally be shadowed from the sun. To help you figure out where your face would be shadowed, stand in a well-lit room with overhead lighting and look for the places that are darker. Here's where you want to apply the dark foundation:

- Right below your hairline at the top of your forehead.
- On the right and left sides of your forehead, near your hairline on either side.
- Along the right and left sides of your nose.
- In the hollows of your cheeks (to find them, suck your cheeks in).
- Along your jawline on both sides, from your ears to the tip of your chin.

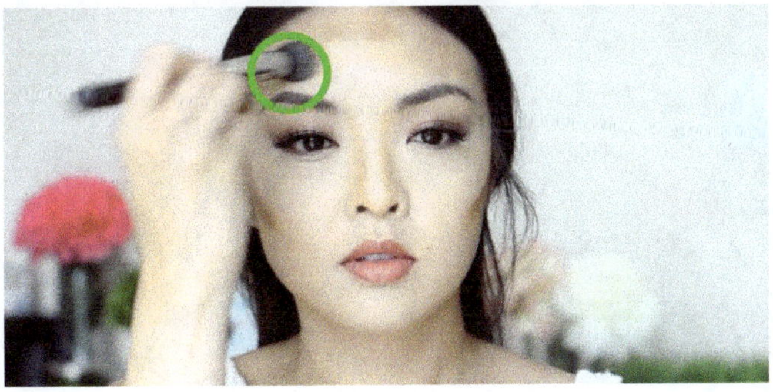

6. Blend your makeup well. Use your fingers or the foundation brush to blend the colors for a nat-

ural finish. Take care not to spread the colors around too much; you want them to stay in the general area where you placed them. Make sure the edges are blended well so that there are no sharp divisions between the lighter and darker foundation.

Part 3

Finishing the Look

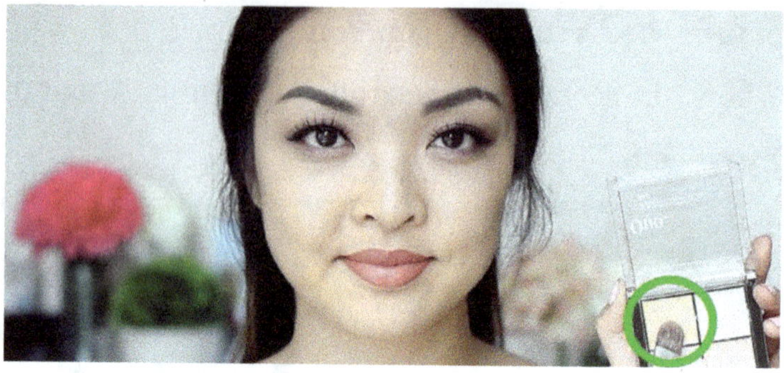

1. Consider adding highlighter. If you want the light areas to stand out even more, add a highlighter product to enhance the look. Cream highlighter is slightly shimmery, so it catches the light more than regular foundation. Apply it in the exact same places where you applied the lighter foundation.

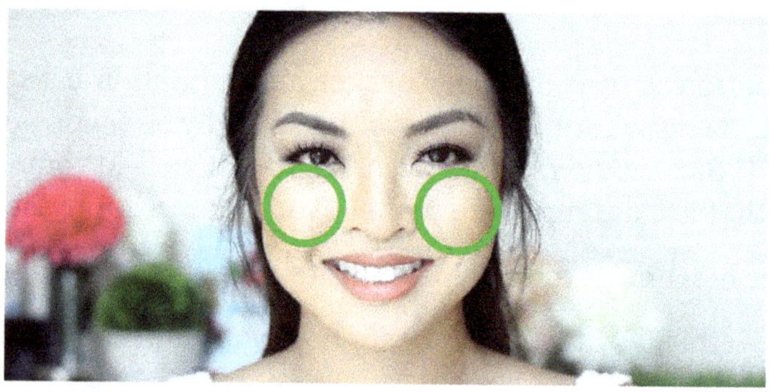

2. Consider applying blush. If you feel your face looks a little wan without some pink color, apply a small amount of blush to the apples of your cheeks. Be sure to blend the blush well with the other products on your face.

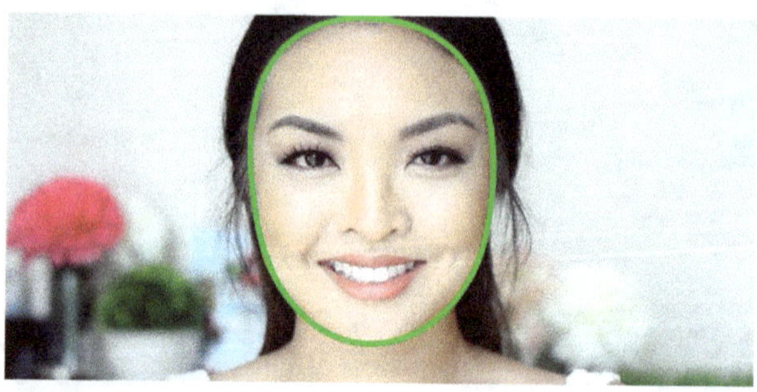

3. Consider using a matte setting powder. Setting powder is helpful to use when your products are

cream-based. It helps to keep everything in place and gives the look a smooth finish. Use a clean powder brush to add a light coating of setting powder over your entire face.

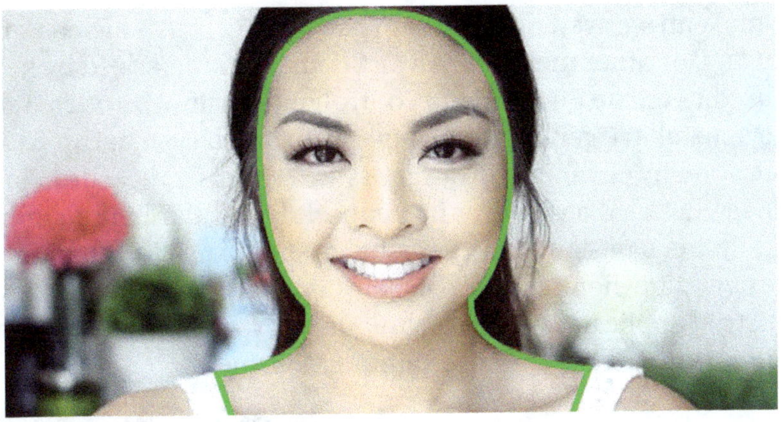

4. Add shimmer for a night out. If you're going out on the town, you may want to add some shimmer and shine. Choose a shimmery, translucent face powder an apply a light layer to your face, focusing on the highlighted areas. Apply a bit to your neck and chest as well.

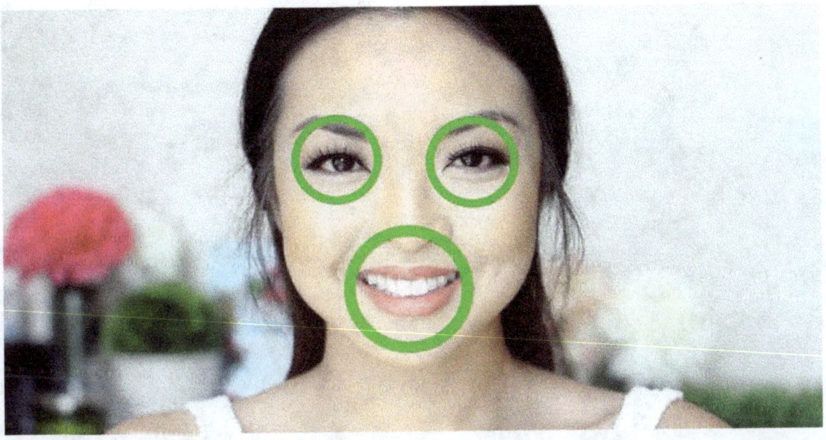

5. Save your eye and lip makeup for last. Make sure everything is completely blended and set before you start applying eye and lip makeup. Contouring is a bold look, so you may want to choose either heavy eye makeup or a bright lip, but not both.

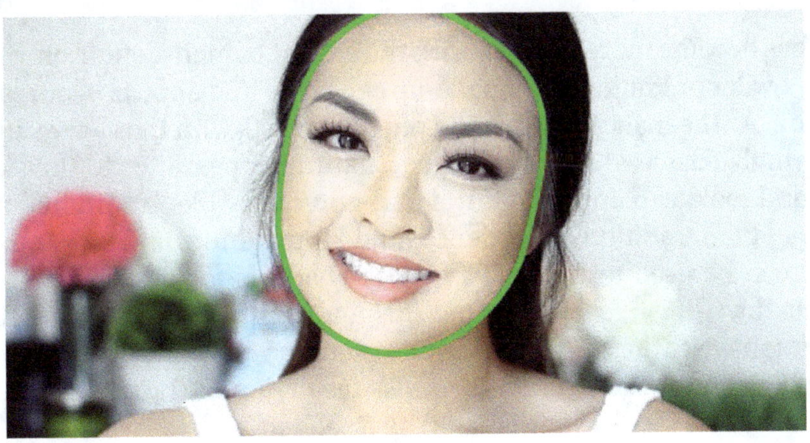

Airbrush Makeup

Airbrush makeup is makeup sprayed onto the skin using an airbrush instead of being applied with sponges, brushes, fingers, or other methods. An airbrush is characterized by 3 major parts. A powered compressor is used to create an even and controllable airflow through a medical grade hose. The hose connects to a metal, trigger-actioned gun. An airbrush system can be altered to suit every type of makeup application by changing the air pressure (typically measured in pounds per square inch) for lighter, heavier, detailed or broader makeups. It is popular in film, theater, bridal makeup and sunless tanning. Systems designed for personal cosmetic use in the home are also available. Airbrush systems designed for home use are usually smaller and work at a lower pressures than systems used in industrial applications. The technique was first used in 1959 on actors in Ben Hur and has since grown in popularity in the entertainment business.

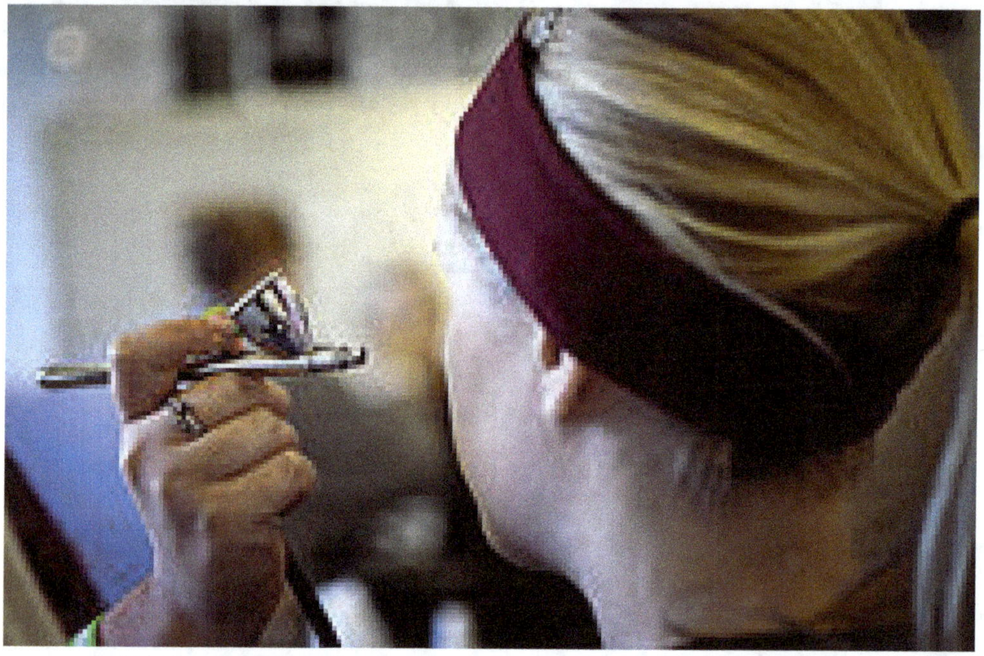

A makeup artist applies foundation to a models face with an airbrush.

Uses

Airbrush makeup has become more popular with the advent of high-definition video and television (HD). Traditional powder or liquid based make-up can settle and appear in pores and wrinkles and be visible on HD film. As the makeup is sprayed on, it connects with the skin as millions of droplets of formula. The formula can create an even, sheer, natural appearance to the skin that, if applied properly for a natural look, can appear natural and non-heavy like traditional makeup. Airbrush makeup wears longer than traditional powder or liquid foundation, and is able to stay put upwards of 12–24 hours. It can be used to cover five o'clock shadows for men. Airbrush makeup is also available for eye shadow, blush, eyebrows and lips and can be layered, shaded, highlighted and contoured. Application wise, the technique is more sanitary than traditional makeup application due the artist never having to touch the skin. It's also faster, if done by a trained artist. Fantasy and special effects are able to be stenciled or created by freehand.

Benefits

Airbrush makeup is characterized by its unique 'globular' application technique. The makeup is dispersed as an extremely fine mist through the airbrush gun. Millions of tiny little dots are created on the skin and when connected and layered together, create somewhat of a net over the entire face. This makes airbrush makeup to be a thin, light layer on the skin that is barely noticeable to the wearer. Certain formulas wear better than others and it is important to choose carefully when deciding what mixture is right for the job. Some airbrush makeups are entirely waterproof unless taken off with a specific remover that breaks down the active ingredient. For instance, silicone-based airbrush fluid is largely waterproof depending on how much, and how you set the makeup. It can be dunked in water (handy for fashion photography or film) or sweat through without removing or dislodging the airbrush base. It does however, take a specific silicone makeup remover to thoroughly take off (but will naturally come off over the course of many hours). In the contemporary makeup scene, airbrush makeup has become a preferred option for bridal and events makeup due to its long wearing and flawless appearance.

Ingredients

Airbrush makeup comes in six different formulas:

- Water based: Finely ground pigments dissipated in water.
- Polymer-water-based: A mix of water, polymers and pigment, when airbrushed on the skin the polymer dries leaving a continuous coating on the skin.
- Polymer-SD40-alcohol based: Instead of using water like the polymer-water-based formula, it uses alcohol which assists with drying of the makeup on the skin.
- Alcohol based: Also called "temporary airbrush inks" alcohol based formulas are generally used when creating fake tattoos.
- Silicone-based: Uses silicone for longer lasting wear and without fading. Silicone-based can be thinned with certain types of formula additives, for lighter coverage.

Airbrush makeup can be removed by using a 50/50 mix of isopropyl alcohol and isopropyl myristate.

Technique

Airbrushing for makeup utilizes a freehand technique to apply makeup while manipulating aspects such as distance and air pressure to produce certain effects and coverage. Airbrush makeup artists will either use a circular motion or forward-back motion with the airgun when applying foundation. Both dual-action and single-action airbrushes can be used for airbrushing makeup and require slightly different techniques.

A dual-action airbrush allows the user to control airflow by depressing the trigger with the index finger and drawing it backwards. This draws air from the compressor. The further the trigger is depressed, the more makeup is released. The advantage to using a dual-action airbrush is that one can use the air as a guide before allowing makeup to pass through the nozzle. Air is also used to dry the makeup after application. Makeup is also mixed in the cup by allowing a small amount of air to flow into it, thereby mixing two pigments. This technique is known as 'back-bubbling'.

A single-action airbrush is generally considered easier to use because depressing the trigger releases a fixed ratio of makeup to air. However, in order to achieve different levels of coverage and detail the nozzle has to be changed between applications.

Generally an airbrush makeup artist will work with a PSI range between 0-35 PSI. Many compressors designed for personal use in the home will not achieve airflow greater than 15 PSI. A low PSI is preferable when airbrushing makeup around the face and eyes while full body application (such as covering blemishes or tanning) is easier and faster with a higher PSI.

Airbrush makeup is applied by layering several passes of makeup. This allows the artists to build upon previous layers to produce subtle changes. When applying foundation between 6-12 drops of makeup are used. The makeup is sprayed onto the face at a distance of 6-12 inches.

Stencils are commonly used to assist the application of difficult areas such as eye-liner. Stencils are also available for body-art and temporary tattoos.

Chapter

2 Makeup Tools for Asian Women

There can be different ways of choosing makeup, as there are different tools for makeup. Companies can have different products for the same purpose. Some of the tools used by Asian women are rouge, eyelash curler, glitter, lotion, kohl and eyelash extensions. Those interested in the field of makeup will be greatly benefited from this section.

How to Shop for Makeup

If you've never shopped for makeup before, the process can seem overwhelming. There are so many different brands, different products and different applications. It's impossible to learn everything in one day, but with a little help, you can successfully shop for makeup that will make you look and feel like a rockstar.

Method 1

Picking the Makeup Products that Work Best for You

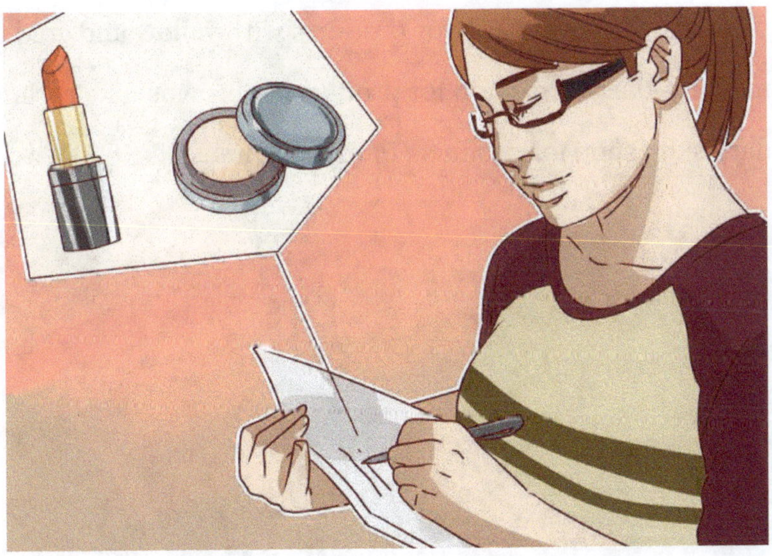

1. Take stock of what you own and use. Buying makeup is a waste of time if you're not going to use it. If you're the kind of person who only wears a little mascara, buying a large quantity of skin products isn't going to help you. Likewise, if you already own four bright red lipsticks, one more isn't going to make a difference.

- Before heading to the store, make a list of products you need or would actually use. Then purchase only these items.
- Go through your makeup and check to see what's already expired. Make a list of any products you need to replenish.

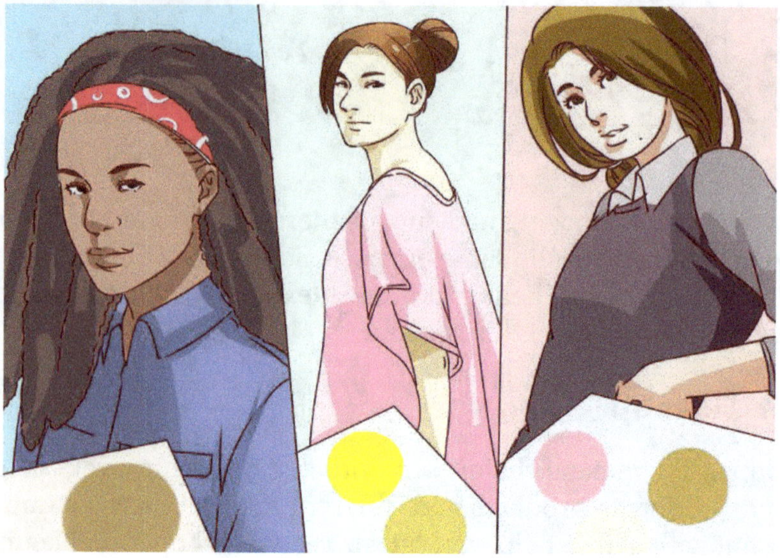

2. Choose the right makeup for your skin-tone. Everyone's coloring is different, and the shade that looks amazing on your best friend might not paint you in the best light. Try going to a department store or specialty makeup store for a color consultation.

- If you have fair skin, shop for products in soft pink, tawny and beige. Avoid orangey reds.
- If you have medium- fair skin, shop for products with yellow and gold undertones.
- If you have medium-dark skin, shop for products in browns, like caramel and honey.
- If you have dark skin, shop for products in metallic hues, like copper or bronze.

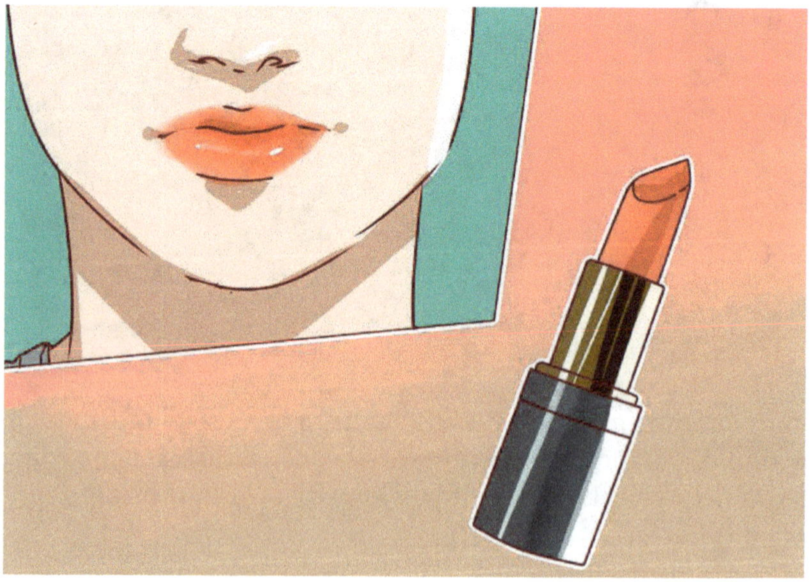

3. Highlight your best assets. The best way to avoid wearing too much makeup (or spending too much money on makeup) is to focus on your best features. Play up the features you're most proud of and let the rest of your makeup be a little more natural.

- If you have amazing eyes, spend your money on eyeliner and eye-shadow.
- If your eyelashes are long, buy an eyelash curler and mascara.
- If you have killer cheekbones, shop for blush, bronzer, and an illuminator.
- If you have a full mouth, shop for lipstick.

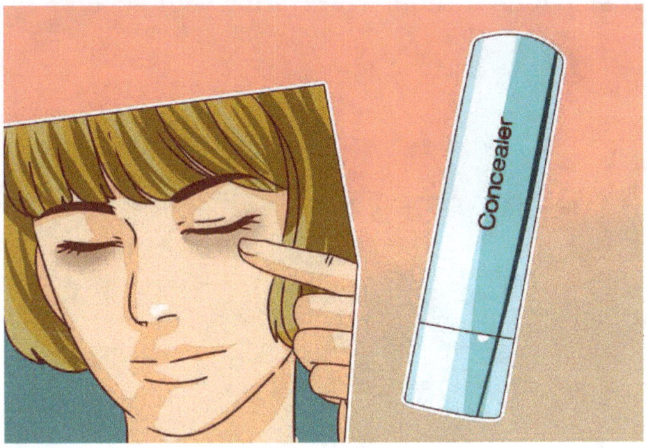

insecure about something on your face, shop for products that will help downplay that insecurity.

- If you get bad under-eye circles, invest in a good concealer.
- If you have bad skin, invest in a good concealer and foundation.
- If you have short or light-colored lashes, look for a mascara that adds length and volume.
- If you have thin eyebrows, shop for eyebrow gel and an eyebrow comb.

Method 2

Shopping for Specific Makeup Products

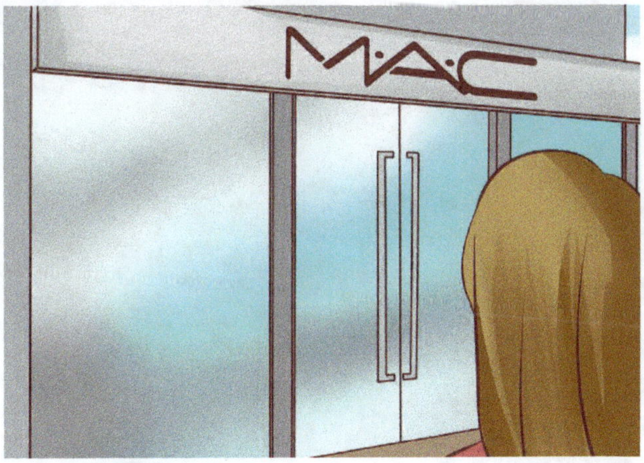

1. Buy your foundation at a specialty store. Drugstores have a good supply of foundation, but what they don't offer is a way to try on the product. Foundation needs to match your skin perfectly, so it's important that you try it on at a store that offers tester strips, like MAC or Sephora.

- Look for foundations with built-in sun protection, so you don't have to apply yours separately.
- If you have to shop at a drugstore, look for a foundation in a neutral tone. Avoid anything with overtones of other colors (yellow, peach, pink, copper, etc).
- If you have bad skin, splurge on the best foundation you can afford. The higher quality will help even out your skin tone without aggravating your acne.

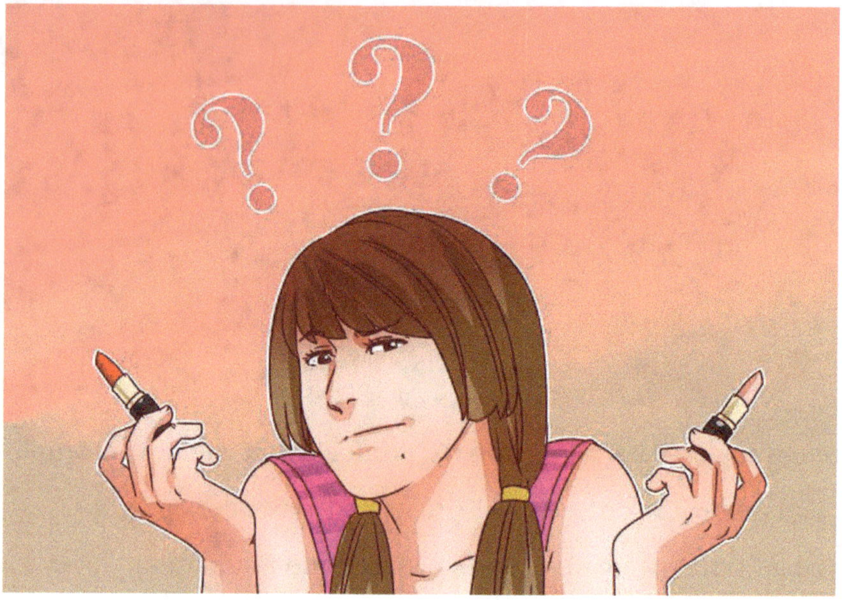

2. Choose a lipstick that looks and feels good. The biggest mistake people make when shopping for lipstick is only considering color. Choosing a lipstick that works with the color of your skin is important, but it's not the only factor that counts.

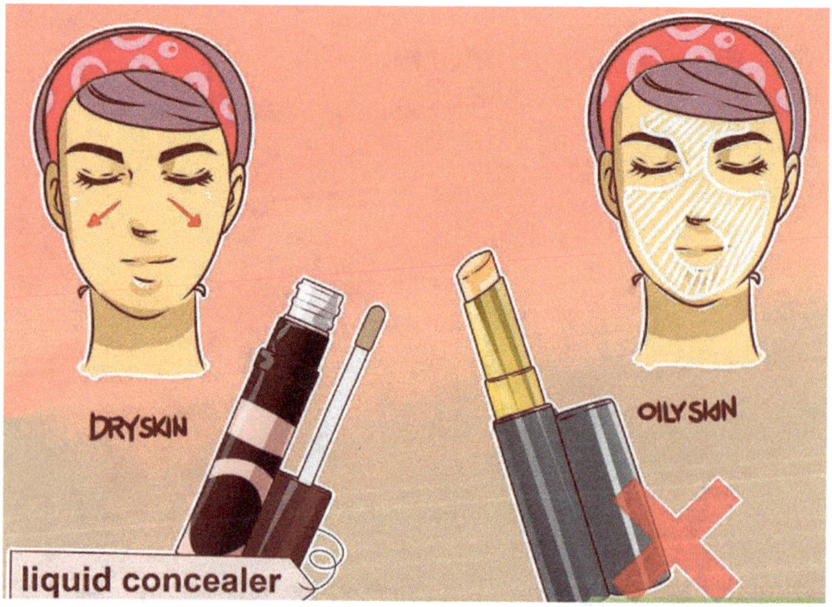

- Walk around the store and see how the color holds up over time.

- Consider how easy or difficult the lipstick is to apply. If it's hard to apply, you won't wear it often.
- Think about if the lipstick feels good on your lips. If it's too dry, it won't be comfortable.
- For a natural lipstick color, choose a color that either matches or is slightly darker than your natural lip shade.

3. Pick your concealer based on what you're concealing. Concealer is meant to conceal small areas, not to be used as an all-over foundation. If you're just evening out a few small blemishes, look for a concealer with light coverage.

- If you have dry skin, steer clear of liquid concealers.
- If you have oily skin or enlarged pores, avoid stick concealers.
- For dark circles, select a concealer with at least medium coverage.

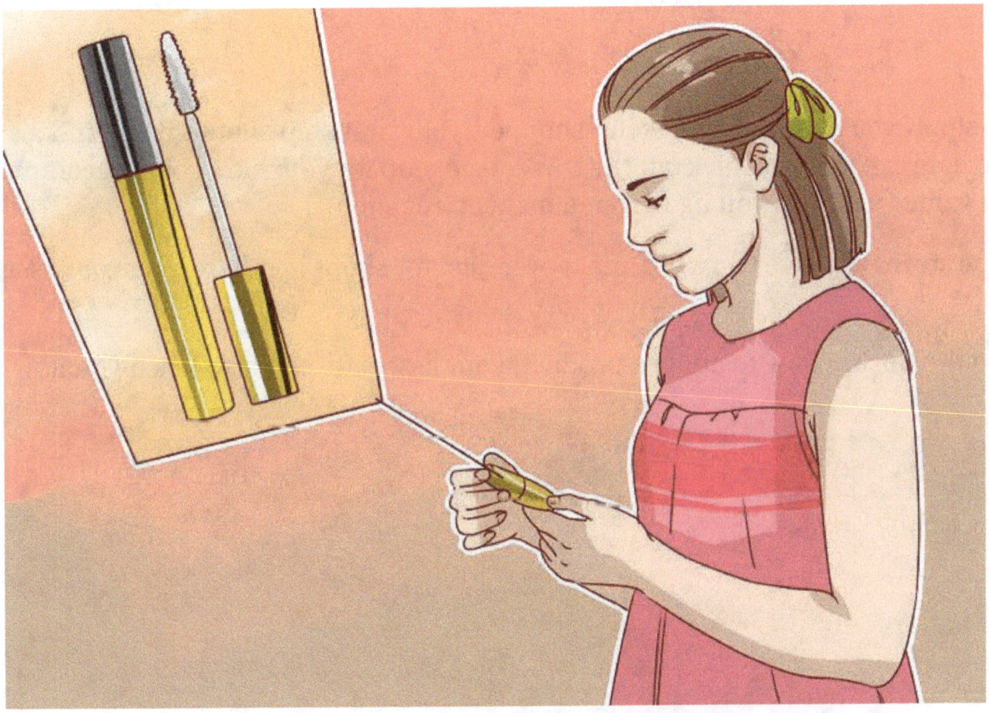

4. Shop for a mascara that works with your lashes. Different types of lashes require different treatments, so it's important to match your mascara with your needs. If you have very straight lashes, you'll also need to invest in an eyelash curler.

- If your lashes are short, look for a mascara with a lengthening formula.
- If you have dry eyes, use a mascara with a wax-based formula.
- Skip the waterproof mascara – it's harder to remove.

Method 3

Shopping for Makeup in Store

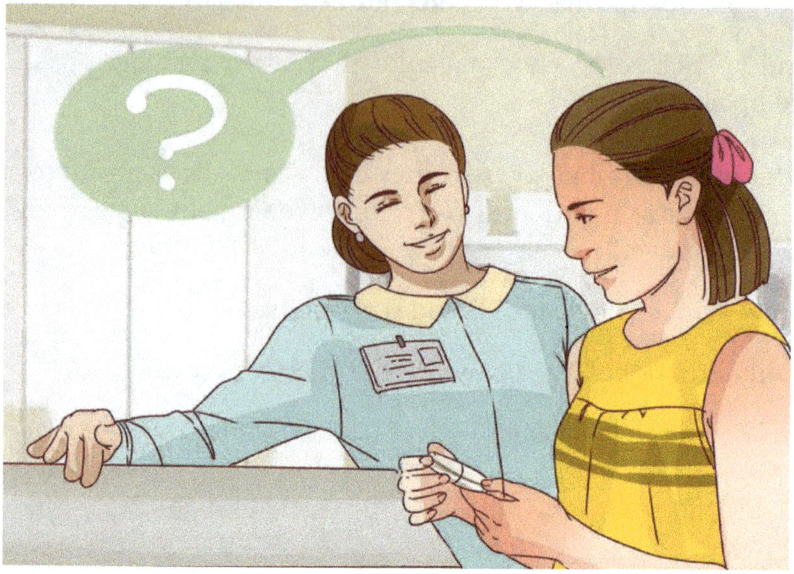

1. Ask for help. If you're a rookie makeup shopper, your first step should be to find a store associate. An associate can help you pick out the correct makeup for your skin color, recommend the best brands and values and help you figure out a makeup regimen.

- Some stores will give you a free makeover, just for shopping there. Ask your associate about this.
- If you're unsure how to apply a product, your associate can also teach you how to do this.

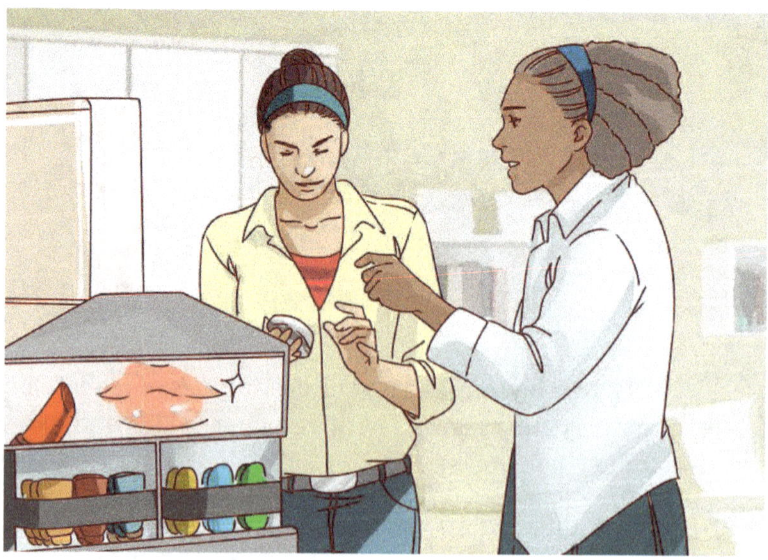

2. Get a second opinion. If you're brand new to shopping for makeup, you may want to bring a friend to the store with you. You friend can weigh in on color options and tell you whether an item is worth purchasing or passing on.

- If you can't find a friend to accompany you, take pictures on your cell-phone. Sometimes, makeup looks different on camera than it does in real life.

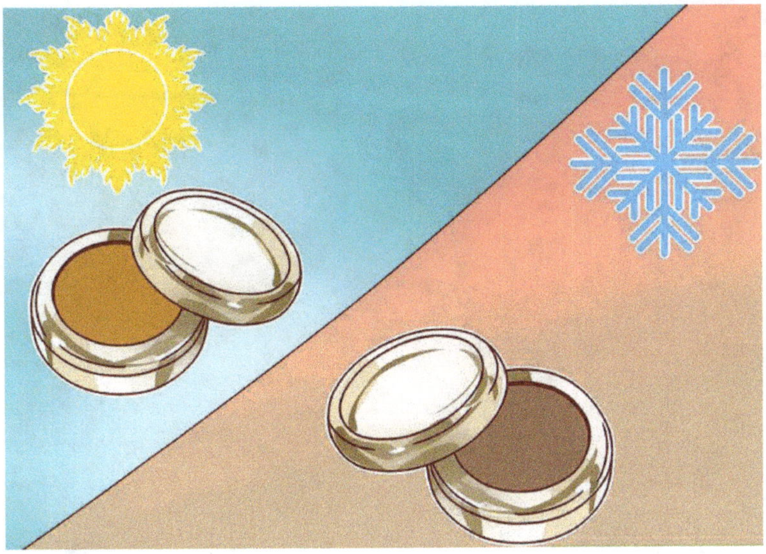

3. Buy different makeup for different seasons. Your skin changes throughout the year, so it stands to reason you should have different makeup for different parts of the year. When you buy bronzer, buy two shades so you can match your skin tone as it changes.

- If you're buying bronzer in the summer, buy an additional shade lighter to use in the winter.
- If you're buying bronzer in the winter, buy an additional shade darker to use in the summer.

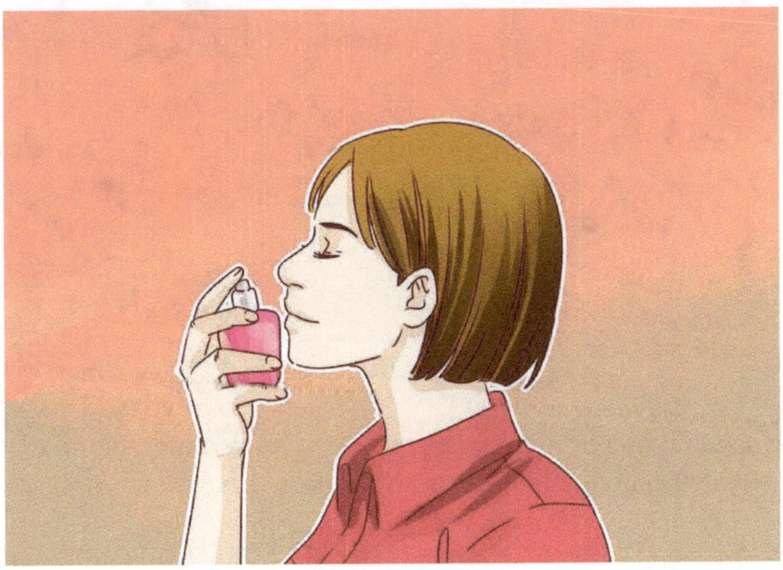

4. Smell your perfume sample twice. Perfume smells different from the time you initially spray it to the time it dries on your body. When testing perfumes, spray a little on your wrist, then wait two minutes before checking the smell.

- If you're going to be testing multiple perfumes, spray the fragrances on tester strips so their scents don't intermingle.

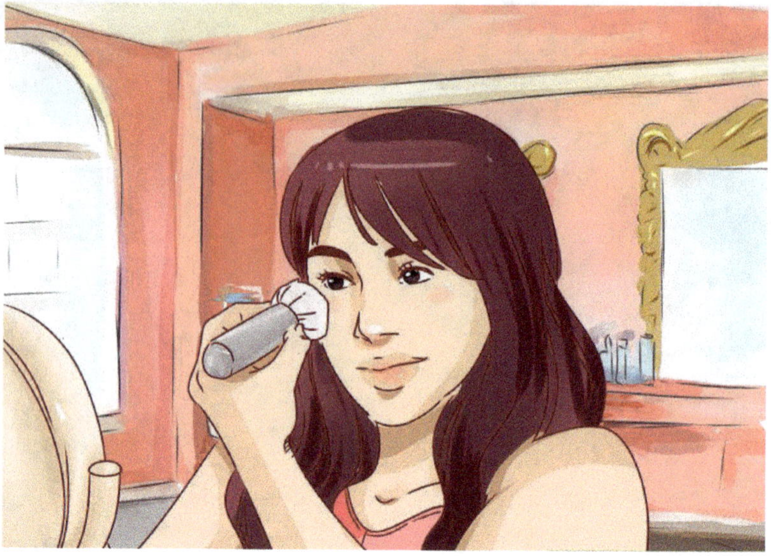

5. Test your makeup in natural light. Lighting affects your makeup significantly, and the way your skin looks in the store may not be the way it looks outside. When shopping for foundation or skin powder, ask for a sample, then try that sample out at home and outside before committing.

- If your store doesn't give samples, try the product on, then head outside to look in a mirror.

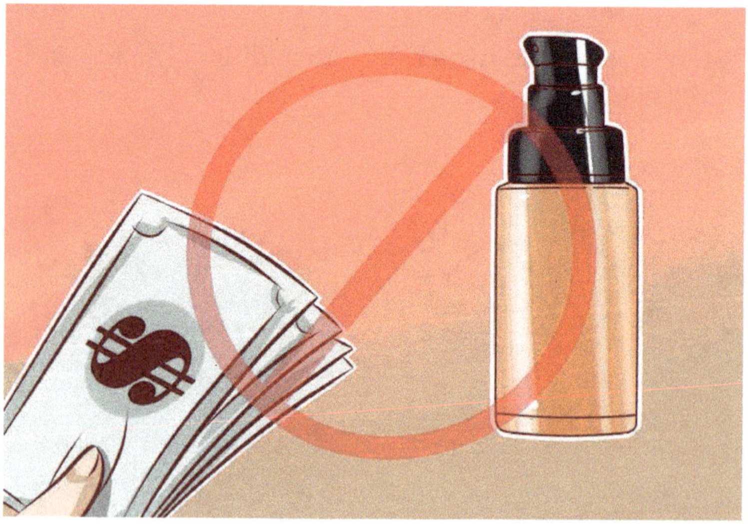

6. Don't buy the big size. If you're purchasing a new-to-you product, buy the smallest option. The biggest bottle may save you money long-term, but if you never wear it, it's a complete waste of money.

- Buy the smallest bottle and upgrade later when you run out.
- If you love something, buy a second travel sized bottle so you can take your products with you on planes.

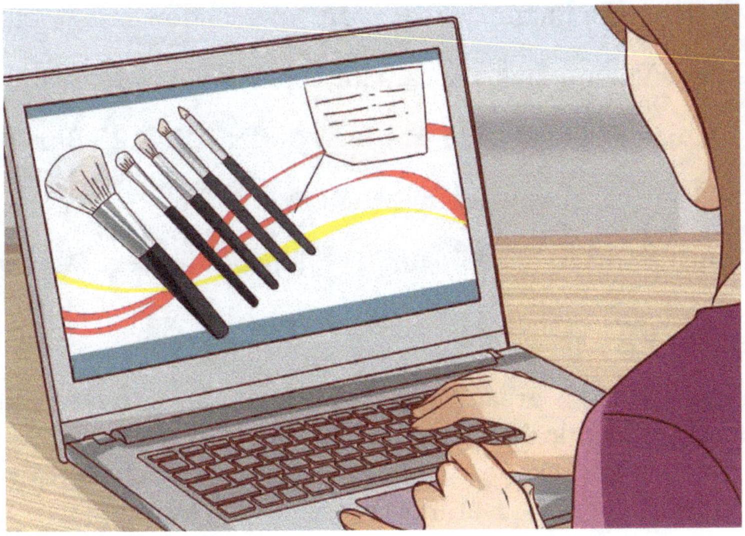

7. Read online reviews. Not everyone will have the same experience with the same product, but reviews will be able to give you some insight into a product's long-term durability and usefulness.

- Do extra research when you're investing in something you'll use for years, like makeup brushes.
- Don't buy new colors of products online. Use online shopping to re-up on items you already know work for you.

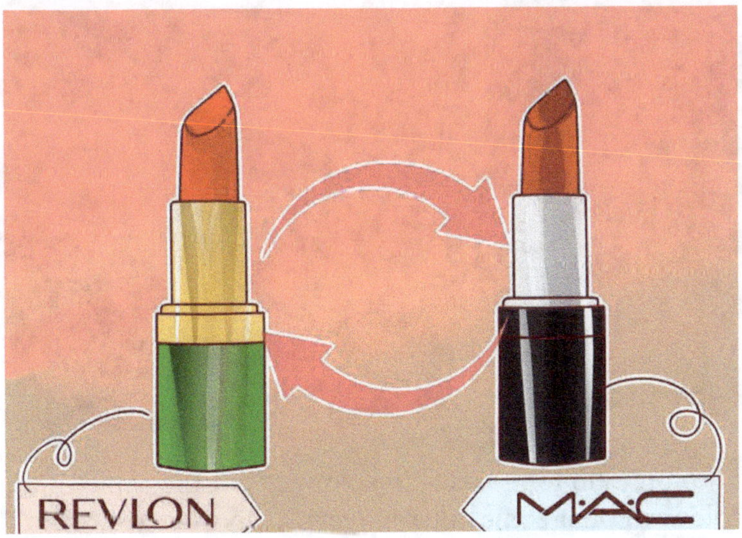

8. Find cheap alternatives for expensive makeup. Most people don't have unlimited amounts of disposable income, and sometimes you can't afford the really quality makeup that you want. Luckily, there are some good affordable options you can use to replace your expensive favorites.

- Swap CoverGirl Nature Luxe Silk Foundation for Giorgio Armani Luminous Silk Foundation.
- Swap Styli-Style Line and Seal Eyes for Giorgio Armani Smooth Silk Eye Pencil.

- Swap NYX Eyeshadow in Champagne for MAC Eyeshadow in All That Glitters.
- Swap L'Oreal Paris Voluminous Mascara for Dior Diorshow Mascara.
- Swap E.L.F. Contouring Blush and Bronzing Powder for NARS Blush/Bronzer Duo
- Swap Ben Nye Translucent Powder for MAC Set Powder.
- Swap Revlon Lipstick in Orange Flip for MAC Lipstick in Lady Danger with Luster.

How to Choose Makeup

You're gloriously unique—which is great, right up until you have to buy makeup. Suddenly, you just wish that everyone were identical so you could spend less time and stress picking out the right foundation or the perfect red lipstick. Fortunately, it's easy to narrow down your choices. You just have to know a little more about those features that make you so unique.

Part 1

Determining Your Skin Tone

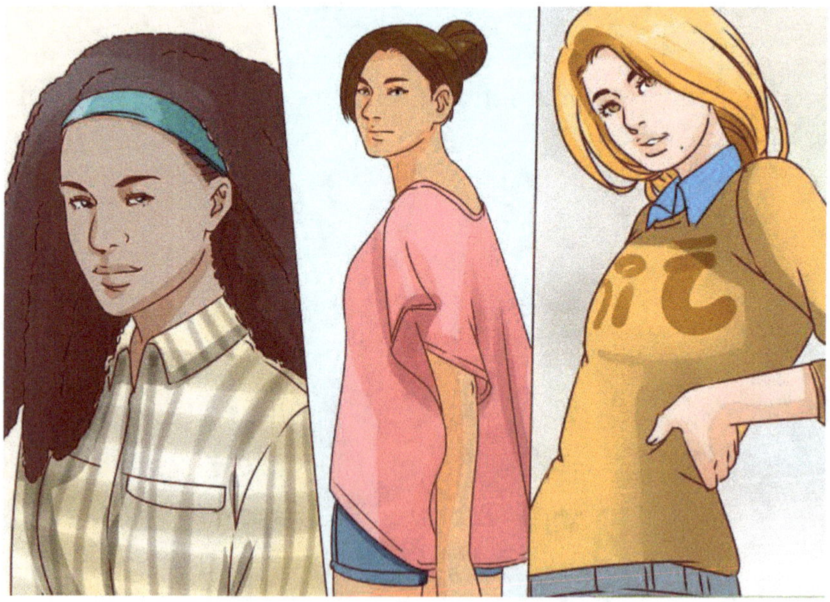

1. Start with your skin color. Skin tone and skin color are not the same thing, but they do overlap in some areas. Skin color can offer some general clues as to what your skin tone may be, and can help you determine the type of makeup to purchase. Skin color should not be your only method of determining tone. While there are some general rules, a variety of factors should be considered to assess your skin tone.

- If you have olive skin, you're highly likely to have a neutral skin tone leaning toward a warm skin tone.
- If you have darker skin, you are probably warm-toned. However, if your skin is a bluish ebony rather than warm brown, you may have a cool skin tone.

- Ruddy, reddish skin is likely to have cooler undertones. If you skin has a lot of reddish patches or discolorations, and tends to flush easily, you likely have ruddy skin. This increases the chances your skin will have a cool undertone.
- Neutral skin is skin with very little undertones of olive, sallow, or pink. If you have neutral skin, with very little color or variations in color, most makeups and foundations will be flattering on you.

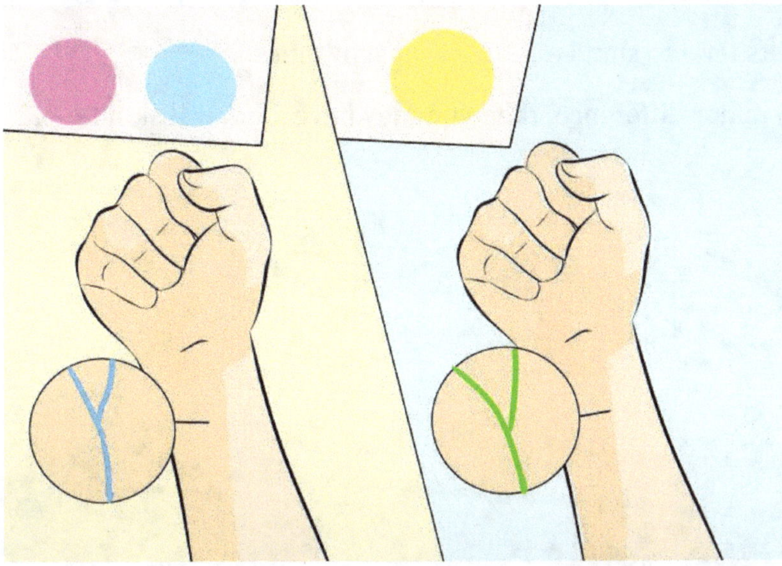

2. Look at your wrist. What color are the veins you see there? This is a quick shortcut that can help you guess at your likely skin tone. However, you should keep in mind that no one indicator can help determine skin tone. You should consider a variety of factors to figure out your tone.

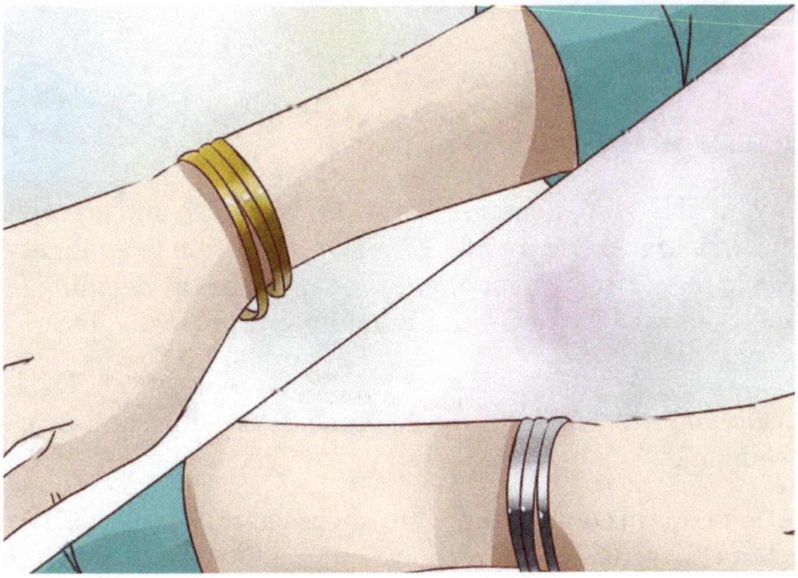

- If they look blue, then you may have a cool skin tone.
- If they look green, then you may have a warm skin tone.

- If some look blue and some look green, or it's hard to tell, then you're likely to have a neutral skin tone.

3. Put a silver bracelet on one wrist and a gold bracelet on the other. Does one of them blend in better? Or does one clearly look better against your skin than the other one does? This can also indicate your probable skin tone.

- Silver bracelets usually look best on cool skin tones.
- Gold bracelets tend to stand out on warm skin tones.
- If there's no major difference, then you may have a neutral skin tone.

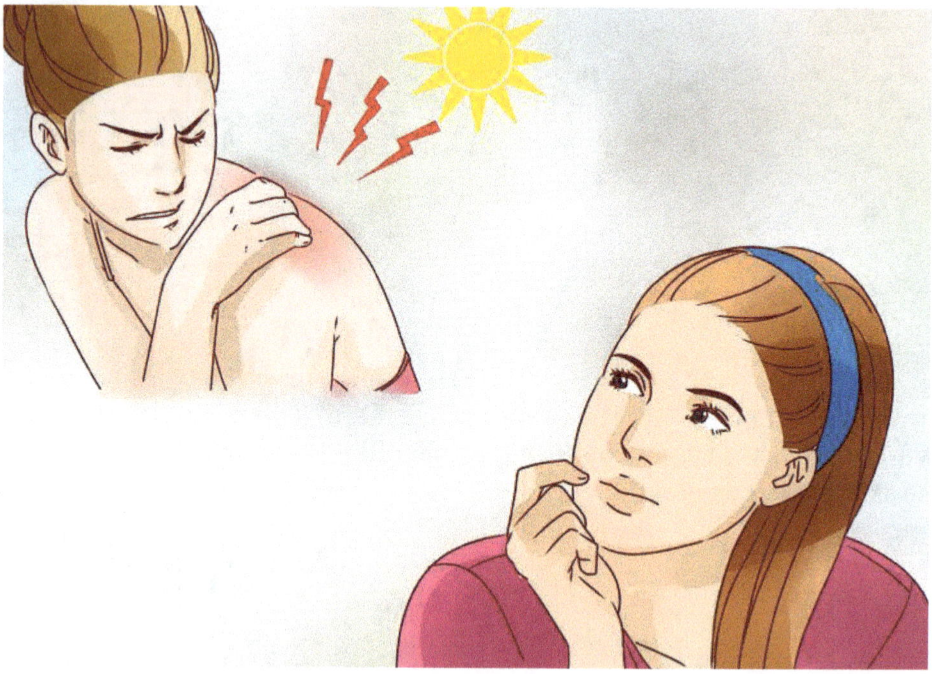

4. Think about how your skin responds to sunlight. Do you flush and even burn easily? Are you already brown by the time May rolls around? Your skin's reaction to sunlight can give you a hint as to your probable skin tone. However, sunlight should not be the deciding factor for determining your skin tone. People with darker skin often do not burn easily, but may still have a cool tone.

- If you tan easily, you may have a warm skin tone. If you flush and/or burn easily, you may have a cool skin tone.
- Make sure to take this in conjunction with other factors. People with dark skin often don't burn easily, but may actually have a cool skin tone. If you are dark-skinned, and you notice other signs of a cool skin tone, you're unlikely to have a warm tone regardless of how your skin responds to the sun. Makeups designed for a warm tone may look off on your skin.

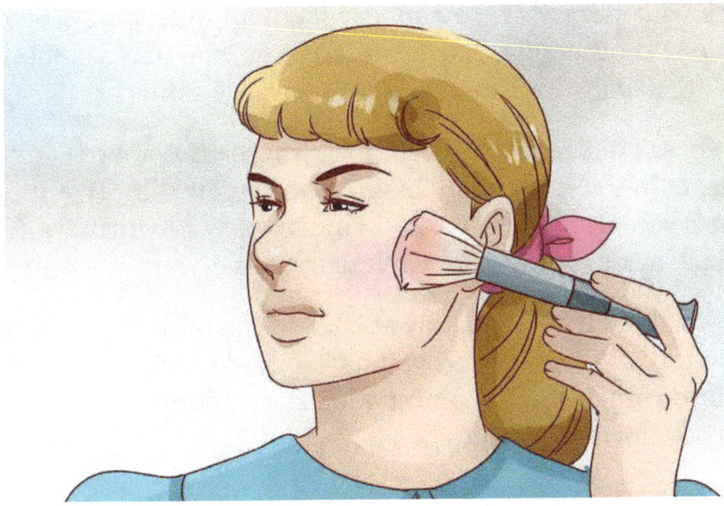

5. Use your skin tone to figure out what colors you should wear. Once you know your skin tone, you can use it to help you pick out foundations, blush, clothes, shades of lipstick, and many other things.

- When it comes to makeup, cool skin tones generally mix best with pink and berry shades. Dark skins with cooler tones may work well with espresso shades.
- Warm tones go well with bronzes, golds, and makeup with yellow undertones.
- Neutral skin tones can wear a wide range of colors and undertones, but they may lean more toward warmer or cooler tones, like a neutral skin tone that leans warm when combined with olive skin color. Experiment with pink and yellow undertones to see which ones work best.

Part 2

Choosing a Foundation

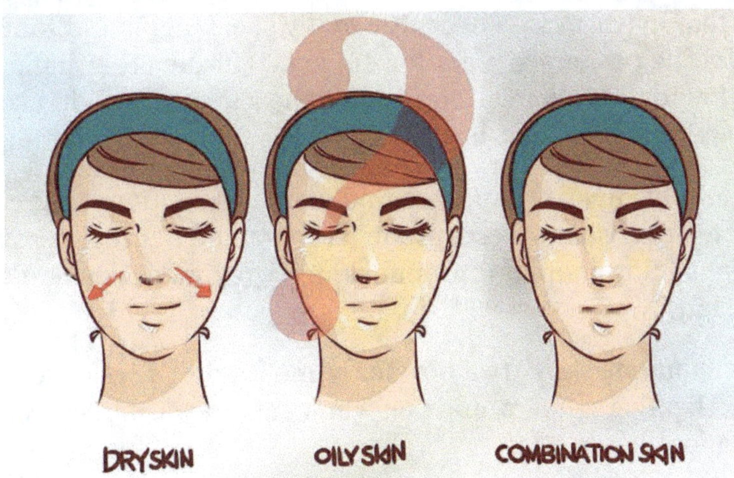

1. Figure out your skin type. Does your skin tend to be oily, dry, or a combination of the two? To determine your skin type, look closely at your skin in the mirror.

- How visible are your pores? If they appear large all over, you probably have oily skin. If some are visible and others are harder to see, you may have combination skin. Small to invisible pores are usually indicative of normal or dry skin.
- Do you tend to break out regularly, and if so, where? If you break out a lot in your T-zone (forehead, nose, chin), you probably have combination skin. If you tend to get break outs all over your face, you probably have oily skin. People with normal and dry skin will also get pimples and blackheads, but with much less frequency.
- How shiny is your skin? If it's not shiny at all, and can even appear dull and scaly, your skin is probably dry. If it's shiny all over, you have oily skin. Normal skin appears smooth and healthy without too much shine. Combination skin is shiny around the forehead, nose, and chin, but looks normal across your cheeks.

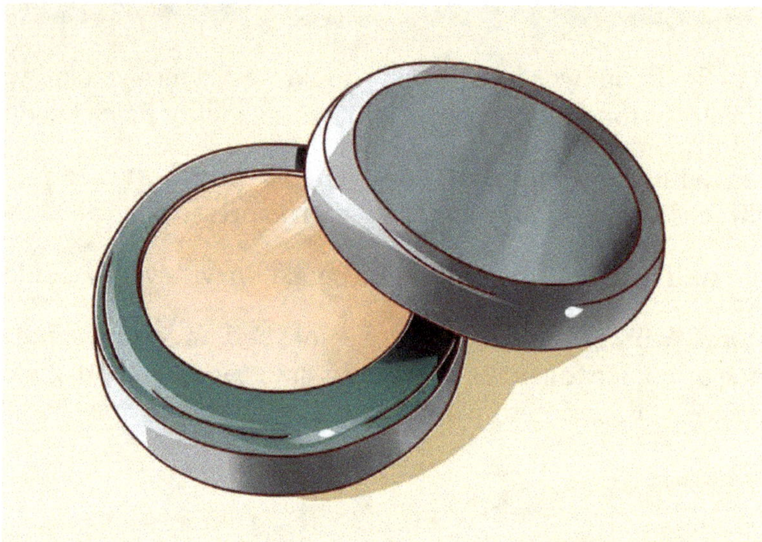

2. Let your skin type determine the type of foundation. Each person's skin has different needs, so go with a foundation that meets those needs. Generally speaking, liquid foundations or creamier foundations with hydrating power are great for dry skin. On the other hand, oily skin looks best with a matte powder foundation that will tone down the shine. If you do use a liquid foundation with oily skin, make sure that it isn't oil-based.

- If you have a lot of acne, you can even find some foundations that contain salicylic acid. However, if you already use several products contained benzoyl peroxide or salicylic acid, be careful about adding another into your skincare regimen. You don't want to end up with acne plus dry skin.
- If you have combination skin, try a powder foundation. It's easier to apply more heavily in some areas and lightly in others, and you won't get awkward lines, which can happen with a liquid foundation.
- If you want a foundation that does everything for you—hydration, sunscreen, packed with nutrients, evening out skin tone—you can use a product called a BB cream. The "BB" stands for "beauty balm" or "blemish balm." Basically, it's an all-in-one product that can be used

for any skin type. It's less specific to a particular skin tone or hue, but it is versatile enough to work as a foundation.

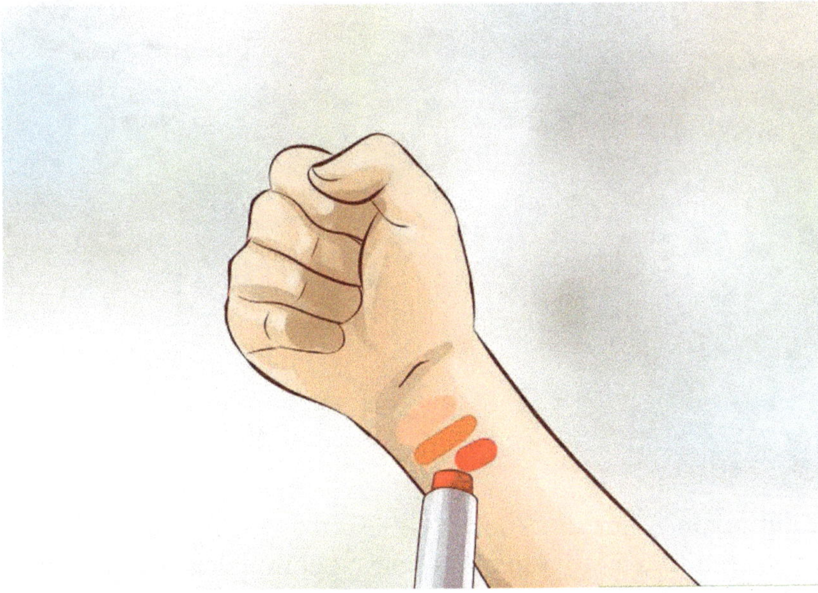

3. Narrow down your color choices by your skin tone. Some foundations have a rosier or bluish undertone. For those with cool skin tones, that's ideal. For those who have warmer skin tones, you should be looking for a similarly warm base, like a yellow or ivory. Neutral skin tones should experiment with both to see what looks best. If you have olive skin, try neutral or warm undertones.

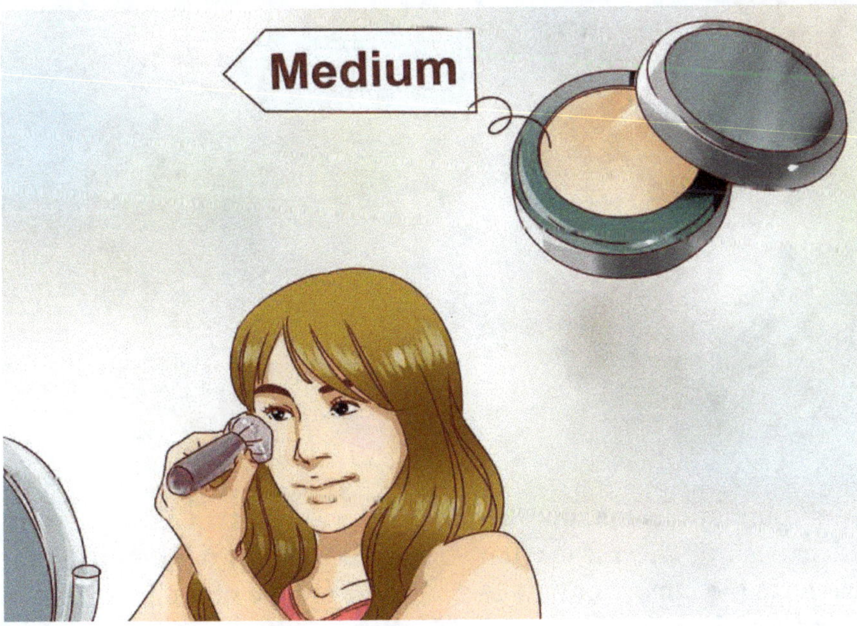

4. Decide how much you want to cover up. If you have major acne, you have the option of using a medium or heavyweight foundation. This will help to even out your skin texture. On the other hand, you might not want much coverage at all. Lightweight options include tinted moisturizers and sheer foundations.

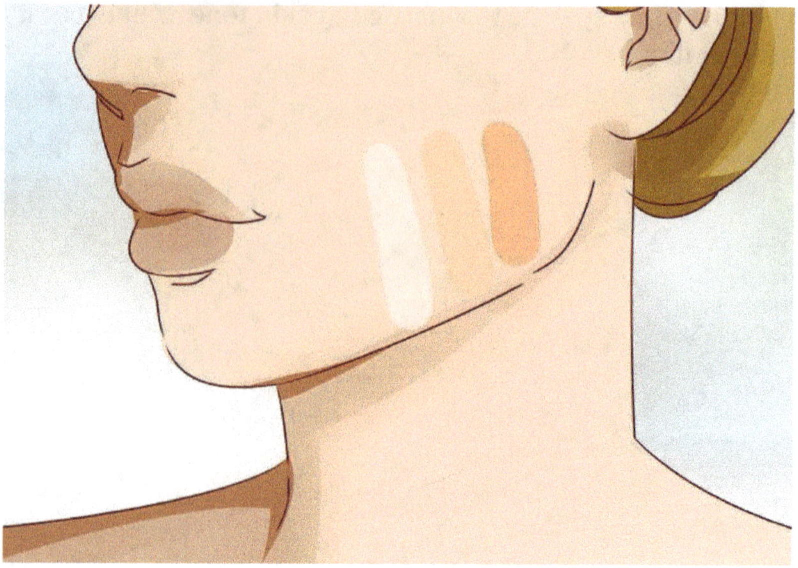

5. Test out the foundation on your skin. You've narrowed down your choices to one or two types of foundation and you've eliminated anything that doesn't complement your skin tone. To found out which one matches your skin color, apply a dab of each one to your neck or upper chest—your face and jawline may be too uneven to get a good match.

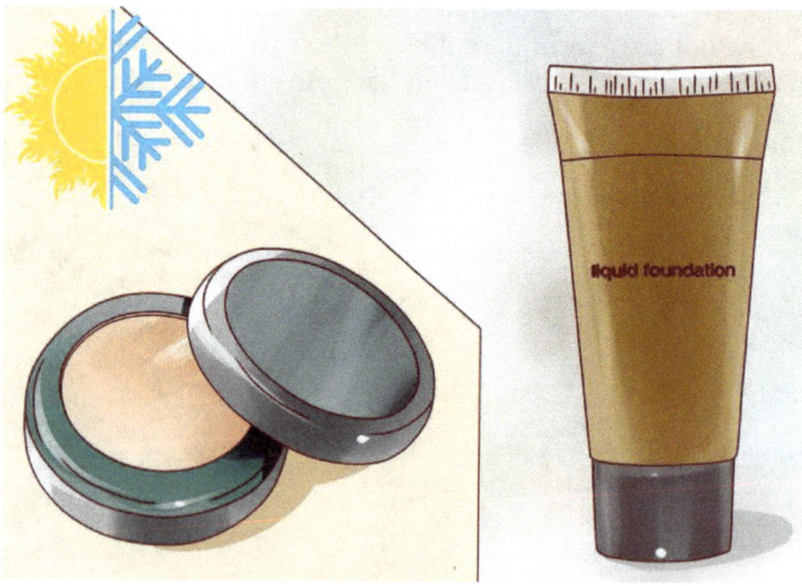

6. Pick out different foundations for summer and winter. Your skin changes from winter to summer, thanks to sun exposure. This means that you should have two different shades of foundation to match. You also have the opportunity to use a different type of foundation if your skin's needs change over the course of the year, like using a foundation with more hydration in winter and one with a higher SPF in summer.

- If you have fairly consistent skin quality from season to season, use the same type of foundation (powder, liquid, crème, etc.) so that you can just mix the summer and winter shades for spring and fall.

Part 3

Finding Your Perfect Color Palette

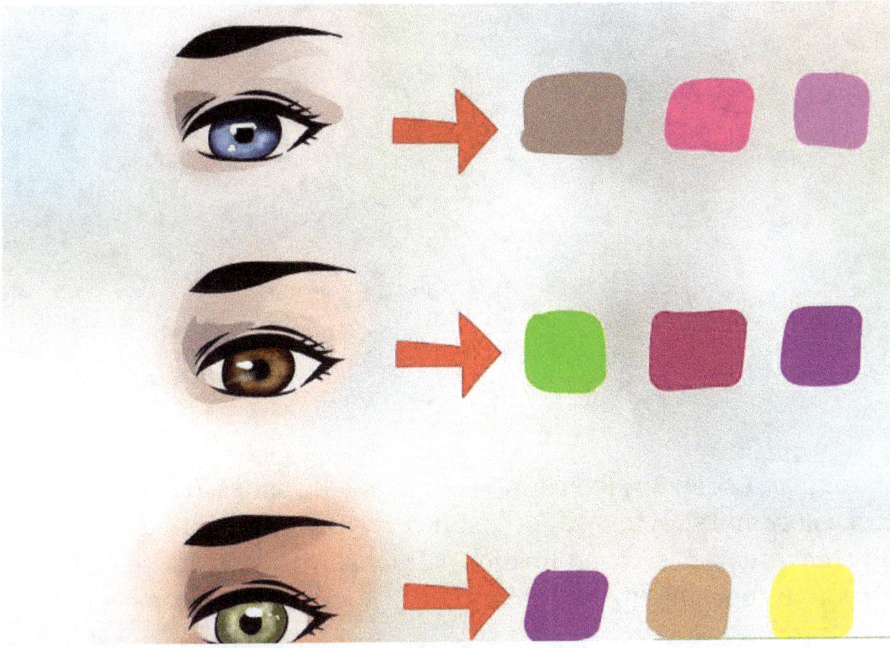

1. Base your eyeshadow selection on the color of your eyes. Are they true blue, gray, green, hazel, or brown? Different eye colors "pop" with different eyeshadow colors.

- Brown eyes don't really have a specific palette. Fortunately, they look good with almost anything. You can add warmth to your eyes with red-browns and metallics, or you can play up your look with darker colors or brighter jewel tones that other eyes can't get away with as easily.
- For blue or gray eyes, the best choices for a little pop are warm copper and brown tones. For drama or to highlight the blue, wear a smoky gray shadow (or liner!). For other colors, generally steer towards pinks and pastels. If you have lighter eyes, colorful eyeshadow that is darker than your eye color can be overpowering.
- For green eyes, purple is your best friend. If you want a little dramatic flair, try a purple that's almost black for double the effect.
- Hazel eyes get a little more variety. If your eyes are greener, opt for the purple palette that makes green eyes look glamorous. If your eyes have more brown or flecks of gold, play that up with warm brown and gold tones.
- Don't forget about your skin tone. If your smoky eye turns out looking more like a bruised eye, then you might need to factor in your skin tone and whether your skin is fair, olive, or dark. Fair skin goes far with light colors, like pastel peaches and pinks, but bright and bold tones are too pronounced, leaving everything else looking washed out. Similarly, darker skin could appear ashy if you use a cool blue or grey. If you're having trouble figuring it out, pick up a cheap palette with a wide array of colors and experiment with your eyes.

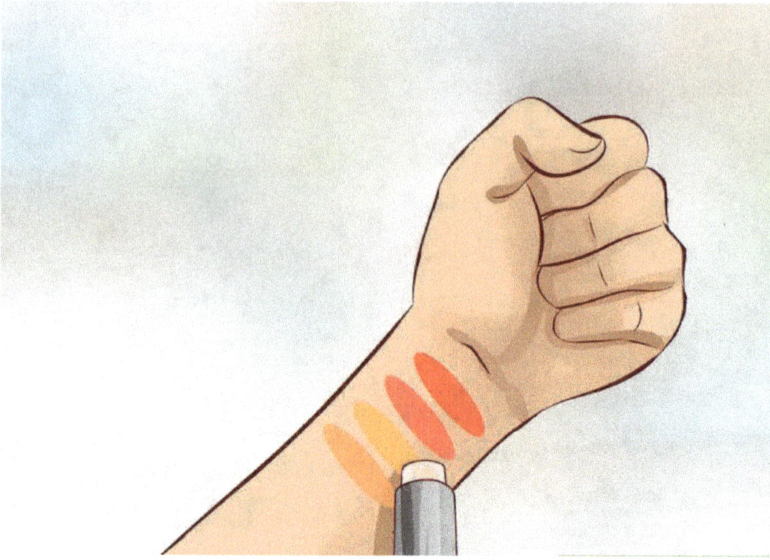

2. Use your skin tone and color to determine your lipstick shades. This is usually pretty easy to figure out for most colors and skin tones. For instance, if you're fair with a cool skin tone, you probably already know that an orange-toned lipstick will make you look strange. There are two things to consider when you're choosing lipstick colors.

- First, use your skin color to guide you toward the right color range. Fair skin plays well with bold and bright colors. Olive, neutral, or medium skin works with most colors, just avoid ones that will look pale. Dark skin pairs with richer, deeper colors, like wine or bright red.
- Second, narrow down your selection by factoring in your skin tone. Warmer skin tones pair well with warm base notes. When you're choosing a red lipstick, for example, you can easily wear a brick red or one with more orange to it. Cooler skin tones work best with pinks, blues, and purples. Your ideal red lipstick is more berry than brick or has a little plum in it.

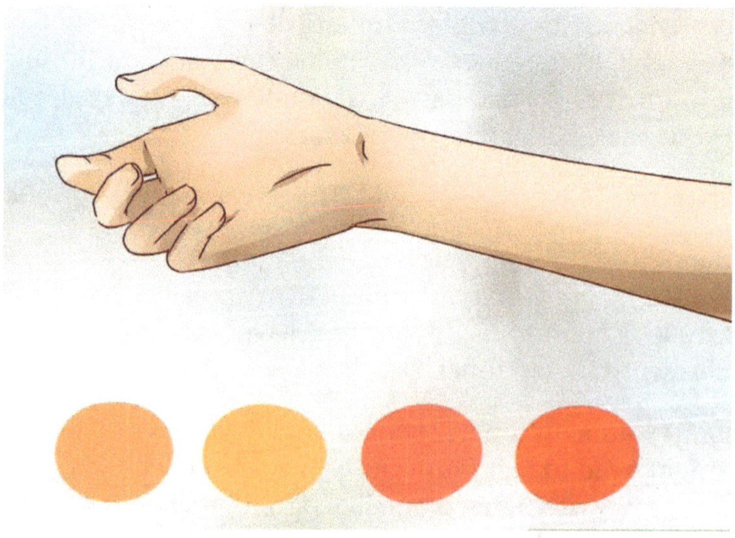

3. Pick a blush using your skin tone. The theme here is that whatever you put on your skin should work with your skin's natural pigmentation. Cool skin tones should wear pink blushes that go

well with their naturally rosier tendencies, or try pinker peach tones. A warm skin tone will shine with golden undertones, more towards the beige, orange peach, and apricot end of the spectrum. If you're lucky enough to have neutral skin tone, play around with different colors depending on your mood.

- If you're unsure how bright or dark to go with the blush, use your skin color as a guide. Fair skin works great with pastel pinks, while dark skin requires rich, bold colors like red-toned browns and oranges. Olive skin has a little more room to play around, but still leans more towards the pink end with room for darker, brighter colors than fair skin.

Part 4

Applying Makeup for Day or Night

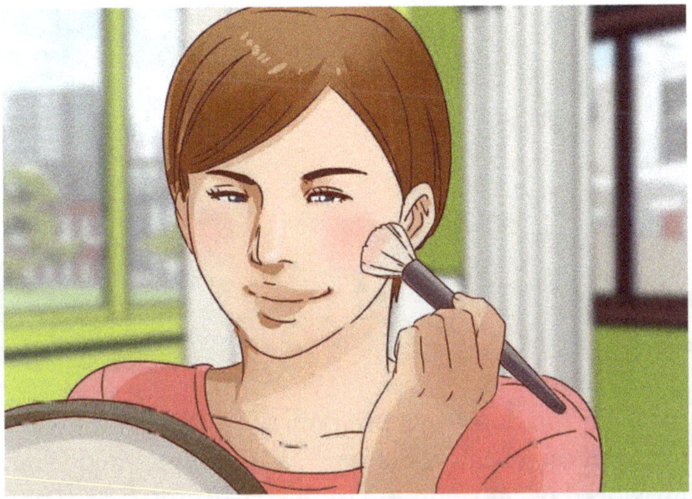

1. Choose neutrals or lighter colors for workplace wear. This is generally true if you work in a workplace with a business or business casual dress code. You might be able to get away with a dark lip color if you have darker skin, but otherwise, avoid dramatic or bright colors. Opt for nudes, beiges, and pastels around your eyes, and apply minimal eyeliner.

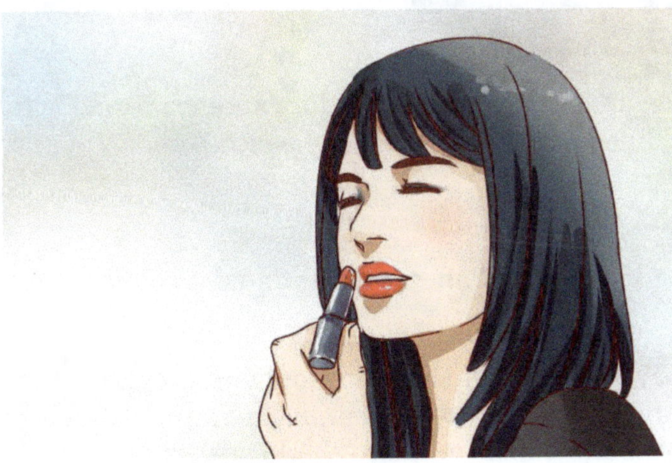

- Do have at least a basic makeup regimen for work. Women are perceived more favorably when they take those extra steps. You never know: some foundation, a bit of eyeshadow, and a sweep of mascara may be the little thing that tilts the balance in your favor.

2. Play with brighter, bolder colors for evenings out. You have less to constrain your style, so why not go for something a bit more astonishing? Break out the bright red lipstick for a kissable confidence boost. Play with a tropical theme for your eyeshadow. Add false eyelashes to take your lash game from good to great.

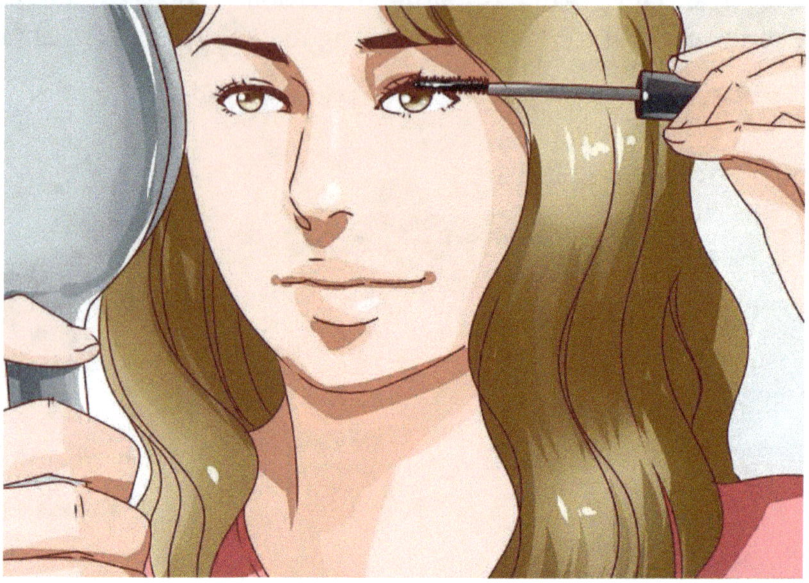

3. Set yourself up for an easy transition. If you're going out after work, start your day with the basics. Line your eyes lightly, put on a coat of mascara, and wear a single shade of eyeshadow. Once you get to the end of your workday, you can pop in the bathroom for extra eyeliner, another shade or two of eyeshadow to complete the effect, and an extra coat (or two) of mascara. Finish it off with a bright touch of lip color and you'll be good to go.

Primer

A cosmetic primer is a cream or lotion applied before another cosmetic to improve coverage and lengthen the amount of time the cosmetic lasts on the face.

Variations

There are different kinds of cosmetic primers such as foundation primer, eyelid primer, lip primer, and mascara primer.

A foundation primer may work like a moisturizer only different, or it may absorb oil with salicylic acid or aid in creating a less oily, more matte appearance. It aids in applying the foundation more evenly and smoothly, and increases the longevity of the foundation. Some contain antioxidants such as A, C, and E, or other ingredients such as grape seed extract and green tea extract. There are water-based and silicon-based foundation primers. Ingredients may include cyclomethicone and dimethicone. Some primers do not contain preservative, oil or fragrance. Some may also have sun protection factor (SPF). Some foundation primers are tinted to even out or improve skin tone or color. Others give a pearlized finish to make the complexion more light reflective. There are also foundation primers which are mineral-based primers, which contain mica and silica.

Eyelid or eye shadow primers are similar, but made specifically for use near the eyes. An eyelid primer may help even the color of the lid and upper eye area, may reduce oiliness, may add shimmer, or inversely may mattify. Eye primers aid in the smooth application of eye shadow, prevent it from accumulating in eyelid creases, and improve its longevity. Eye shadow primers are applied to the eyelid and lower eye area prior to the application of eye shadow. They even out the skin tone of the eyelids hide eyelid veins, and smooth out the skin of the eyelids. Eye shadow primers help with the application of eye shadows. They intensify the color of the eye shadows and keep them from smearing or creasing by reducing the oiliness of the lids. The effect of eye shadow primers is not limited to eye shadows. They also work for eye liners and eye shadow bases.

Mascara primer is sometimes colorless. It usually thickens and/or lengthens the lashes before the application of mascara for a fuller finished look. It may also help keep mascara from smudging or flaking, and some claim to improve the health of the lashes.

Lip primers are intended to smooth the lips and help improve the application of lipstick or lip gloss, although exfoliating the lips is often recommended before applying. They also are intended to increase the longevity of lip color, and to prevent lipstick from "feathering", that is, smearing past the lip vermilion, and especially from migrating into any fine lines around the lips.

Rouge

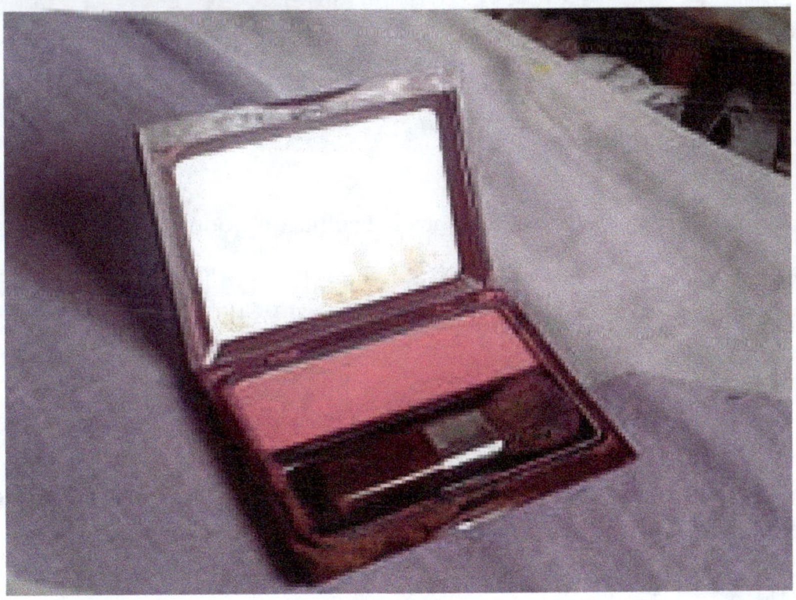

A rouge compact containing a mirror and brush

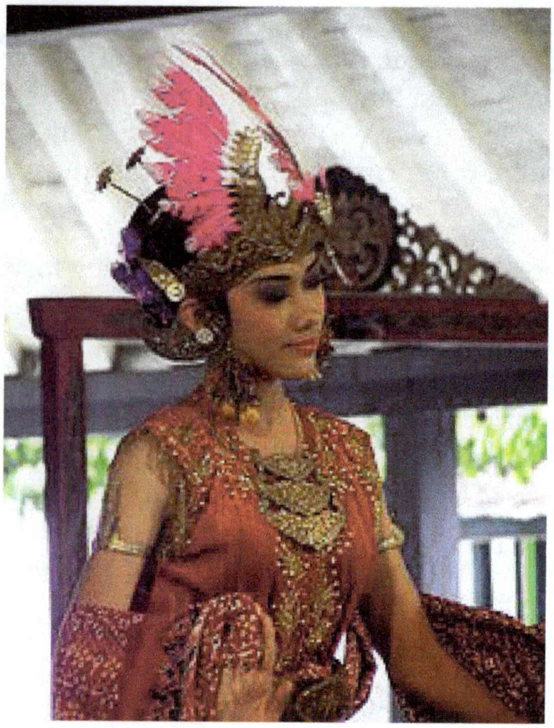

A dancer wearing rouge

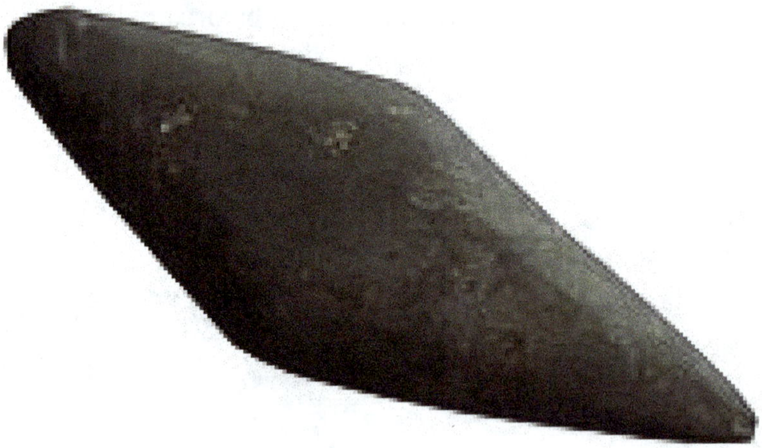

Shale rouge palette of the Naqada I culture, c. 4000–3500 BCE

Rouge, also called blush or blusher, is a cosmetic typically used by women to redden the cheeks so as to provide a more youthful appearance, and to emphasize the cheekbones.

Contemporary

Modern rouge generally consists of a red-coloured talcum-based powder that is applied with a brush to the cheek. The colouring is usually either the substance of safflor (the petals of safflower), or a solution of carmine in ammonium hydroxide and rosewater perfumed with rose oil. A cream-based variant of rouge is schnouda, a colourless mixture of Alloxan with cold cream, which also colours the skin red.

Types of Blush

Pressed-powder

The majority of blushes found in drugstore or high-end stores are in the form of pressed-powder. The blush lies flat on the pan, unlike baked blushes. These are best suited for people with oily skin. Using a pressed-powder blush for people with dry skin is not recommended because the powder might cling to dry patches of their skin. Pressed-powder blushes usually last long on the skin, are easily blended and are very buildable. For these reasons, pressed powder blushes are usually used by makeup artists during special occasions like weddings or events that project harsh lighting. Pressed-powder blushes come in many finishes, including matte, shimmer and satin.

Cream

Cream blushes usually come in a short, round container, much like a lip balm or solid perfume. These blushes are best suited for people with dry skin. Cream blush is typically blended using fingers or a stippling brush. Since the nature of the blush is a cream, it can be layered with a powder blush to improve longevity of use.

Mineral Baked

Mineral baked blush can be differentiated from pressed-powder blushes mainly because of its appearance on the pan. It is luminous, has shimmery veins and shaped like a dome. Mineral baked blushes are made from a liquid that is baked into solid form. This means that there is less talc and more pigment. Because it is originally liquid form, spraying the pan with water can make the blush creamy and more opaque. However, it does change back to its solid form when it dries. Mineral baked powder is very sheer when applied, but is buildable and can be the perfect choice for someone who is going for a more flushed and natural look.

Blush Brushes

- Stippling brush: suitable for softening out harsh lines and blend together blush, bronzer and highlight. It is most suitable for applying cream blush.
- Fluffy brush: suitable for dispersing the colour of the blush, creating a natural flushed look.
- Flat brush: The type of brush included with many, especially drugstore, blushes. Used to achieve a more dramatic look, as this type of brush is not well suited for blending.

Kohl

Kohl is an ancient eye cosmetic, traditionally made by grinding stibnite (Sb_2S_3) - for similar purposes to charcoal used in mascara. It is widely used in South Asia, the Middle East, North Africa, the Horn of Africa, and parts of West Africa as eyeliner to contour and/or darken the eyelids and as mascara for the eyelashes. It is worn mostly by women, but also by some men and children.

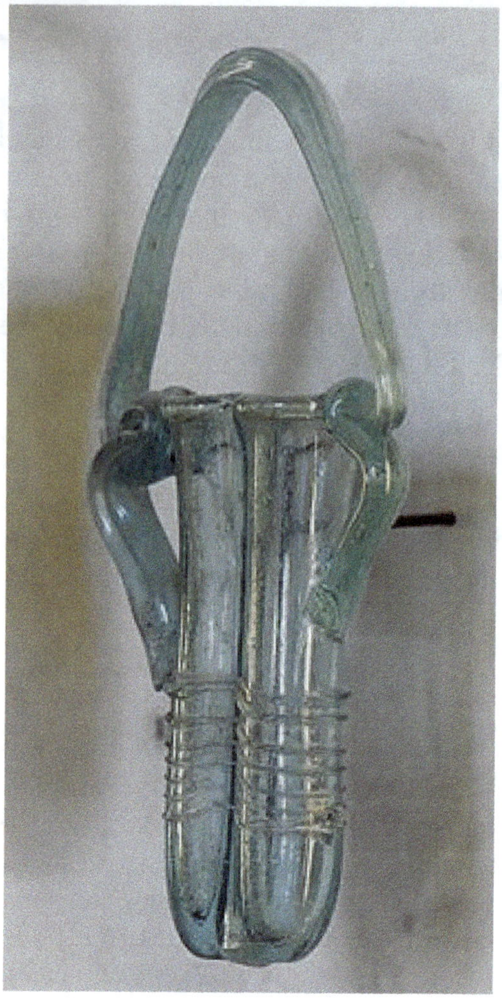

A double cosmetic tube for kohl from the Louvre Museum in Paris.

Kohl has also been used in India as a cosmetic for a long time. In addition, mothers would apply kohl to their infants' eyes soon after birth. Some did this to "strengthen the child's eyes", and others believed it could prevent the child from being cursed by the evil eye.

Preparation

Preparation of homemade kajal begins with dipping a clean, white, thin muslin cloth, about four by four inches square, in sandalwood paste or the juice of Alstonia scholaris (Manjal karisilanganni), which is then dried in the shade. This dip and dry process is done all day long. After sunset, a wick is made out of the cloth, which is then used to light a mud lamp filled with castor oil. A brass vessel is kept over the lamp, leaving a little gap, just enough for the oxygen to aid the burning of the lamp. This is left burning overnight. In the morning, one or two drops of pure ghee (clarified cow's butter) or castor oil are added to the soot which now lines the brass vessel. It is then stored in a clean dry box.

All the ingredients used in this preparation (sandalwood/Manjal karsilanganni, castor oil, ghee) are believed to have medicinal properties. They are still used in Indian therapies like ayurveda and Siddha medicines.

In rural Bengal, kajal is made from the "Monosha" plant, a type of succulent spurge (*Euphorbia neriifolia*). The leaf of Monosha is covered with oil and is kept above a burning diya (mud lamp). Within minutes the leaf is covered with creamy soft black soot which is so safe and sterile that it is even applied to infants.

Eyelash Curler

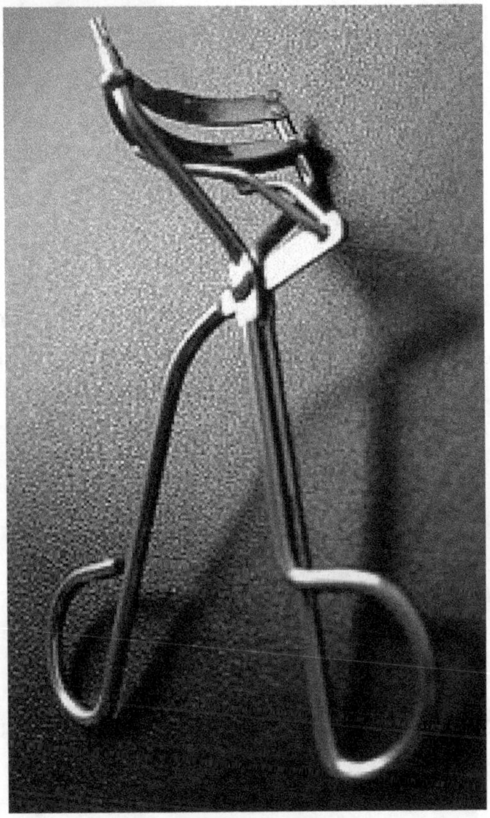

Eyelash curler

An eyelash curler is a hand-operated mechanical device for curling eyelashes for cosmetic purposes. Usually only the upper eyelashes are curled. Before using, the device can be heated for a short time with a hair dryer, but not to the extent to burn the delicate skin above the eyes. Self-heating, battery-operated units are available.

The first known patent for the eyelash curler states that it was filed by Charles Stickel and William McDonell from Rochester, New York. A further review of the 1931 Eyelash Curler patent shows that it was invented by William McDonell.

William Beldue and his Kurlash Company held patents in Canada, the United States and Great Britain for the eyelash curler and improvements to it.

Eyelash curlers are usually made of metal, and often have rubber pads where the curlers make contact with the lashes. Manufacturers include ForteBellezza, Shiseido and Shu Uemura.

Usage

There are two ways of using an eyelash curler. It can be either used after warming up with a hair dryer or without warming. To get the best results, it is recommended to use it after warming up with a hair dryer because it lasts longer. When using heated eyelash curlers, it is very important to be cautious of the temperature the curler is heated to. To avoid the risk of burning the eyelid with the hot metal curlers, many companies have introduced plastic based curlers. Some companies are looking into introducing self-heated curlers to control the temperature and completely eliminate the risk of a burn.

To begin, warm up the curler and then curl the eyelashes for 10 to 15 seconds. Continue curling them until you have the desired shape. Next, apply more coats of mascara and curl the eyelashes once more for the final look. Repeat the application of mascara and curling of the lashes until the desired length reached. Due to varying eyelash length, some users might have to apply mascara and curl the eyelashes more times.

Advantages

It is a good makeup kit tool because it gives the illusion of bigger and brighter eyes and helps lengthen the eyelashes. When it is applied using different tactics such going heavier on the outer corner eyelashes, it gives a different and well-defined shape to the eyes. It is easy to use without professional training and is not very expensive to purchase. Additionally, it is not a very big tool, so it can be comfortably placed in the makeup bag.

Eyelid Glue

Eyelid glue, commonly called eye putti, is a type of eye make-up used in East Asia designed to change the monolid (eyelid without a crease). Eyelid glue is a water-soluble adhesive that can be easily removed.

Use

Double eyelids are considered a sign of feminine beauty in East Asia. Some women opt for a temporary solution by wearing eyelid glue. The glue is painted on the upper eyelid, which is then pushed upward with a plastic prong and held in place by the adhesive. The glue needs to dry for a minute before holding the fold. This method creates or enhances a fold in the eyelid ("double eyelid") that opens up the eye exposing the eyelashes. The use of eyelid glue also exists amongst men.

The glue does not last and must be reapplied after a few hours. Eyelid glue may also cause irritation.

Variant

A variant called eyelid tape or crease tape comes in a fibrous elastic strip that is trimmed to shape and placed on the eyelid. The tape creates a crease that stays on the eyelid. The tape does not last and must be reapplied after a few hours.

Makeup Brush

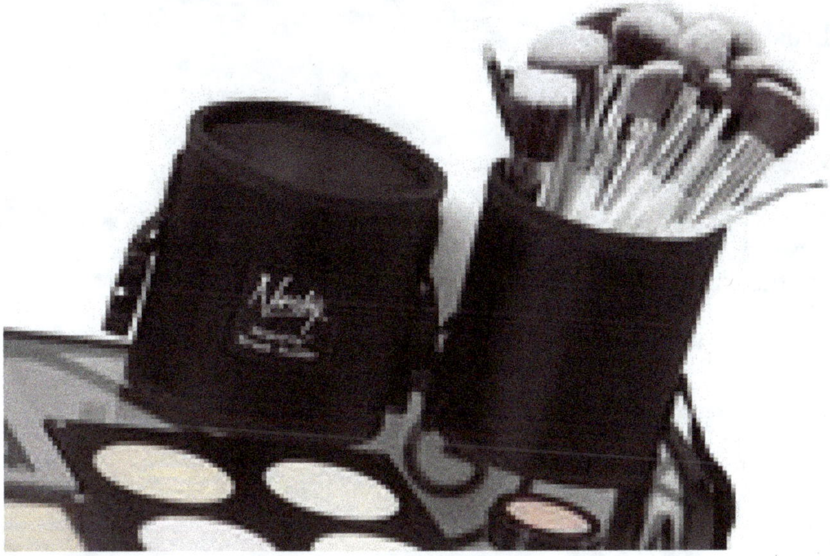

Make-up brushes

A makeup brush is a tool with bristles, used for the application of make up or face painting. The bristles could be made out of natural or synthetic materials, while the handle is usually made out of plastic or wood. When cosmetics are applied using the appropriate brush they blend better into the skin.

There is a large variety of shapes and sizes of make up brushes, depending on the face area where make up will be applied, the cosmetic product and the wanted result. For example, the shape of the brush tip can be chiseled, straight, angular, round, flat or tapered.

Types of Makeup Brushes (by Area of Application)

Face

- Foundation brush - long, flat bristles and tapered tip
- Powder brush - fluffy bristles; soft, full and rounded
- Fan brush - similar to a fan painting brush, used for light touches
- Blush brush - fine bristles and rounded head
- Concealer brush - soft and flat with a pointed tip and a wide base
- Kabuki brush - very thick and rounded with a short handle
- Duo fiber multipurpose brush - flat, circular and feathery head
- Mineral powder brush - thick and rounded
- Face Contour Brush - Slanted and rounded for cheekbones

- Face Sponge - Varied Shape, Sponge Texture

Eyes

- Eyeshadow brushes
- basic eyeshadow brush
- crease brush
- lid brush
- contour brush/blending brush
- Angle eyeshadow brush - small, soft and rounded angled tip
- Eyeliner brush - very thin and fine with soft bristles
- Blending eyeshadow brush - long with a round head
- Smudge brush - flat and soft
- Mascara (usually comes with the mascara)
- Eyebrow brush - long, thin with tougher bristles
- Slanted Eyebrow Definer Brush - Stiff and Angeled
- Spiral brush

Lips

- Lipstick brush - fine, soft and tapered
- Lip gloss brush (usually comes with the lip gloss)

Types of Makeup Brush Bristles

Makeup application can alter due to the materials used to create a makeup brush. Bristles of a makeup brush can either be synthetic or natural. The brush itself is important to the application of makeup as it can densely pack on product or loosely pack on product.

Synthetic Bristles

Synthetic bristles are the most common material used in a makeup brush. They are widely found in drugstores and makeup specific stores. The bristles are made out of plastic, and are often dyed to get some color on the bristles. Synthetic bristles are often used with liquid and cream products, as they tend to blend out products more easily and will not absorb product as much compared to a natural bristle brush. Synthetic are cruelty-free. The bristles are usually made from nylon or other synthetic fibers. The longevity of synthetic brushes are usually longer than natural haired bristles as they do not degrade or breakdown and are not as fragile.

Natural Bristles

Natural bristles are made from real hair as opposed to plastic. Many prefer to use natural bristles, since they could be less abrasive to the skin. Although natural bristles are more preferred in the cosmetic industry, the bristles themselves can cause allergic reactions because of the animal fur/hair. Natural bristles may be easier to control the product when blending out or even packing on a product. Natural bristles do have hair cuticles which is why it is easier for the brush to pick up more product and blending it out.

Types of Natural Bristle Brushes

- Sable
- Goat
- Badger
- Pony
- Squirrel

Kabuki Brush

A kabuki brush (sometimes called mushroom brush) is a makeup brush with a short stem and dense bristles. The brush head is most often rounded, though it can also be flat. Traditionally, the bristles are made of natural materials like animal hair (e.g., goat or horse hair), but most brushes available now on the market have synthetic bristles.

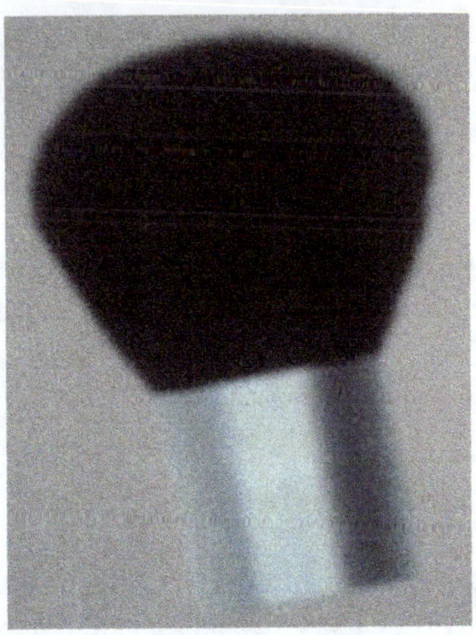

Kabuki Brush

Modern Usage

Usually, a kabuki brush is used to apply loose powdered make-up on large surfaces of the face (e.g., foundation, face powder, blush). Because of its design, the brush blends powdered make up evenly on the skin and creates a very natural looking coverage. The brush's popularity is also due to the convenience of being able to replace a series of brushes (foundation, powder, blush and mineral powder brushes).

Glitter

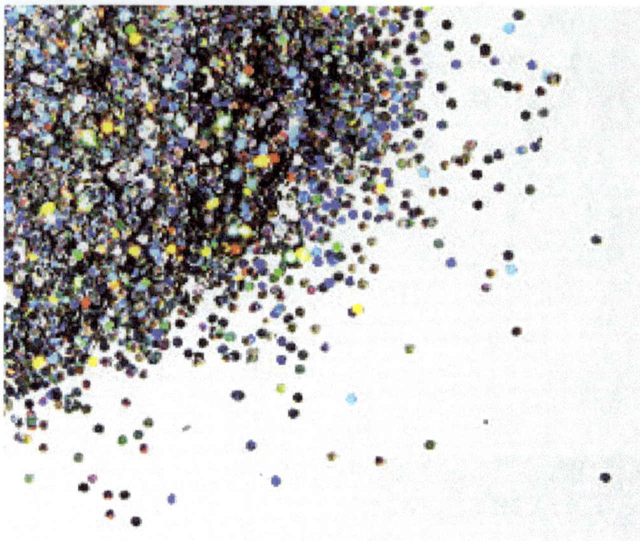

Close-up of glitter

Glitter describes an assortment of small, flat, reflective particles. Glitter particles reflect light at different angles, causing the surface to sparkle or shimmer. Glitter is like confetti, sparkles, or sequins, but somewhat smaller. Since prehistoric times, glitter has been made and used as decoration, from many different materials including stones such as malachite, galena, and mica, as well as insects and glass. Modern glitter is usually manufactured from plastic.

Modern Glitter

The first production of modern plastic glitter is credited to the American machinist Henry Ruschmann, who found a way to cut plastic or mylar sheets into glitter in 1934. During World War II with German glass glitter unavailable, Ruschmann found a market for scrap material ground into glitter made of plastics. He founded Meadowbrook Inventions, Inc. in Bernardsville, New Jersey, the company is still a producer of industrial glitter. Decades later he filed a patent for a mechanism for cross-cutting films as well as other related inventions.

Today over 20,000 varieties of glitter are manufactured in a vast number of different colors, sizes, and materials. Over 10,000,000 pounds (4,500,000 kg) of glitter was purchased between the years of 1989 and 2009 alone. Commercial glitter ranges in size from 0.002 square inches (1.3 mm^2) to 0.25 square inches (160 mm^2). First, flat multi-layered sheets are produced combining plastic, coloring, and reflective material such as aluminium, titanium dioxide, iron oxide, and bismuth oxychloride. These sheets are then cut into tiny particles of many shapes including squares, rectangles, and hexagons.

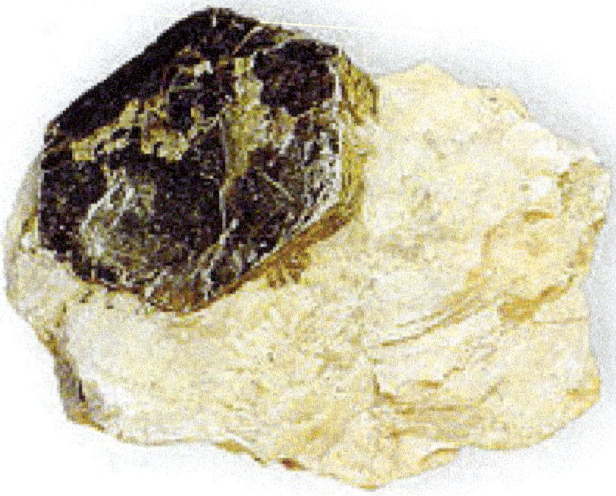

Mica

Glittering surfaces have been found to be used since prehistoric times in the arts and in cosmetics. The modern word "glitter" comes from *glitra* in Old Norse through Middle English. However, as early as 30,000 years ago, mica flakes were used to give cave paintings a glittering appearance. Prehistoric humans are believed to have used cosmetics, made of powdered hematite, a sparkling mineral.

8,000 years ago people of the Americas were using powdered galena a form of lead, to produce a bright greyish-white glittering paint used for objects of adornment. The collecting and surface mining of galena was prevalent in the Upper Mississippi Valley region by the Cahokia native peoples, for regional trade both raw and crafted into beads or other objects.

Over 6,000 years ago, ancient Egyptians produced glittering cosmetics from the iridescent shells of beetles as well as finely ground green malachite crystal. Researchers believe Mayan temples were sometimes painted with red, green, and grey glitter paint made from mica dust, based on infrared scans of the remnants of paint still found on the structures in present-day Guatemala.

Prior to modern plastics, particles of glass were used to create glittering surfaces and glass glitter is still produced commercially.

Uses

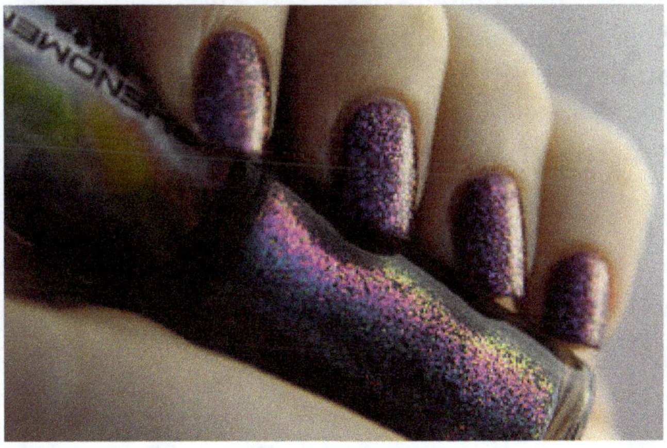

Glitter nail polish

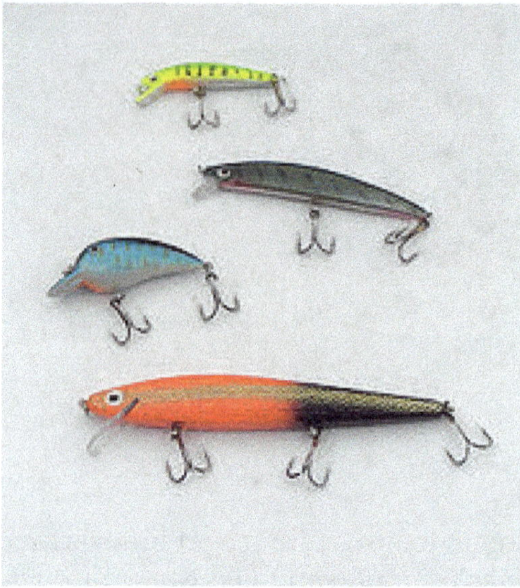

Iridescent fishing lures

Prior to fabrics made with modern glitter, sequins were sewn or woven on to fabric to give it a glittering appearance. Edible glitter made from gum arabic and other ingredients is even used by culinary artists.

Glitter is used in cosmetics to make the face and nails appear more shiny or sparkly. Additionally, it is used in children's arts and crafts to color and texture items. The small, brightly colored particles often stick to clothing, skin, and furniture, and can be a hassle to remove.

Glitter coatings or finishes are frequently used on fishing lures to draw attention by simulating the scales of prey fish.

Due to its unique characteristics, glitter has also proven to be useful forensic evidence. Because of the tens of thousands of different commercial glitters, identical glitter particles can be compelling evidence that a suspect has been at a crime scene. Glitter particles are easily transferred through the air or by touch, yet cling to bodies and clothing, often unnoticed by suspects.

Glitter is also used for glitter bombing, which is an act of protest in which activists throw glitter on people at public events. Glitter bombers have frequently been motivated by, though not limited to, their targets' opposition to same-sex marriage. Some legal officials argue glitter bombing is technically assault and battery. It is possible for glitter to enter the eyes or nose and cause damage to the cornea or other soft tissues potentially irritating them or leading to infection, depending on the size of the glitter. Whether a prosecutor would pursue the charges depends on a number of factors.

Eyelash Extensions

Applying extensions to the eyelashes is a practice that enhances the length, thickness and fullness of natural eyelashes. The extensions may consist of silk, mink, synthetic hair, or human hair. The main method of applying eyelash extensions is individually adhering them to the lash line one-by-one because it prevents the lashes from sticking together. False eyelashes and *eyelash extensions* are not the same.

Types of Lashes

Although false eyelashes and eyelash extensions both enhance the length of eyelashes, they differ in various ways. Furthermore, false eyelashes and eyelash extensions are also referred to as temporary false lashes and semi-permanent lashes, respectively.

Temporary False Lashes

Temporary false lashes are any lashes designed to be worn for a short period of 1–2 days. They can be made with a variety of materials and are not designed to be worn when showering, sleeping or swimming. They are applied with lash glue designed specifically for temporary lashes; the technique is called one-by one-application.

Semi-permanent Lashes

Semi-permanent lashes, also known as individual eyelash extensions, are eyelashes applied with an FDA approved adhesive with a stronger bond. The adhesive for lash extensions consists mainly of cyanoacrylate. There are various types of cyanoacrylates including ethyl, methyl, butyl, octyl and more. Different types of cyanoacrylates are designed for bonding to different surfaces. For example, lash adhesives are made from methyl-2 cyanoacrylate which is designed to bond a smooth surface (the eyelash extension) to a porous surface (the natural eyelash). Lash adhesive (methyl-2 cyanoacrylate) is designed to be used *around* the eyes and on the natural lashes, this is to ensure that it doesn't touch the skin as it may cause irritation. All cyanoacrylate adhesives are made using the same properties and ingredients found in medical-grade adhesives. Eyelash extensions are waterproof and give the appearance of having mascara on without the messy clumps and smudging of makeup. Generally, a single lash is applied to each natural lash. When applied properly, neither the extension lash nor the glue should touch the eyelid. The bond is designed to last until the lashes naturally fall out. Eyelash extensions create lashes that remain on for approximately 3–4 weeks with their natural growth and shedding cycle. However, the extensions may fall out faster if oil-based eye makeup remover is used, as oil weakens the bond between the glue and the lash. Moreover, rubbing one's eyes regularly also causes the extensions to fall out faster. To maintain one's lashes, one should avoid rubbing their eyes or wearing any mascara. Instead, one should use oil-free make up removal wipes and eyelid cleanser. To keep the eyelashes full, they must be refilled bi-monthly.

Eyelash extensions come in various types, lengths, colors, curves and thicknesses, from natural-looking, to glamorous, as well as dramatic.

Process

In the United States, eyelash extension services can range from $100 to $500, depending on:

- the type and number of lashes used,

- the skill level of the cosmetician,
- and the venue where the extensions are applied.

It usually takes one to two hours to attach a full, new set. An average person might have anywhere from thirty to eighty lashes per eye. The variance in the number of lashes accounts for the difference in how long it takes to apply them. Eyelash extensions usually last around 3–4 weeks, after which they start falling out or thinning. Maintaining a full set of lashes requires a refill service approximately every 3–4 weeks.

Training and Certification

Professionals trained in Lash Artistry go by various titles including "Lash Technicians", "Lash Artists", and "Lash Stylists". There are various companies that provide training and certification for potential Eyelash Extensions Technicians. In the UK, the Guild of Professional Beauty Therapists accredit courses for the safe application of semi-permanent individual eyelash extensions. The value of the course content can be judged by the number of CPD (Continued Professional Development) points that the course is awarded.

Tweezers

Tweezers are small tools used for picking up objects too small to be easily handled with the human hands. They are probably derived from tongs, pincers, or scissors-like pliers used to grab or hold hot objects since the dawn of recorded history. In a scientific or medical context they are normally referred to as forceps.

Tweezers make use of two third-class levers connected at one fixed end (the fulcrum point of each lever), with the pincers at the others.

People commonly use tweezers mainly for tasks such as plucking hair from the face or eyebrows, often using the term eyebrow tweezers. Other common uses for tweezers are as a tool to manipulate small objects, including for example small, particularly surface-mount, electronic parts, and small mechanical parts for models and precision mechanisms. Stamp collectors use tweezers (stamp tongs) to handle postage stamps which, while large enough to pick up by hand, could be damaged by handling; the jaws of stamp tongs are smooth. One example of a specialised use is picking out flakes of gold in gold panning. Tweezers are also used in kitchens for food presentation to remove bones from fillets of fish in a process known as pin boning.

Types

Tweezers come in a variety of tip shapes and sizes. Blunt tip tweezers have a rounded end which can be used when a pointed object may get entangled, when manipulating cotton swabs, for example. Flat tip tweezers, pictured at right, have an angled tip which may be used for removing splinters. Some tweezers have a long needle-like tip which may be useful for reaching into small crevices. Triangular tip tweezers have larger, wider tips useful for gripping larger objects. Tweezers with curved tips also exist, sometimes called bent forceps. Microtweezers have an extremely small, pointed tip used for manipulating tiny electronic components and the like.

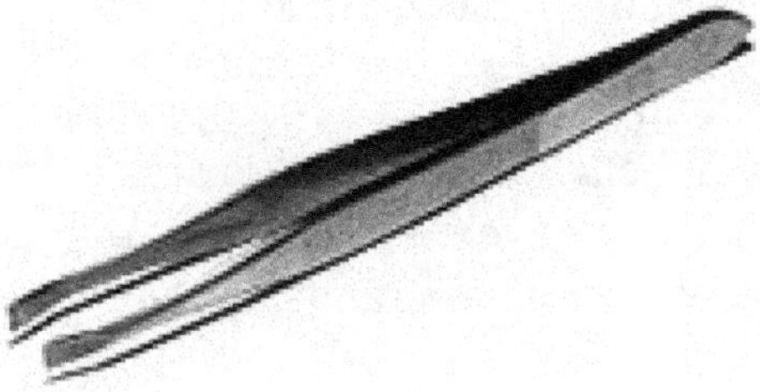

Flat tip conventional tweezers

There are two common forms of construction for tweezers: two fused, angled pieces of metal, or one piece of metal bent in half. The bent tweezer is cheaper to manufacture, but gives weaker grip. The fused tweezer is more expensive, but allows for a stronger grip. The width between the tips of the tweezers when no force is applied also affects how powerful the grip is.

Classification by Usage

Applications:

- in lead type
- in dealing with stamps
- in dealing with smaller coins, to protect the coins these are wrapped at the tips with plastic
- in electronics
- for hair removal (eyebrow tweezers)
- in semiconductor technology in the form of wafer tweezers
- in cosmetics
- in medicine (Forceps and Tissue Forceps)
- in the household
- in jewelery
- In the textile industry as iron nubs
- in soldering
- in science, laboratory
- in aquatics at planting e.g. Aquascaping
- in watchmaker usage

- There are also other tweezers, for example, so-called optical tweezers and vacuum tweezers to the tweezers.

The original tweezers for mechanical gripping have given rise to a number of tools with similar action or purpose but not dependent upon mechanical pressure, including

- Optical tweezers use light to manipulate microscopic objects as small as a single atom. The momentum transfer from a focused laser beam is able to trap small particles. In the biological sciences, these instruments have been used to apply forces in the pico Newton range and to measure displacements in the nm range of objects ranging in size from 10 nm to over 100 mm.
- Magnetic tweezers use magnetic forces to manipulate single molecules (such as DNA) via paramagnetic interactions. In practice it is an array of magnetic traps designed for manipulating individual biomolecules and measuring the ultra-small forces that affect their behavior.

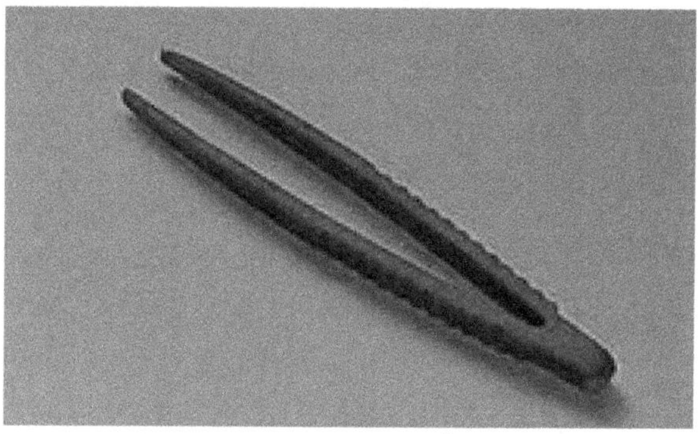

Plastic tweezers used in first aid kit

- Electric tweezers deliver an electrical signal through the tip, intended for depilation by damaging hair roots to prevent new hair from growing from the same root.
- Vacuum tweezers use differences in atmospheric pressure to grasp items from 100 micrometres in size up to parts weighing several pounds. Special vacuum tweezer tips are manufactured to handle a wide variety of items such as surface-mount electronics, optics, biological material, stamps and coins. They may be used to handle parts that are so small that conventional mechanical tweezers may cause parts to be damaged or dropped and lost.
- Molecular tweezers are noncyclic host molecules that have two arms capable of binding guests molecules through non-covalent bonding.
- Hot, or soldering, tweezers combine the squeezing action of mechanical tweezers with heating, to grip small surface-mount electronic devices while simultaneously heating them, for soldering or desoldering.
- Tweezer probes are a pair of electrical test probes fixed to a tweezer mechanism to measure voltages or other electronic circuit parameters between closely spaced pins.
- Tweezers integrated with an electronic measuring device for evaluation of electrical parameters of small-size electronic components.

- Carbon nano-tweezers have been fabricated by deposition of MWNT bundles on isolated electrodes deposited on tempered glass micropipettes.Those nanotube bundles can be mechanically manipulated by electricity and can be used to manipulate and transfer micro- and nano-structures. The nanotube bundles used for tweezers are about 50 nm in diameter and 2 μm in lengths. Under electric bias, two close sets of bundles are attracted and can be used as nanoscale tweezers.

Other uses of the same principle are named tweezers; although such terms are not necessarily widely used their meaning is clear to people in the relevant field. E.g., Raman tweezers, which combine Raman spectroscopy with optical tweezers.

Artificial Nails

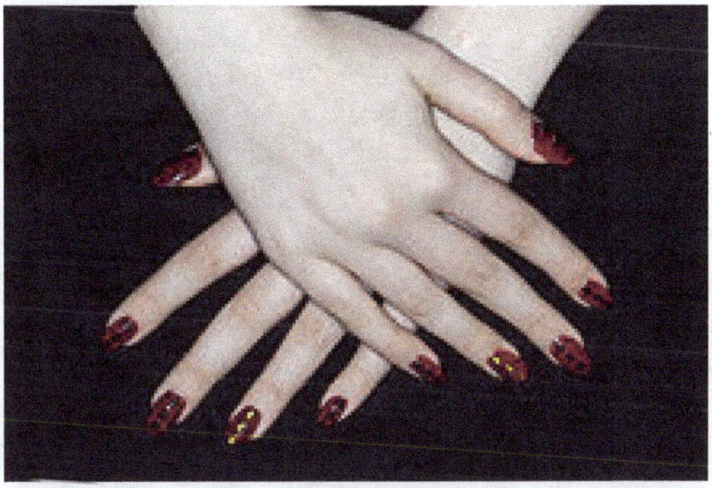

Artificial nails

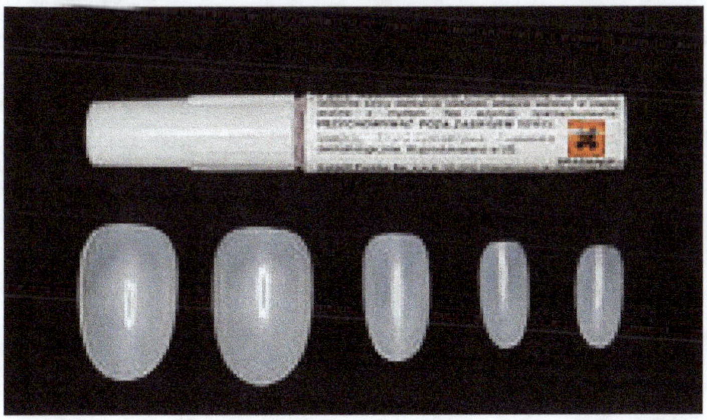

Artificial nails and glue

Artificial nails, also known as fake nails, false nails, fashion nails, nail enhancements, nail wraps or nail extensions, are coverings placed over fingernails as fashion accessories. Some artificial nails attempt to mimic the appearance of real fingernails as closely as possible, while other designs may deliberately stray in appearance from real fingernails. Artificial nails are made from a wide variety of materials.

Types

The artificial nails are not a replacement, but an extension for natural nails. There are two main approaches to creating artificial nails—*tips* and *forms*. Tips are made of lightweight plastic plates that are "nail"-shaped. They are glued on the end of the natural nail and acrylic or gel or a combination of both is then applied over the entire nail. Tips are now available in many different colors and designs, ranging from simple colors such as yellow or blue to flamboyant designs such as animal prints and mixed metallic colors. Forms are fitted over the nail and then an artificial nail is sculpted out of acrylic or gel and the form is removed and then properly shaped and buffed to a shine.

One popular material commonly called "Polymethyl methacrylate acrylics" is a mixture of a polymer powder and a liquid monomer (e.g. ethyl methacrylate). The mixture starts to harden in 20–30 seconds after application and continues to harden to final hardness typically within fifteen minutes. Powder and liquid acrylics can be removed by using a variety of solvents (usually acetone is used). Usually it takes 20 to 30 minutes to remove the nail while using a nail file to help take off each layer of the artificial nail.

Another material, commonly called "UV Top Coat" (in correct chemical terms a polymer resin) cures under ultraviolet light. Depending on brand these can show a broader variety of quality and properties (flexibility, strength, etc.) but may be more expensive. They generally cannot be removed by organic solvents, but only be removed by filing (or left to grow out with the natural nail). There are, however, a variety of soak off UV gels which can be quickly and easily removed using acetone.

Another popular alternative to acrylic or gel preparations are fiberglass or silk wraps. They are done by cutting pieces of actual fiberglass or silk fabric to fit on the surface of the nail or tip and then it is sealed down with a resin or glue. These are a possible alternative for those who are allergic to chemicals used in the acrylic or gel process. These sort of treatments are commonly used to protect the nails if they have been broken. The silk or fiberglass overlay acts as a false layer of nail and thus protects the nail plate from splitting or becoming damaged any further.

Other materials can be used, as well as combinations of them. There are also temporary, cheaper flexible tips that can be quickly glued at home without help from a professional.

Acrylic nail powders are available in a variety of colours and can use "special effects" such as contours, sparkles and the very popular French manicure (pink or tan and white appearance)

Concealer

A concealer or colour corrector is a type of cosmetic that is used to mask dark circles, age spots, large pores, and other small blemishes visible on the skin. It is similar to foundation, but thicker and used to hide different pigments by blending the imperfection into the surrounding skin tone. It is normally applied after primer, after foundation and used on the face.

Both concealer and foundation are typically used to make skin appear more uniform in color, and make a clean base for all the other cosmetics. These two types of cosmetics differ in that concealers tend to be more heavily pigmented, though they are available in a wide range of opacity. It also comes in different forms from liquid to solid. Also, foundation is usually applied to larger areas. The first commercially available concealer was Max Factor's *Erace*, launched in 1954. Concealer can be used alone or with foundations. Camouflage makeup is a much heavier pigmented form of concealer. It is used to cover serious skin discolorations such as birthmarks, scars and vitiligo. An example of a modern camouflage makeup is Colortration, which is a liquid cover makeup.

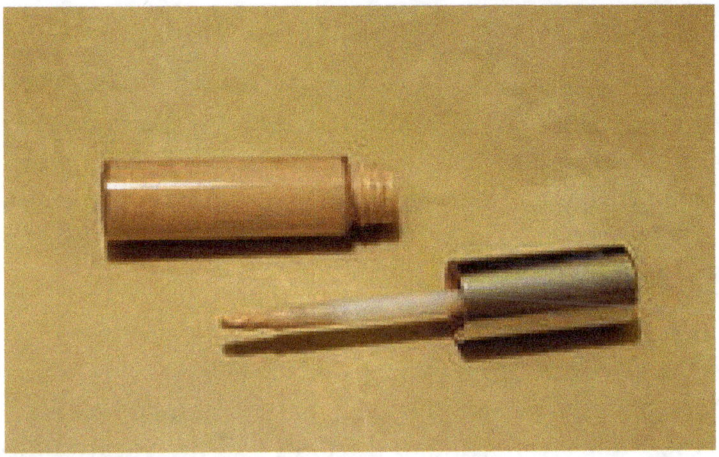

Liquid concealer

Concealer is available in a variety of shades, from lightest to deepest. When picking a concealer, people tend to choose one or two shades lighter than their skin tone to better hide their blemishes and dark circles under the eye. Some colors are intended to look like a natural skin tone, while others are meant to contrast with a particular type of blemish. Concealers with yellow undertones are used to hide dark circles. Green and blue can counteract red patches on the skin, such as those caused by pimples, broken veins, or rosacea. A purple-tinted concealer can make sallow complexions look brighter. Colored concealers such as these are usually applied sparingly beneath a concealer or foundation that matches the wearer's skin tone. Skin-toned concealers are not only the most common type, but are often sufficient on their own at hiding or blurring imperfections.

Cleanser

A cleanser is a facial care product that is used to remove make-up, dead skin cells, oil, dirt, and other types of pollutants from the skin of the face. This helps to unclog pores and prevent skin conditions such as acne. A cleanser can be used as part of a skin care regimen together with a toner and moisturizer.

Using a cleanser to remove dirt is considered to be a better alternative to bar soap or another form of skin cleanser not specifically formulated for the face for the following reasons:

- Bar soap has a high pH (in the area of 9 to 10), and the skin's surface pH is on average 4.7. This means that soap can change the balance present in the skin to favor the overgrowth of some types of bacteria, increasing acne.

- Bar cleansers have thickeners that allow them to assume a bar shape. These thickeners can clog pores, leading to acne.
- Using bar soap on the face can remove natural oils from the skin that form a barrier against water loss. This causes the sebaceous glands to subsequently overproduce oil, a condition known as reactive seborrhoea, which will lead to clogged pores. In order to prevent drying out the skin, many cleansers incorporate moisturizers.

Types of Facial Cleansers

Different types of cleansers have been developed for people with different skin types. Active cleansers are more suitable for oily skins to prevent breakouts. But they may overdry and irritate dry skin, this may make the skin appear and feel worse. Very dry skin may require a creamy lotion-type cleanser. These are normally too gentle to be effective on oily or even normal skin, but dry skin requires much less cleansing power. It may be a good idea to select a cleanser that is alcohol-free for use on dry, sensitive, or dehydrated skin.

Some cleansers may incorporate fragrance or essential oils. However, for some people, these cleansers may irritate the skin and often provoke allergic responses. People with such sensitivity should find cleansers that are pH-balanced cosmetic balanced, contain fewer irritants, suit many variating skin types, and do not make the skin feel dehydrated directly after cleansing. Tight, uncomfortable skin is often dehydrated and may appear shiny after cleansing, even when no sebum is present. This is due to the taughtening and 'stripping' effect some cleaners can have on the skin. One should discontinue use of a cleanser that upsets the balance of the skin; cleansers should work with the skin not against it. Finding the right cleanser can involve some trial-and-error.

Lotion

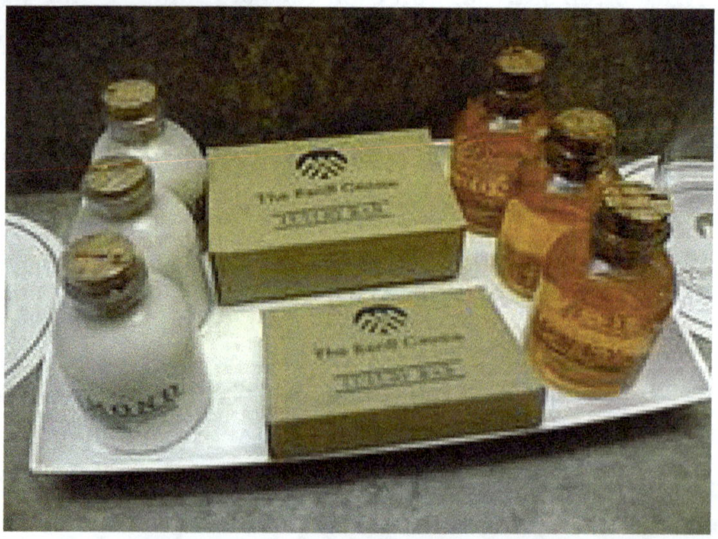

Lotion and shampoo at the Banff Centre

A lotion is a low-viscosity topical preparation intended for application to unbroken skin. By contrast, creams and gels have higher viscosity.

Lotions are applied to external skin with bare hands, a brush, a clean cloth, cotton wool, or gauze. While lotion may be used as a medicine delivery system, many lotions, especially hand lotions and body lotions are meant instead to simply smooth, moisturize and soften the skin. These may be used in anti-aging lotions, which can also be classified as a cosmetic in many cases, and may contain fragrances. The Food and Drug Administration voiced concern about lotions not classified as drugs that advertise anti-aging or anti-wrinkle properties.

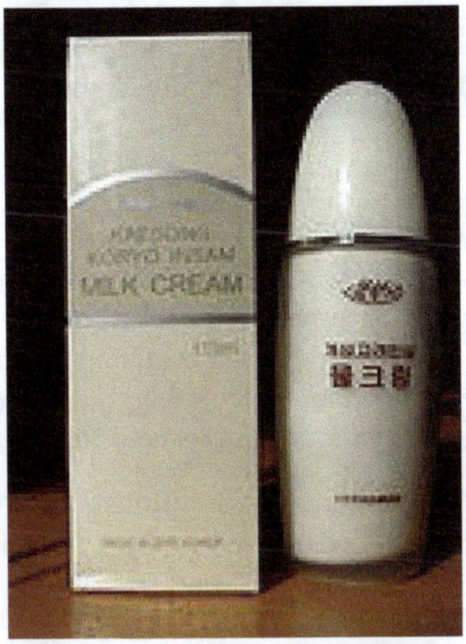

Ginseng hand cream from North Korea

Medicine Delivery

Dermatologists can prescribe lotions to treat or prevent skin diseases. It is not unusual for the same drug ingredient to be formulated into a lotion, cream and ointment. Creams are the most convenient of the three but are inappropriate for application to regions of hairy skin such as the scalp, while a lotion is less viscous and may be readily applied to these areas (many medicated shampoos are in fact lotions). Historically, lotions also had an advantage in that they may be spread thinly compared to a cream or ointment and may economically cover a large area of skin, but product research has steadily eroded this distinction. Non-comedogenic lotions are recommended for use on acne prone skin.

Lotions can be used for the delivery to the skin of medications such as:

- Antibiotics
- Antiseptics
- Antifungals
- Corticosteroids

- Anti-acne agents
- Soothing, smoothing, moisturizing or protective agents (such as calamine)

Occupational Use

Since health care workers must wash their hands frequently to prevent disease transmission, hospital grade lotion is recommended to prevent skin dermatitis caused by frequent exposure to cleaning agents in the soap. A 2006 study found that application of hospital grade lotion after hand washing significantly reduced skin roughness and dryness.

Care must be taken not to use consumer lotions in a hospital environment, as the perfumes and allergens may be a danger to those who are immunodeficient.

Production

Most lotions are oil-in-water emulsions using a substance such as cetearyl alcohol to keep the emulsion together, but water-in-oil lotions are also formulated. The key components of a skin care lotion, cream or gel emulsion (that is mixtures of oil and water) are the aqueous and oily phases, an emulgent to prevent separation of these two phases, and, if used, the drug substance or substances. A wide variety of other ingredients such as fragrances, glycerol, petroleum jelly, dyes, preservatives, proteins and stabilizing agents are commonly added to lotions.

Since thickness and consistency are key factors in lotions and creams, it is important to understand the manufacturing process that determines viscosity.

Manufacturing lotions and creams can be completed in two cycles:

1. Emollients and lubricants are dispersed in oil with blending and thickening agents.
2. Perfume, color and preservatives are dispersed in the water cycle. Active ingredients are broken up in both cycles depending on the raw materials involved and the desired properties of the lotion or cream.

A typical oil-in-water manufacturing process might go like this:

- Step 1: Add flake/powder ingredients to the oil being used to prepare the oil phase.
- Step 2: Disperse active ingredients.
- Step 3: Prepare the water phase containing emulsifiers and stabilizers.
- Step 4: Mix the oil and water to form an emulsion. (Note: This is aided by heating to between 110-185 F (45-85 C) depending on the formulation and viscosity desired.)
- Step 5: Continue mixing until the end product is completed

Careful note should be taken in choosing the right mixing equipment for lotion manufacturing to avoid agglomerates and long processing times. It can make all the difference in manufacturing time and costs. Conventional agitators can present a number of problems including agglomerates and longer processing times. On the other hand, high shear in-line mixers can produce quality lotions and creams without many of the complications encountered with conventional mixers. Sonolation is also a process that is growing in popularity.

Shampoo

Shampoo is a hair care product, typically in the form of a viscous liquid, that is used for cleaning hair. Less commonly, shampoo is available in bar form, like a bar of soap. Shampoo is used by applying it to wet hair, massaging the product into the hair, and then rinsing it out. Some users may follow a shampooing with the use of hair conditioner.

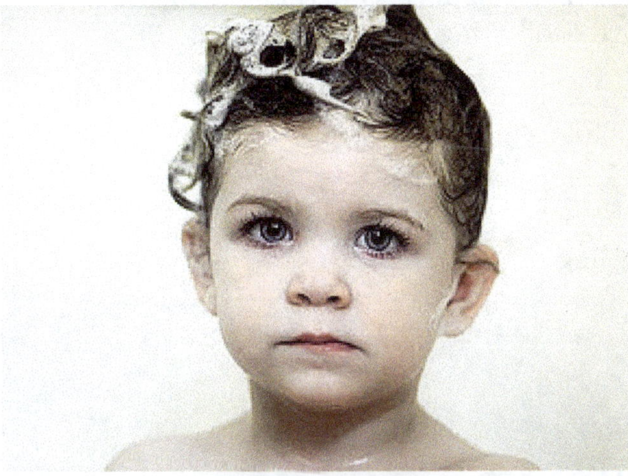

Shampoo lather in hair

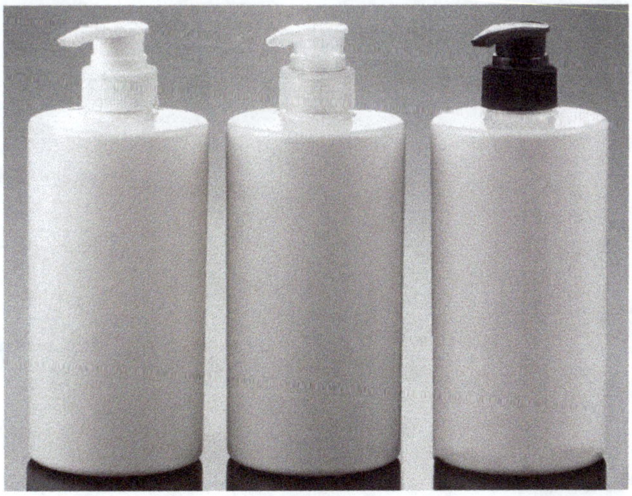

The goal of using shampoo is to remove the unwanted build-up in the hair without stripping out so much sebum as to make hair unmanageable. Shampoo is generally made by combining a surfactant, most often sodium lauryl sulfate or sodium laureth sulfate, with a co-surfactant, most often cocamidopropyl betaine in water.

Specialty shampoos are available for people with dandruff, color-treated hair, gluten or wheat allergies, an interest in using an "all-natural", "organic", "botanical" or "plant-derived" product, and infants and young children ("baby shampoo" is less irritating). There are also shampoos intended for animals that may contain insecticides or other medications to treat skin conditions or parasite infestations such as fleas.

Composition

Shampoo is generally made by combining a surfactant, most often sodium lauryl sulfate or sodium laureth sulfate, with a co-surfactant, most often cocamidopropyl betaine in water to form a thick, viscous liquid. Other essential ingredients include salt (sodium chloride), which is used to adjust the viscosity, a preservative and fragrance. Other ingredients are generally included in shampoo formulations to maximize the following qualities:

- pleasing foam
- ease of rinsing
- minimal skin and eye irritation
- thick or creamy feeling
- pleasant fragrance
- low toxicity
- good biodegradability
- slight acidity (pH less than 7)
- no damage to hair
- repair of damage already done to hair

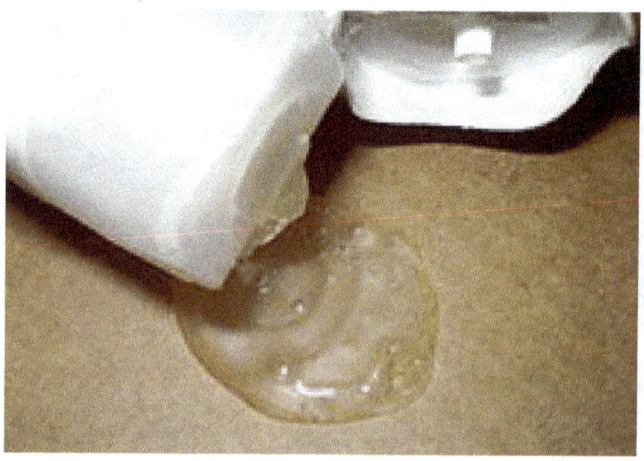

Typical liquid shampoo

Many shampoos are pearlescent. This effect is achieved by addition of tiny flakes of suitable materials, e.g. glycol distearate, chemically derived from stearic acid, which may have either animal or vegetable origins. Glycol distearate is a wax. Many shampoos also include silicone to provide conditioning benefits.

Commonly used Ingredients

- Ammonium Chloride
- Ammonium lauryl sulfate
- Glycol
- Sodium laureth sulfate is derived from coconut oils and is used to soften water and create a lather. There was some concern over this particular ingredient circa 1998 as evidence suggested it might be a carcinogen, and this has yet to be disproved, as many sources still describe it as irritating to the hair and scalp.
- Sodium lauryl sulfate
- Sodium lauroamphoacetate is naturally derived from coconut oils and is used as a cleanser and counter-irritant. This is the ingredient that makes the product tear-free.
- Polysorbate 20 (abbreviated as PEG(20)) is a mild glycol-based surfactant that is used to solubilize fragrance oils and essential oils; meaning it causes liquid to spread across and penetrate the surface of a solid (i.e. your hair).
- Polysorbate 80 (abbreviated as PEG(80)) is a glycol used to emulsify (or disperse) oils in water (so the oils do not float on top like Italian salad dressing).
- PEG-150 distearate is a simple thickener.
- Citric acid is produced biochemically and is used as an antioxidant to preserve the oils in the product. While it is a severe eye-irritant, the sodium lauroamphoacetate counteracts that property. Citric acid is used to adjust the pH down to approximately 5.5. It is a fairly weak acid which makes the adjustment easier. Shampoos usually are at pH 5.5 because at slightly acidic pH, the scales on a hair follicle lie flat, making the hair feel smooth and look shiny. It also has a small amount of preservative action. Citric acid as opposed to any other acid will prevent bacterial growth.
- Quaternium-15 is used as a bacterial and fungicidal preservative.
- Polyquaternium-10 has nothing to do with the chemical quaternium-15; it acts as the conditioning ingredient, providing moisture and fullness to the hair.
- Di-PPG-2 myreth-10 adipate is a water-dispersible emollient that forms clear solutions with surfactant systems
- Methylisothiazolinone, or MIT, is a powerful biocide and preservative.

Ingredient and Functional Claims

In the USA, the Food and Drug Administration (FDA) mandates that shampoo containers accurately list ingredients on the products container. The government further regulates what shampoo manufacturers can and cannot claim as any associated benefit. Shampoo producers often use these regulations to challenge marketing claims made by competitors, helping to enforce these regulations. While the claims may be substantiated however, the testing methods and details of such claims are not as straightforward. For example, many products are purported to protect hair from damage due to ultraviolet radiation. While the ingredient responsible for this protection does block UV, it is not often present in a high enough concentration to be effective. The North American Hair Research Society has a program to certify functional claims based on third party testing. Shampoos made for treating medical conditions such as dandruff, itchy scalp are regulated as OTC drugs in the US marketplace. In other parts of the world such as the EU, there is a requirement for the anti-dandruff claim to be substantiated, but it is not considered to be a medical problem.

Specialized Shampoos

Dandruff

Cosmetic companies have developed shampoos specifically for those who have dandruff. These contain fungicides such as ketoconazole, zinc pyrithione and selenium sulfide, which reduce loose dander by killing *Malassezia furfur*. Coal tar and salicylate derivatives are often used as well.

Despite a big success of medicated shampoos there are also other alternatives for people who dislike using a lot of chemicals. Organic, natural shampoos can be a suitable alternative. These shampoos often use tea tree oil, essential oils and extracts.[w]

Colored Hair

Many companies have also developed color-protection shampoos suitable for colored hair; many of these shampoos contain gentle cleansers, or so the companies claim.

Gluten-free or Wheat-free

Many people suffer from eczema on their palms and their head. Some find that wheat or gluten (the protein found in many grains including wheat) is the cause, particularly if they are sensitive to this in food; e.g. celiac disease wheat allergy. Shampoo can often go into the mouth, particularly for children, so all individuals who are on gluten-free diets may prefer to find a gluten-free shampoo. Shampoo manufacturers are starting to recognize this and there are now gluten-free and wheat-free products available.

Wheat derivatives and ingredients from the other gluten grains are commonly used as binders to help the shampoo stick together and are also used as emollients in the form of oils. Following is a list of grain-derived shampoo ingredients. Most of these ingredients do not theoretically contain any intact wheat proteins, but may do so due to incomplete processing or contamination.

- Triticum vulgare (wheat), hordeum vulgare (barley), secale cereale (rye), or avena sativa (oats), including any oil, protein, hydrosylate, or other extract from any part of the plant.
- Tocopherol/Tocopheryl acetate (Vitamin E), which may be derived from wheat
- Hydrolyzed wheat protein or hydrolyzed wheat starch, also sometimes listed as hydrolyzed vegetable protein, stearyldimoniumhydroxypropyl or hydroxypropyltrimonium

- Cyclodextrin, which may be produced from starch by means of enzymatic conversion
- Amino peptide complex
- Maltodextrin, dextrin, dextrin palmitate, or (hydrolyzed) malt extract
- Phytosphingosine extract
- Amino peptide complex
- prolamine
- Beta glucan
- Disodium wheat Germamido PEG-2-Sulfosuccinat
- Fermented grain extract
- AMP-Isostearoyl
- PG-Propyl Silanetriol
- PVP crosspolymer
- Ethyldimonium ethosulfate
- Yeast extract
- Phytospingosine extract
- "Fragrance" is a broad category that may contain many chemicals that are otherwise unlisted on the label.

All-natural

Some companies use "all-natural", "organic", "botanical", or "plant-derived" ingredients (such as plant extracts or oils), combining these additions with one or more typical surfactants. The use of the term "natural" is not regulated in any form, leading many companies to "green-wash" consumers into buying shampoos with harsh, stripping surfactants without their knowledge. A company may also slightly change the name of a surfactant to another acceptable form in order to fool unwitting customers.

Baby

Shampoo for infants and young children is formulated so that it is less irritating and usually less prone to produce a stinging or burning sensation if it were to get into the eyes. For example, Johnson's Baby Shampoo advertises under the premise of "No More Tears". This is accomplished by one or more of the following formulation strategies.

1. dilution, in case the product comes in contact with eyes after running off the top of the head with minimal further dilution

2. adjusting pH to that of non-stress tears, approximately 7, which may be a higher pH than that of shampoos which are pH adjusted for skin or hair effects, and lower than that of shampoo made of soap
3. use of surfactants which, alone or in combination, are less irritating than those used in other shampoos
4. use of nonionic surfactants of the form of polyethoxylated synthetic glycolipids and polyethoxylated synthetic monoglycerides, which counteract the eye sting of other surfactants without producing the anesthetizing effect of alkyl polyethoxylates or alkylphenol polyethoxylates

The distinction in 4 above does not completely surmount the controversy over the use of shampoo ingredients to mitigate eye sting produced by other ingredients, or the use of the products so formulated. The considerations in 3 and 4 frequently result in a much greater multiplicity of surfactants being used in individual baby shampoos than in other shampoos, and the detergency or foaming of such products may be compromised thereby. The monoanionic sulfonated surfactants and viscosity-increasing or foam stabilizing alkanolamides seen so frequently in other shampoos are much less common in the better baby shampoos.

Solid

Solid shampoos or shampoo bars use as their surfactants soaps or other surfactants formulated as solids. They have the advantage of being spill-proof. They are easy to apply; one may simply rub the bar over wet hair, and work the soaped hair into a low lather.

Jelly and Gel

Stiff, non-pourable clear gels to be squeezed from a tube were once popular forms of shampoo, and can be produced by increasing a shampoo's viscosity. This type of shampoo cannot be spilled, but unlike a solid, it can still be lost down the drain by sliding off wet skin or hair.

Paste and Cream

Shampoos in the form of pastes or creams were formerly marketed in jars or tubes. The contents were wet but not completely dissolved. They would apply faster than solids and dissolve quickly.

Antibacterial

Antibacterial shampoos are often used in veterinary medicine for various conditions, as well as in humans before some surgical procedures.

No Poo Movement

Closely associated with environmentalism, the "no poo" movement consists of people rejecting the societal norm of frequent shampoo use. Some adherents of the no poo movement use baking soda or vinegar to wash their hair, while others use diluted honey. Other people use nothing, rinsing their hair only with conditioner.

Perfume

Perfume is a mixture of fragrant essential oils or aroma compounds, fixatives and solvents - used to give the human body, animals, food, objects, and living-spaces "a pleasant scent".

Ancient texts and archaeological excavations show the use of perfumes in some of the earliest human civilizations. Modern perfumery began in the late 19th century with the commercial synthesis of aroma compounds such as vanillin or coumarin, which allowed for the composition of perfumes with smells previously unattainable solely from natural aromatics alone.

How to Apply Perfume

Perfume may be just the thing to finish off your outfit, even if it's a T-shirt and your favorite jeans. Applying perfume can liven up a date night, and help attract your desired partner. However, there are some misconceptions as to how to apply perfume, where to apply it, and what types of perfumes to buy. The difference between applying perfume correctly and incorrectly is dramatic, and can change the course of how your evening goes. Luckily, the steps to correctly apply perfume are easy and simple.

Part 1

Preparing to Apply Your Perfume

1. Find your perfect perfume. Do not just wear something because it is a designer perfume. Make sure you absolutely love the perfume's top notes and bottom notes.

- The top notes are what you smell initially right when you get near the spray bottle. These are usually citrus, fruit, and herb smells. They often wear off very quickly, so it is important to check the bottom notes as well.

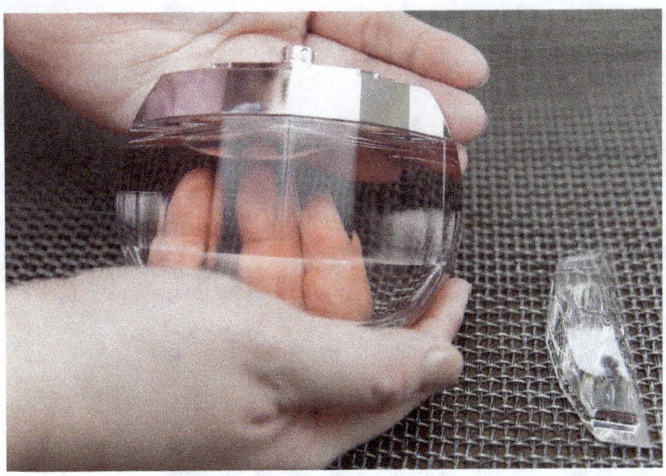

- The bottom notes are generally wood and natural smells. To find out if you like the bottom notes, spray a little of the perfume on the back of your wrist, wait 20 minutes and smell the perfume again.

- You can also filter your decision by going to an actual perfume store (like Bath and Body, or at a perfume counter at a department store) and ask for help.

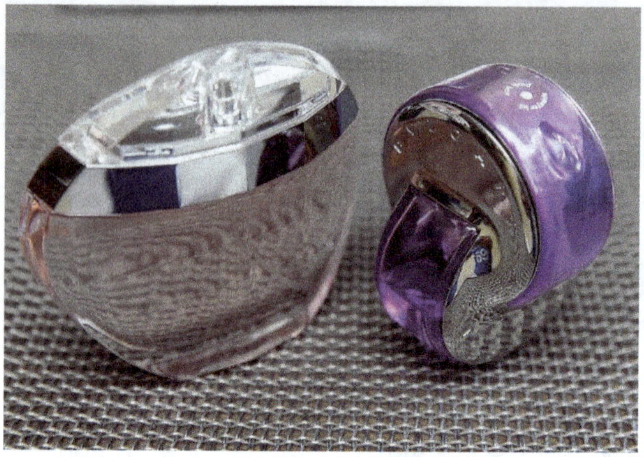

2. Choose a daytime or nighttime fragrance. If you are simply going out on the town, going to work, or visiting the beach, try a daytime fragrance. If you are planning a date, or going out to dinner, you might try a nighttime fragrance instead.

- Look for labels on the packaging. They will usually say either "daytime" or nighttime." If they do not say explicitly, you can usually tell by the color of the packages. Bright yellows, and oranges mean springtime, and are generally daytime fragrances. Dark blues, reds, and purples suggest a nighttime fragrance.
- Nighttime fragrances are generally sprayed on, or near the neck area. This is because they do not last as long, and you will want a more immediate impact. In that case, apply a little extra moisturizer to the area of choice to hold the fragrance better.
- Daytime fragrances are generally sprayed down by the hips or knees. This is because they rise as the day goes by, and last longer. Therefore, use some extra moisturizer near the area of choice in order for the fragrance to hold on better.

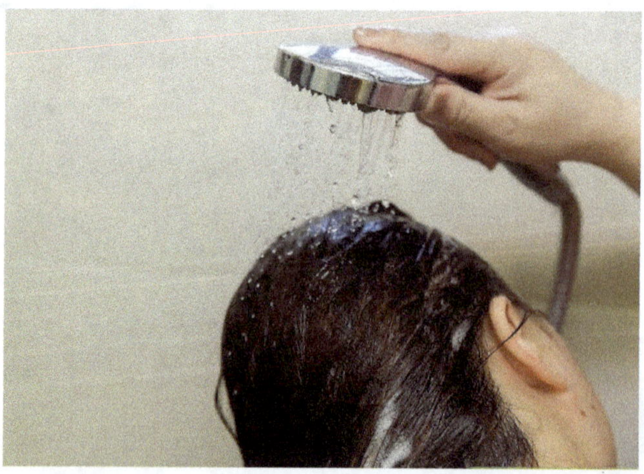

3. Take a shower or bath. Your skin absorbs perfume better after it is nice and warm. Make sure when you take your shower or bath that the water is hot, so that your pores can open.

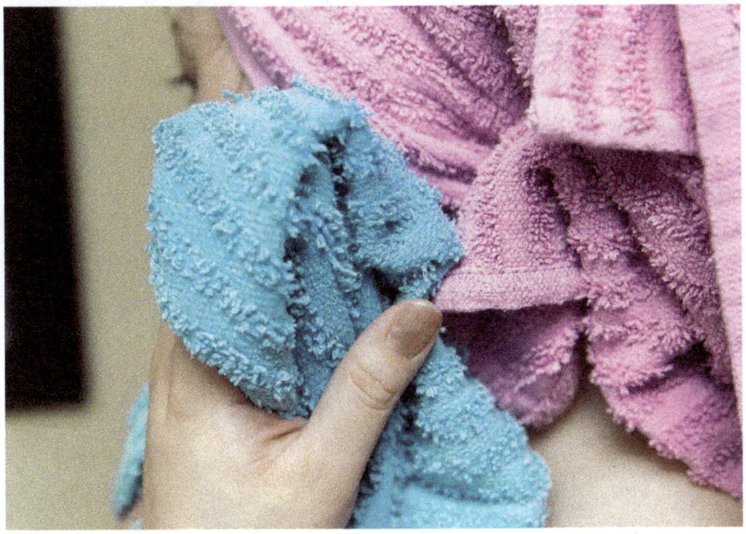

- Use a body wash or soap that is unscented, or has very little scent. You do not want your perfume to clash with the smell.
- This is also a great time to moisturize your skin. Use a cream or oil so that your skin becomes more openly receptive to the perfume.
- Washing your hair can also help out if you plan on using the perfume in your hair. Make sure to use conditioner so that your hair if soft, and receptive of the perfume.

4. Dry your skin off. After you take a warm shower or bath, make sure your skin is dry. If you do not, when you spray the perfume on it will not stick. Specifically, get the hard to reach places like the back of your knees, your neckline, and your hair. These are what are called "pulse points," or places where your perfume goes on, and acts at it's highest level.

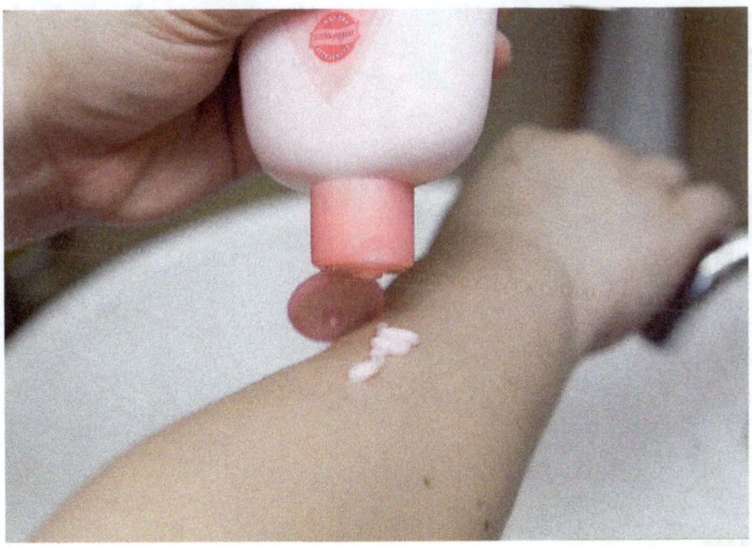

5. Hydrate your skin. If you did not apply moisturizer during your shower, definitely do this after

you dry off. The perfume has a much better chance to lock on to your skin if it is smooth and soft, rather than dry and rough.

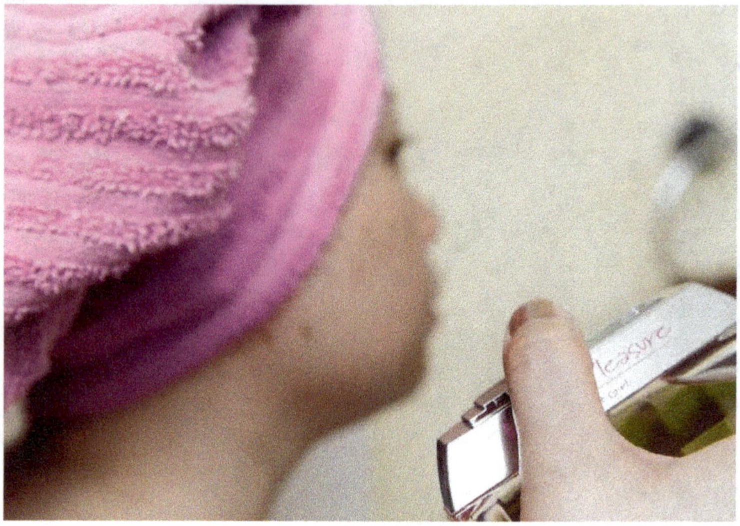

- A lotion or body oil work best. Apply a small amount to your hands and rub it between them. Then take your hands and apply the lotion/oil to the rest of your skin.
- Another great option is petroleum jelly. The perfume will stick to the jelly molecules, rather than the pores, thereby keeping the fragrance alive longer. Apply small dabs and smooth them out on your skin.
- The key is to hit the "pulse points." These include, but are not limited to: feet, knees, elbows, collarbone, and neck. These places are where you will apply the perfume, and where the perfume will be most effective.

6. Apply the perfume before you put your clothes on. Perfume sprayed directly onto clothes can cause water marks which look unseemly, particularly if you are going out to a nice dinner date. Perfume also works much better on "pulse points" rather than clothes, because the molecules interact with direct contact with skin.

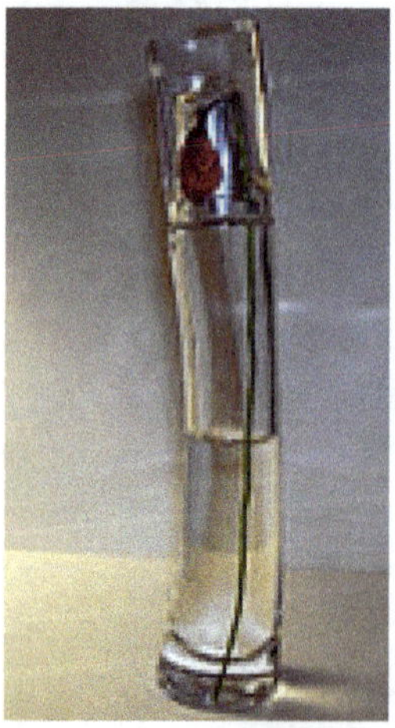

Flower from Kenzo

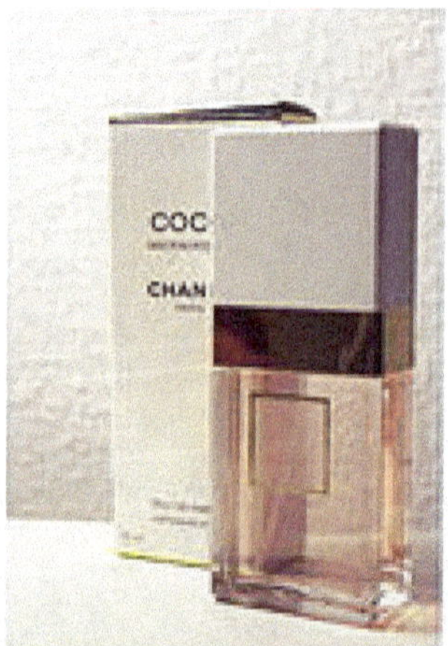

Coco Mademoiselle from Chanel

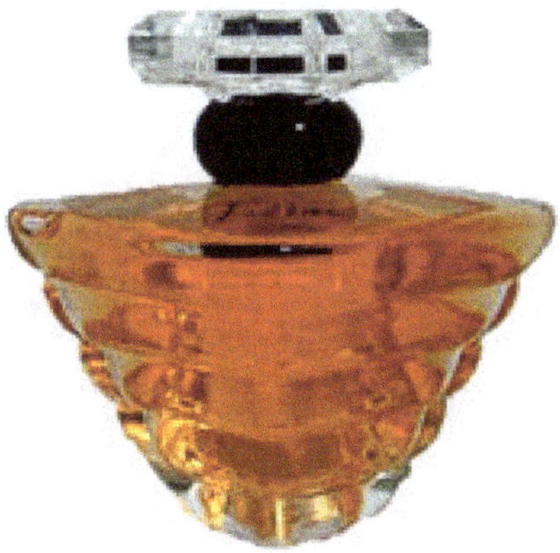

Tresor from Lancôme

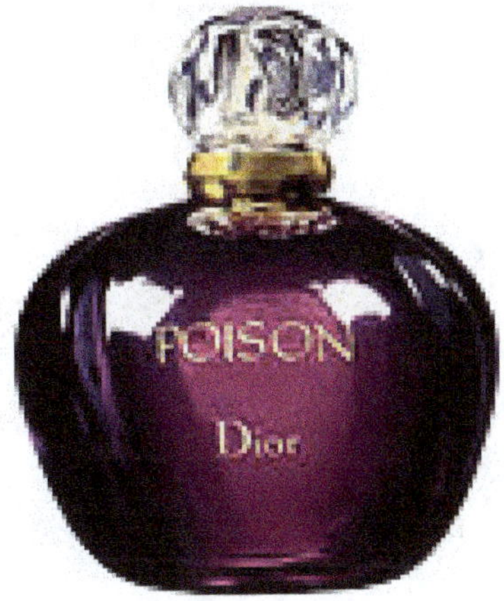

Poison from Dior

Solvent Types

Perfume oils are often diluted with a solvent, though this is not always the case, and its necessity is disputed. By far the most common solvent for perfume oil dilution is an alcohol solution typically a mixture of ethanol and water or a rectified spirit. Perfume oil can also be diluted by means of neutral-smelling oils such as fractionated coconut oil, or liquid waxes such as jojoba oil.

Applying Fragrances

The conventional application of pure perfume (parfum extrait) in Western cultures is at pulse points, such as behind the ears, the nape of the neck, and the insides of wrists, elbows and knees, so that the pulse point will warm the perfume and release fragrance continuously. According to perfumer Sophia Grojsman behind the knees is the ideal point to apply perfume in order that the scent may rise. The modern perfume industry encourages the practice of layering fragrance so that it is released in different intensities depending upon the time of the day. Lightly scented products such as bath oil, shower gel, and body lotion are recommended for the morning; eau de toilette is suggested for the afternoon; and perfume applied to the pulse points for evening. Cologne fragrance is released rapidly, lasting around 2 hours. Eau de toilette lasts from 2 to 4 hours, while perfume may last up to six hours.

A variety of factors can influence how fragrance interacts with the wearer's own physiology and affect the perception of the fragrance. Diet is one factor, as eating spicy and fatty foods can increase the intensity of a fragrance. The use of medications can also impact the character of a fragrance. The relative dryness of the wearer's skin is important, since dry skin will not hold fragrance as long as skin with more oil.

Describing a Perfume

The precise formulae of commercial perfumes are kept secret. Even if they were widely published, they would be dominated by such complex ingredients and odorants that they would be of little use in providing a guide to the general consumer in description of the *experience* of a scent. Nonetheless, connoisseurs of perfume can become extremely skillful at identifying components and origins of scents in the same manner as wine experts.

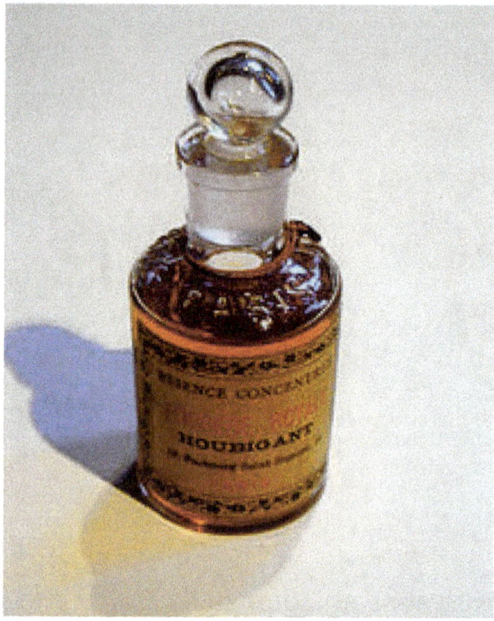

An original bottle of *Fougère Royale* by Houbigant. Created by Paul Parquet in 1884, it is one of the most important modern perfumes and inspired the eponymous Fougère class of fragrances.

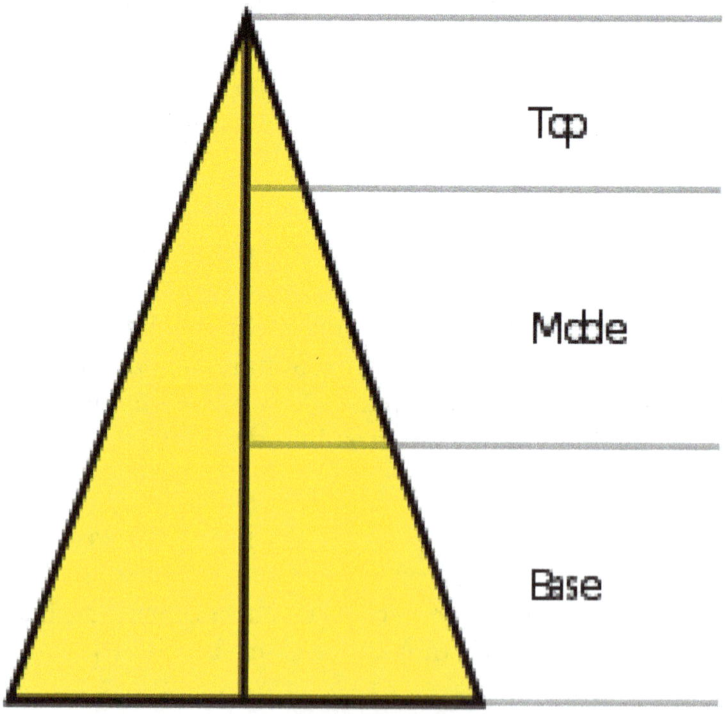

Fragrance pyramid

The most practical way to start describing a perfume is according to the elements of the *fragrance notes* of the scent or the "family" it belongs to, all of which affect the overall impression of a perfume from first application to the last lingering hint of scent.

The trail of scent left behind by a person wearing perfume is called its *sillage*, after the French word for "wake", as in the trail left by a boat in water.

Olfactive Families

Grouping perfumes can never be a completely objective or final process. Many fragrances contain aspects of different families. Even a perfume designated as "single flower", however subtle, will have undertones of other aromatics. "True" unitary scents can rarely be found in perfumes as it requires the perfume to exist only as a singular aromatic material.

Classification by olfactive family is a starting point for a description of a perfume, but it cannot by itself denote the specific characteristic of that perfume.

Traditional

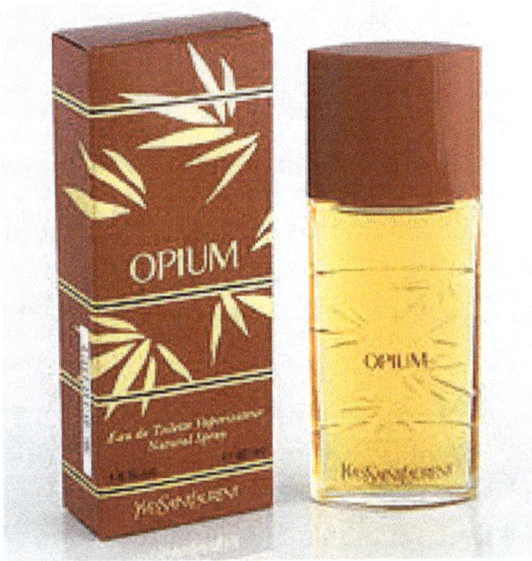

Opium by YSL, of amber or oriental fragrance class

The traditional classification which emerged around 1900 comprised the following categories:

- Single Floral: Fragrances that are dominated by a scent from one particular flower; in French called a *soliflore*. (e.g. Serge Lutens' *Sa Majeste La Rose*, which is dominated by rose.)
- Floral Bouquet: Is a combination of fragrance of several flowers in a perfume compound. Examples include *Quelques Fleurs* by Houbigant and *Joy* by Jean Patou.
- Amber or "Oriental": A large fragrance class featuring the sweet slightly animalic scents of ambergris or labdanum, often combined with vanilla, tonka bean, flowers and woods. Can be enhanced by camphorous oils and incense resins, which bring to mind Victorian era imagery of the Middle East and Far East. Traditional examples include Guerlain's *Shalimar*, Yves Saint Laurent's *Opium* and Chanel's *Coco Mademoiselle*.
- Woody: Fragrances that are dominated by woody scents, typically of agarwood, sandalwood, cedarwood, and vetiver. Patchouli, with its camphoraceous smell, is commonly found in these perfumes. A traditional example here would be Myrurgia's *Maderas De Oriente* or Chanel *Bois des Îles*. A modern example would be Balenciaga *Rumba*.
- Leather: A family of fragrances which features the scents of honey, tobacco, wood and wood tars in its middle or base notes and a scent that alludes to leather. Traditional examples include Robert Piguet's *Bandit* and Balmain's *Jolie Madame*.

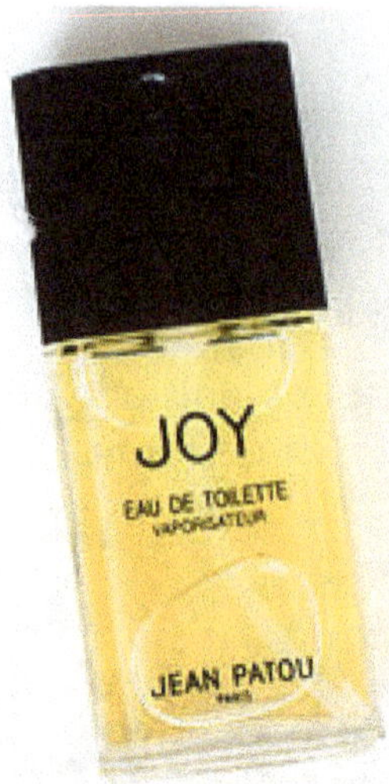

A floral bouquet, Joy from Jean Patou

- Chypre: Meaning *Cyprus* in French, this includes fragrances built on a similar accord consisting of bergamot, oakmoss, and labdanum. This family of fragrances is named after the eponymous 1917 perfume by François Coty, and one of the most famous extant examples is Guerlain's *Mitsouko*.

- Fougère (IPA:: Meaning *fern* in French, built on a base of lavender, coumarin and oakmoss. Houbigant's *Fougère Royale* pioneered the use of this base. Many men's fragrances belong to this family of fragrances, which is characterized by its sharp herbaceous and woody scent. Some well-known modern fougères are Fabergé *Brut* and Guy Laroche *Drakkar Noir*.

Modern

Since 1945, due to great advances in the technology of perfume creation (i.e., compound design and synthesis) as well as the natural development of styles and tastes, new categories have emerged to describe modern scents:

- Bright Floral: combining the traditional Single Floral & Floral Bouquet categories. A good example would be Estée Lauder's *Beautiful*.

- Green: a lighter and more modern interpretation of the Chypre type, with pronounced cut grass, crushed green leaf and cucumber-like scents. Examples include Estée Lauder's *Aliage*, Sisley's *Eau de Campagne*, and Calvin Klein's *Eternity*.

- Aquatic, Oceanic, or Ozonic: the newest category in perfume history, first appearing in 1988 Davidoff *Cool Water* (1988), Christian Dior's *Dune* (1991), and many others. A clean smell reminiscent of the ocean, leading to many of the modern androgynous perfumes. Generally contains calone, a synthetic scent discovered in 1966, or other more recent synthetics. Also used to accent floral, oriental, and woody fragrances.

- Citrus: An old fragrance family that until recently consisted mainly of "freshening" eau de colognes, due to the low tenacity of citrus scents. Development of newer fragrance compounds has allowed for the creation of primarily citrus fragrances. A good example here would be Faberge *Brut*.

- Fruity: featuring the aromas of fruits other than citrus, such as peach, cassis (black currant), mango, passion fruit, and others. A modern example here would be Ginestet *Botrytis*.
- Gourmand: scents with "edible" or "dessert"-like qualities. These often contain notes like vanilla, tonka bean and coumarin, as well as synthetic components designed to resemble food flavors. A sweet example is Thierry Mugler's *Angel*.

Fragrance Wheel

The Fragrance wheel is a relatively new classification method that is widely used in retail and in the fragrance industry. The method was created in 1983 by Michael Edwards, a consultant in the perfume industry, who designed his own scheme of fragrance classification. The new scheme was created in order to simplify fragrance classification and naming scheme, as well as to show the relationships between each of the individual classes.

The five standard families consist of *Floral, Oriental, Woody, Aromatic Fougère*, and *Fresh*, with the first four families borrowing from the classic terminology and the last consisting of newer bright and clean smelling citrus and oceanic fragrances that have arrived in the past generation due to improvements in fragrance technology. Each of the families are in turn divided into subgroups and arranged around a wheel. In this classification scheme, *Chanel No.5*, which is traditionally classified as an aldehydic floral, would be located under the Soft Floral sub-group, and amber scents would be placed within the Oriental group. As a class, chypre perfumes are more difficult to place since they would be located under parts of the Oriental and Woody families. For instance, Guerlain's *Mitsouko* is placed under Mossy Woods, but Hermès *Rouge*, a chypre with more floral character, would be placed under Floral Oriental.

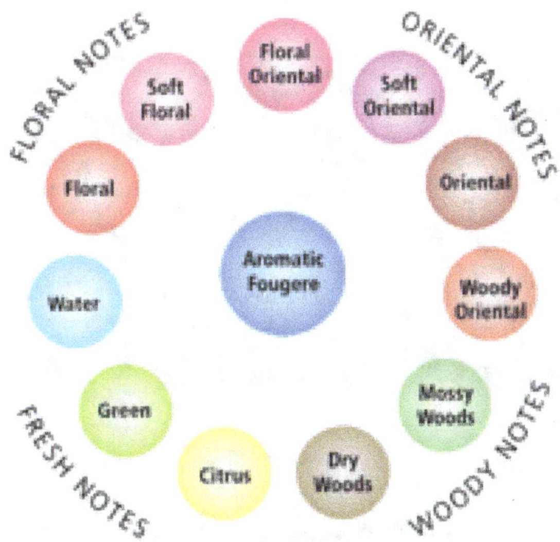

Fragrance Wheel perfume classification chart, ver. 1983

Aromatics Sources

Plant Sources

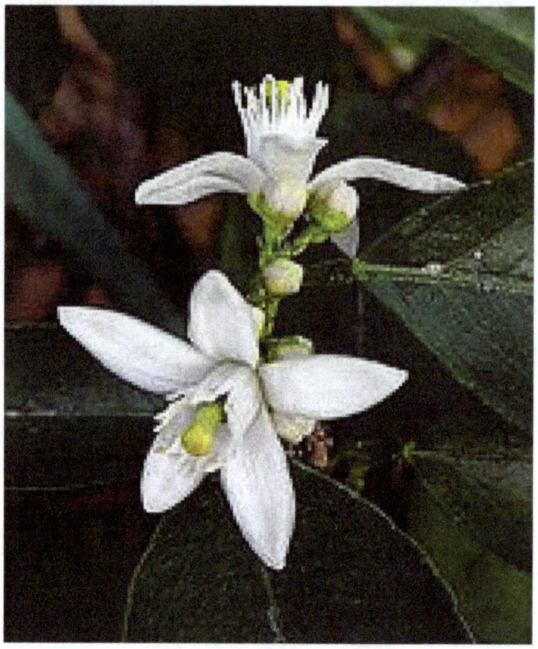

Citrus tree blossom

Plants have long been used in perfumery as a source of essential oils and aroma compounds. These aromatics are usually secondary metabolites produced by plants as protection against herbivores, infections, as well as to attract pollinators. Plants are by far the largest source of fragrant compounds used in perfumery. The sources of these compounds may be derived from various parts of a plant. A plant can offer more than one source of aromatics, for instance the aerial portions and seeds of coriander have remarkably different odors from each other. Orange leaves, blossoms, and fruit zest are the respective sources of petitgrain, neroli, and orange oils.

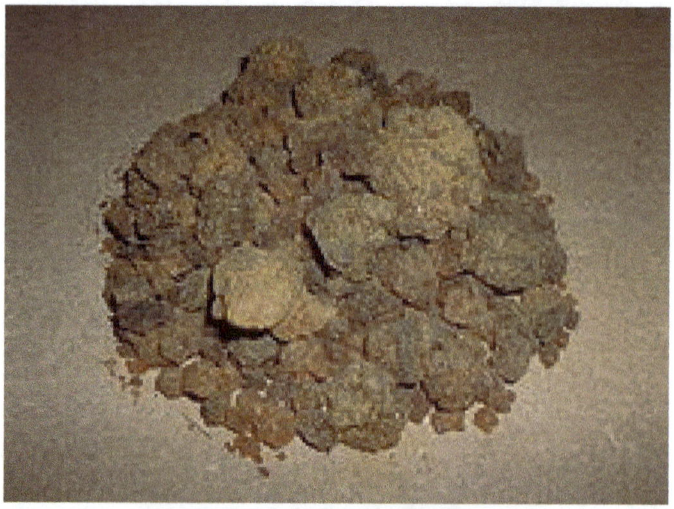

Resins in perfumery include myrrh

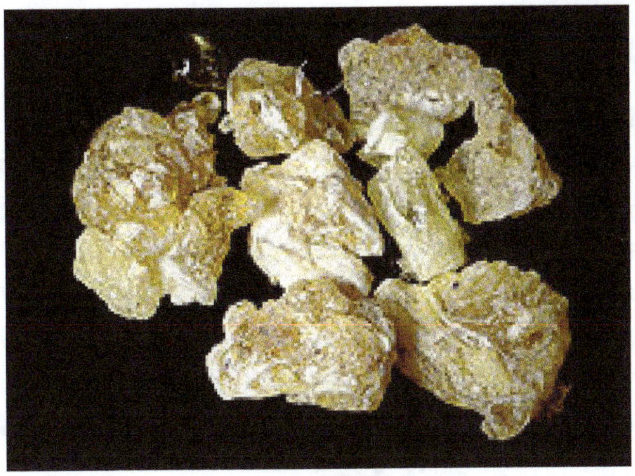

Frankincense

Bark: Commonly used barks include cinnamon and cascarilla. The fragrant oil in sassafras root bark is also used either directly or purified for its main constituent, safrole, which is used in the synthesis of other fragrant compounds.

- Flowers and blossoms: Undoubtedly the largest and most common source of perfume aromatics. Includes the flowers of several species of rose and jasmine, as well as osmanthus, plumeria, mimosa, tuberose, narcissus, scented geranium, cassie, ambrette as well as the blossoms of citrus and ylang-ylang trees. Although not traditionally thought of as a flower, the unopened flower buds of the clove are also commonly used. Most orchid flowers are not commercially used to produce essential oils or absolutes, except in the case of vanilla, an orchid, which must be pollinated first and made into seed pods before use in perfumery.
- Fruits: Fresh fruits such as apples, strawberries, cherries rarely yield the expected odors when extracted; if such fragrance notes are found in a perfume, they are more likely to be of synthetic origin. Notable exceptions include blackcurrant leaf, litsea cubeba, vanilla, and juniper berry. The most commonly used fruits yield their aromatics from the rind; they include citrus such as oranges, lemons, and limes. Although grapefruit rind is still used for aromatics, more and more commercially used grapefruit aromatics are artificially synthesized since the natural aromatic contains sulfur and its degradation product is quite unpleasant in smell.
- Leaves and twigs: Commonly used for perfumery are lavender leaf, patchouli, sage, violets, rosemary, and citrus leaves. Sometimes leaves are valued for the “green” smell they bring to perfumes, examples of this include hay and tomato leaf.
- Resins: Valued since antiquity, resins have been widely used in incense and perfumery. Highly fragrant and antiseptic resins and resin-containing perfumes have been used by many cultures as medicines for a large variety of ailments. Commonly used resins in perfumery include labdanum, frankincense/olibanum, myrrh, balsam of Peru, benzoin. Pine and fir resins are a particularly valued source of terpenes used in the organic synthesis of many other synthetic or naturally occurring aromatic compounds. Some of what is called amber and copal in perfumery today is the resinous secretion of fossil conifers.
- Roots, rhizomes and bulbs: Commonly used terrestrial portions in perfumery include iris rhizomes, vetiver roots, various rhizomes of the ginger family.

- Seeds: Commonly used seeds include tonka bean, carrot seed, coriander, caraway, cocoa, nutmeg, mace, cardamom, and anise.
- Woods: Highly important in providing the base notes to a perfume, wood oils and distillates are indispensable in perfumery. Commonly used woods include sandalwood, rosewood, agarwood, birch, cedar, juniper, and pine. These are used in the form of macerations or dry-distilled (rectified) forms.
- Rom terpenes. Orchid scents

Animal Sources

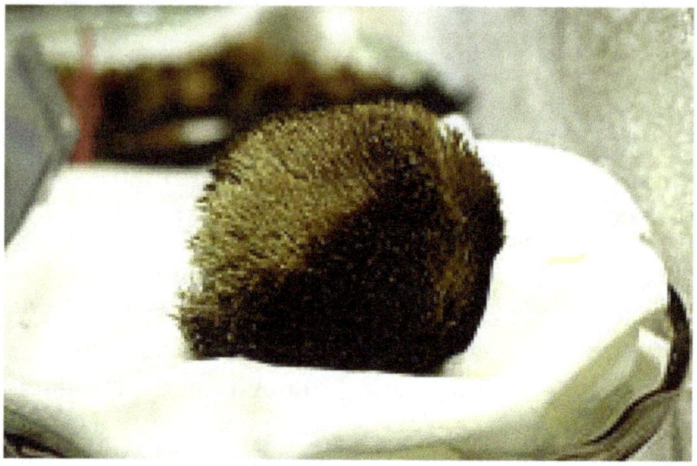

A musk pod. Extensive hunting of male musk deer for their pods in recent history has resulted in the detriment of the species.

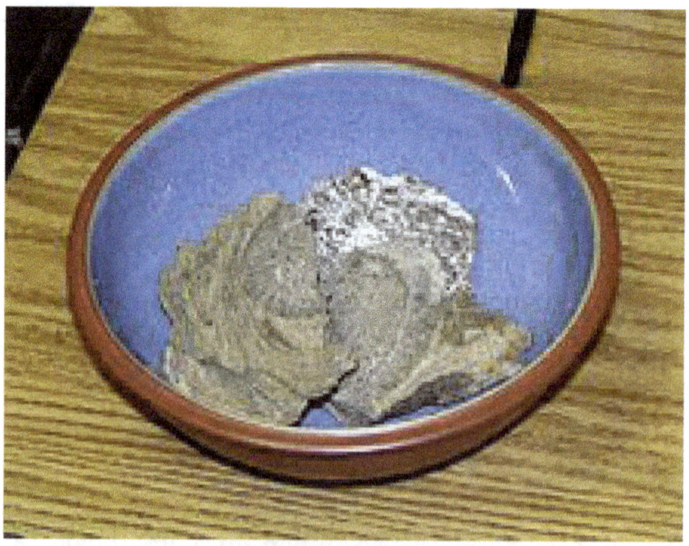

Ambergris

- Ambergris: Lumps of oxidized fatty compounds, whose precursors were secreted and expelled by the sperm whale. Ambergris should not be confused with yellow amber, which is used in jewelry. Because the harvesting of ambergris involves no harm to its animal source, it remains one of the few animalic fragrancing agents around which little controversy now exists.

- Castoreum: Obtained from the odorous sacs of the North American beaver.
- Civet: Also called civet musk, this is obtained from the odorous sacs of the civets, animals in the family *Viverridae*, related to the mongoose. World Animal Protection investigated African civets caught for this purpose.
- Hyraceum: Commonly known as "Africa stone", is the petrified excrement of the rock hyrax.
- Honeycomb: From the honeycomb of the honeybee. Both beeswax and honey can be solvent extracted to produce an absolute. Beeswax is extracted with ethanol and the ethanol evaporated to produce beeswax absolute.
- Musk: Originally derived from a gland (sac or pod) located between the genitals and the umbilicus of the Himalayan male musk deer Moschus moschiferus, it has now mainly been replaced by the use of synthetic musks sometimes known as "white musk".

Other Natural Sources

- Lichens: Commonly used lichens include oakmoss and treemoss thalli.
- "Seaweed": Distillates are sometimes used as essential oil in perfumes. An example of a commonly used seaweed is *Fucus vesiculosus*, which is commonly referred to as bladder wrack. Natural seaweed fragrances are rarely used due to their higher cost and lower potency than synthetics.

Synthetic Sources

Many modern perfumes contain synthesized odorants. Synthetics can provide fragrances which are not found in nature. For instance, Calone, a compound of synthetic origin, imparts a fresh ozonous metallic marine scent that is widely used in contemporary perfumes. Synthetic aromatics are often used as an alternate source of compounds that are not easily obtained from natural sources. For example, linalool and coumarin are both naturally occurring compounds that can be inexpensively synthesized from terpenes. Orchid scents (typically *salicylates*) are usually not obtained directly from the plant itself but are instead synthetically created to match the fragrant compounds found in various orchids.

One of the most commonly used classes of synthetic aromatics by far are the white musks. These materials are found in all forms of commercial perfumes as a neutral background to the middle notes. These musks are added in large quantities to laundry detergents in order to give washed clothes a lasting "clean" scent.

The majority of the world's synthetic aromatics are created by relatively few companies. They include:

- International Flavors and Fragrances (IFF)
- Givaudan
- Firmenich

- Takasago
- Symrise

Each of these companies patents several processes for the production of aromatic synthetics annually.

Characteristics

Natural and synthetics are used for their different odor characteristics in perfumery

	Naturals	Synthetics
Variance	Natural scents will vary from each supplier based on when and where they are harvested, how they are processed, and the extraction method itself. This means that a certain flower grown in Morocco and in France will smell different, even if the same method is used to grow, harvest, and extract the scent. As such, each perfumer will prefer flowers grown in one country over another, or one extraction method to the next. However, due to a natural scent's mixed composition, it is easy for unscrupulous suppliers to adulterate the actual raw materials by changing its *source* (adding Indian jasmine into Grasse jasmine) or the *contents* (adding linalool to rosewood) to increase their profit margin.	Much more consistent than natural aromatics. However, differences in organic synthesis may result in minute differences in concentration of impurities. If these impurities have low smell (detection) thresholds, the differences in the scent of the synthetic aromatic will be significant.
Components	Contains many different organic compounds, each adding a different note to the overall scent. These naturally derived substances have a history of use, therefore it is easy to determine whether they are safe or not. Possible allergenic compounds.	Depending on purity, consists primarily of one chemical compound. Sometimes chiral mixtures of isomers, such as in the case of Iso E Super. Due to the almost pure composition of one chemical compound, the same molecules found diluted in nature will have a different scent and effect on the body, if used undiluted.
Scent uniqueness	Reminiscent of its originating material, although extraction may capture a different "layer" of the scent, depending on the how the extraction method denatures the odoriferous compounds.	Similar to natural scents yet different at the same time. Some synthetics attempt to mimic natural notes, while others explore the entire spectrum of scent. Novel scent compounds not found in nature will often be unique in their scent.
Scent complexity	Deep and complex fragrance notes. Soft, with subtle scent nuances. Highly valued for ideal composition.	Pure and pronounced fragrance notes. Often monotonous in nature, yet reminiscent of other natural scents.

Price	Dependent on extraction method. More expensive, but not always, as prices are determined by the labor and difficulty of properly extracting each unit of the natural materials, as well as its quality. Typically the relationship between, longevity of a perfume, cost and the concentration of essential oils follows the graph below: 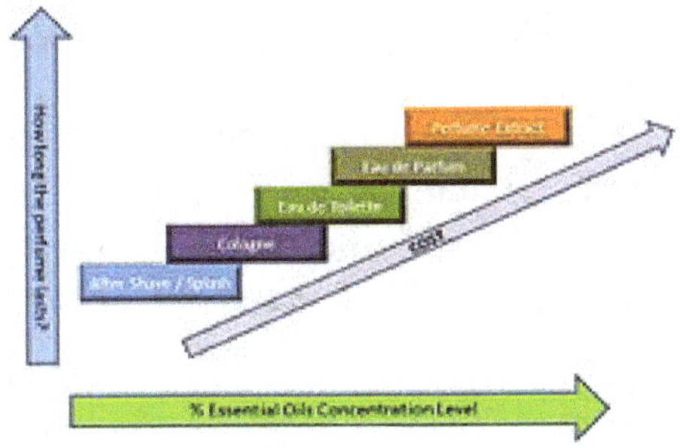 This chart shows the typical relationship between price of perfume, its longevity and the concentration of essential oils.	Dependent on synthesis method. Generally cheaper, but not necessarily. Synthetic aromatics are not necessarily cheaper than naturals, with some synthetics being more costly than most natural ingredients due to various factors such as the long synthesis routes, low availability of precursor chemicals, and low overall yield. However, due to their low odor threshold, they should be diluted when making a perfume.

Obtaining Natural Odorants

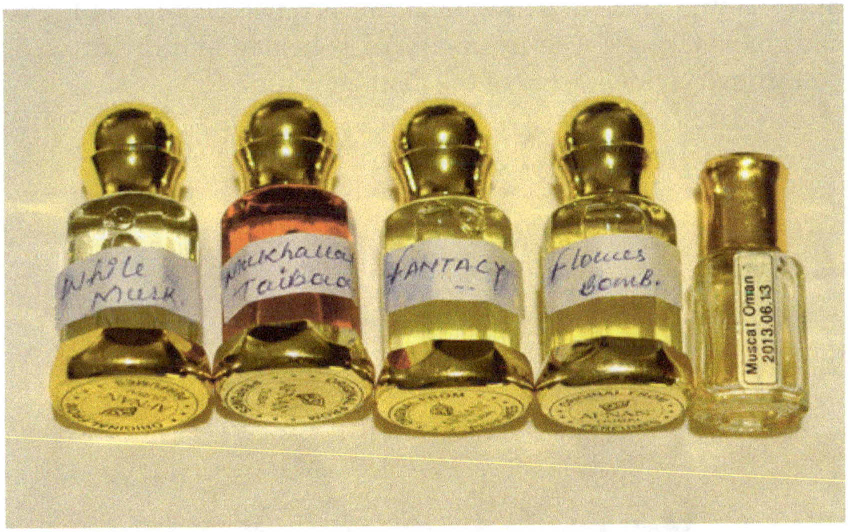

Before perfumes can be composed, the odorants used in various perfume compositions must first be obtained. Synthetic odorants are produced through organic synthesis and purified. Odorants from natural sources require the use of various methods to extract the aromatics from the raw materials. The results of the extraction are either essential oils, absolutes, concretes, or butters, depending on the amount of waxes in the extracted product.

All these techniques will, to a certain extent, distort the odor of the aromatic compounds obtained from the raw materials. This is due to the use of heat, harsh solvents, or through exposure to oxygen in the extraction process which will denature the aromatic compounds, which either change their odor character or renders them odorless.

- Maceration/Solvent extraction: The most used and economically important technique for extracting aromatics in the modern perfume industry. Raw materials are submerged in a solvent that can dissolve the desired aromatic compounds. *Maceration* lasts anywhere from hours to months. Fragrant compounds for woody and fibrous plant materials are often obtained in this manner as are all aromatics from animal sources. The technique can also be used to extract odorants that are too volatile for *distillation* or easily denatured by heat. Commonly used solvents for *maceration/solvent extraction* include ethane, hexane, and dimethyl ether. The product of this process is called a "concrete."
    - o *Supercritical fluid extraction*: A relatively new technique for extracting fragrant compounds from a raw material, which often employs Supercritical CO_2. Due to the low heat of process and the relatively nonreactive solvent used in the extraction, the fragrant compounds derived often closely resemble the original odor of the raw material.
    - o *Ethanol extraction*: A type of solvent extraction used to extract fragrant compounds directly from dry raw materials, as well as the impure oily compounds materials resulting from solvent extraction or enfleurage. Ethanol extraction from fresh plant materials contain large quantities of water, which will also be extracted into the ethanol.
- Distillation: A common technique for obtaining aromatic compounds from plants, such as orange blossoms and roses. The raw material is heated and the fragrant compounds are re-collected through condensation of the distilled vapor.

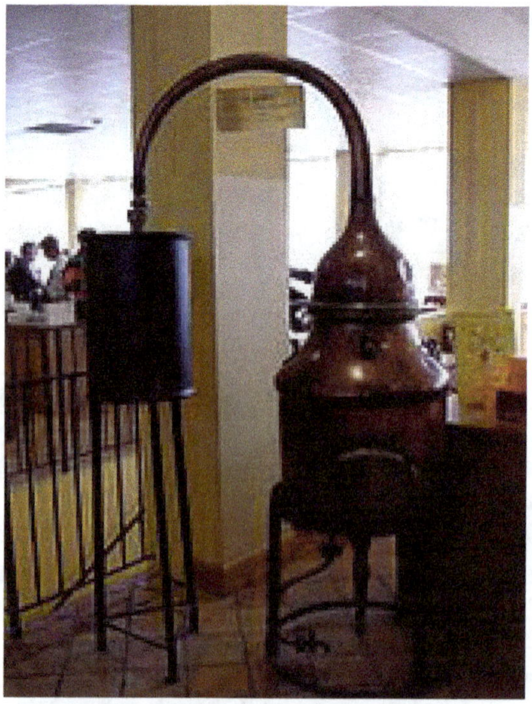

An old perfume still on display at Fragonard

- o *Steam distillation*: Steam from boiling water is passed through the raw material, which drives out their volatile fragrant compounds. The condensate from distillation are settled in a Florentine flask. This allows for the easy separation of the fragrant oils from the water. The water collected from the condensate, which retains some of the fragrant compounds and oils from the raw material is called hydrosol and sometimes sold. This is most commonly used for fresh plant materials such as flowers, leaves, and stems.

- o *Dry/destructive distillation*: The raw materials are directly heated in a still without a carrier solvent such as water. Fragrant compounds that are released from the raw material by the high heat often undergo anhydrous pyrolysis, which results in the formation of different fragrant compounds, and thus different fragrant notes. This method is used to obtain fragrant compounds from fossil amber and fragrant woods where an intentional "burned" or "toasted" odor is desired.

- o *Fractionation*: Through the use of a fractionation column, different fractions distilled from a material can be selectively excluded to modify the scent of the final product. Although the product is more expensive, this is sometimes performed to remove unpleasant or undesirable scents of a material and affords the perfumer more control over their composition process.

- Expression: Raw material is squeezed or compressed and the essential oils are collected. Of all raw materials, only the fragrant oils from the peels of fruits in the citrus family are extracted in this manner since the oil is present in large enough quantities as to make this extraction method economically feasible.

- Enfleurage: Absorption of aroma materials into solid fat or wax and then extraction of odorous oils with ethyl alcohol. Extraction by enfleurage was commonly used when distillation was not possible because some fragrant compounds denature through high heat. This technique is not commonly used in the modern industry due to prohibitive costs and the existence of more efficient and effective extraction methods.

Fragrant Extracts

Although fragrant extracts are known to the general public as the generic term "essential oils", a more specific language is used in the fragrance industry to describe the source, purity, and technique used to obtain a particular fragrant extract. Of these extracts, only *absolutes*, *essential oils*, and *tinctures* are directly used to formulate perfumes.

- Absolute: Fragrant materials that are purified from a *pommade* or *concrete* by soaking them in ethanol. By using a slightly hydrophilic compound such as ethanol, most of the fragrant compounds from the waxy source materials can be extracted without dissolving any of the fragrantless waxy molecules. Absolutes are usually found in the form of an oily liquid.

- Concrete: Fragrant materials that have been extracted from raw materials through *solvent extraction* using volatile hydrocarbons. Concretes usually contain a large amount of wax due to the ease in which the solvents dissolve various hydrophobic compounds. As such concretes are usually further purified through distillation or ethanol based solvent extraction. Concretes are typically either waxy or resinous solids or thick oily liquids.

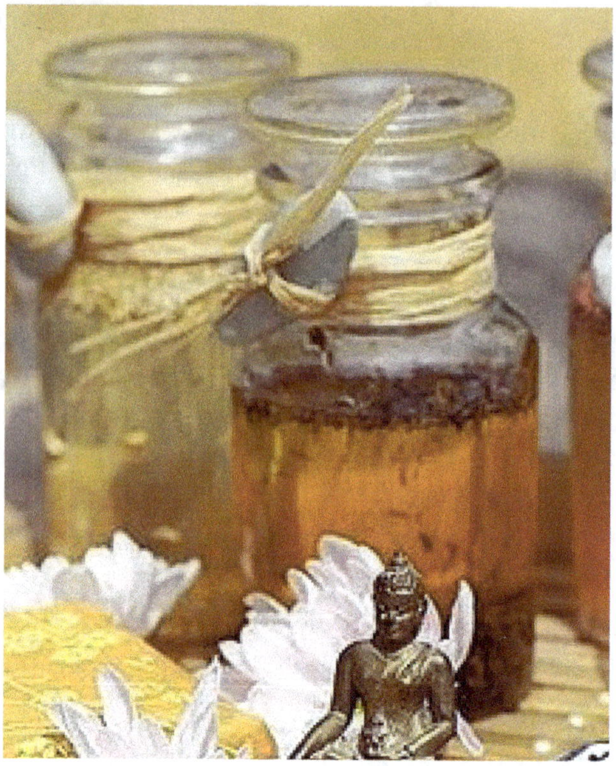

Essential oil

- Essential oil: Fragrant materials that have been extracted from a source material directly through *distillation* or *expression* and obtained in the form of an oily liquid. Oils extracted through expression are sometimes called *expression oils.*
- Pomade: A fragrant mass of solid fat created from the *enfleurage* process, in which odorous compounds in raw materials are adsorbed into animal fats. Pommades are found in the form of an oily and sticky solid.
- Tincture: Fragrant materials produced by directly soaking and infusing raw materials in ethanol. Tinctures are typically thin liquids.

Products from different extraction methods are known under different names even though their starting materials are the same. For instance, orange blossoms from *Citrus aurantium* that have undergone solvent extraction produces "orange blossom absolute" but that which have been steam distilled is known as "neroli oil".

Composing Perfumes

Perfume compositions are an important part of many industries ranging from the luxury goods sectors, food services industries, to manufacturers of various household chemicals. The purpose of using perfume or fragrance compositions in these industries is to affect customers through their sense of smell and entice them into purchasing the perfume or perfumed product. As such there is significant interest in producing a perfume formulation that people will find aesthetically pleasing.

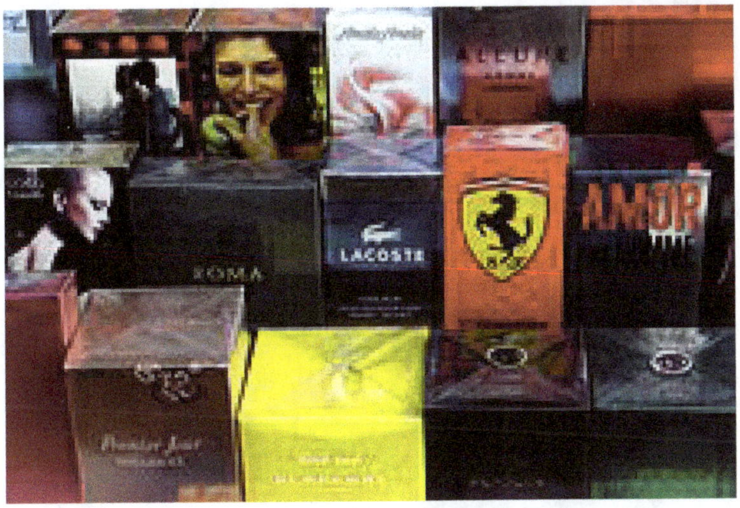

Counterfeit perfumes

The Perfumer

The job of composing perfumes that will be sold is left up to an expert on perfume composition or known in the fragrance industry as the *perfumer*. They are also sometimes referred to affectionately as a "*Nez*" (French for *nose*) due to their fine sense of smell and skill in smell composition.

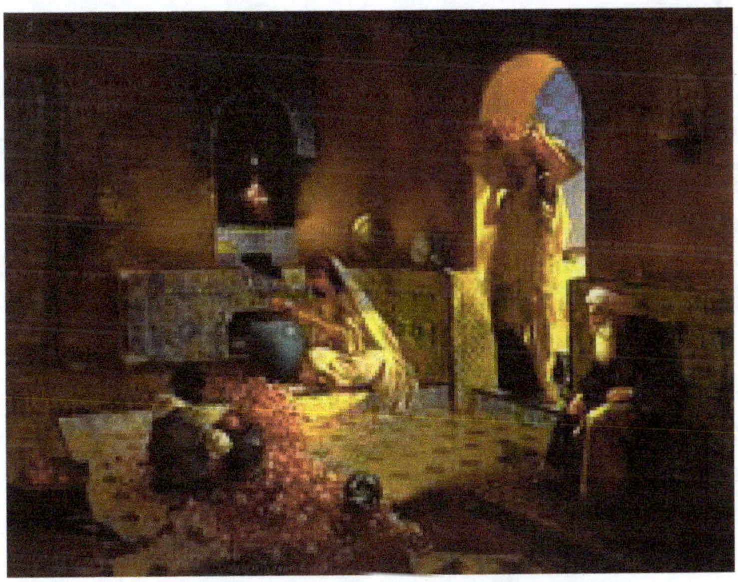

The Perfume Maker, by Rodolphe Ernst

The composition of a perfume typically begins with a *brief* by the perfumer's employer or an outside customer. The customers to the perfumer or their employers, are typically fashion houses or large corporations of various industries. The perfumer will then go through the process of blending multiple perfume mixtures and sell the formulation to the customer, often with modifications of the composition of the perfume. The perfume composition will then be either used to enhance another product as a *functional fragrance* (shampoos, make-up, detergents, car interiors, etc.), or marketed and sold directly to the public as a *fine fragrance*.

Technique

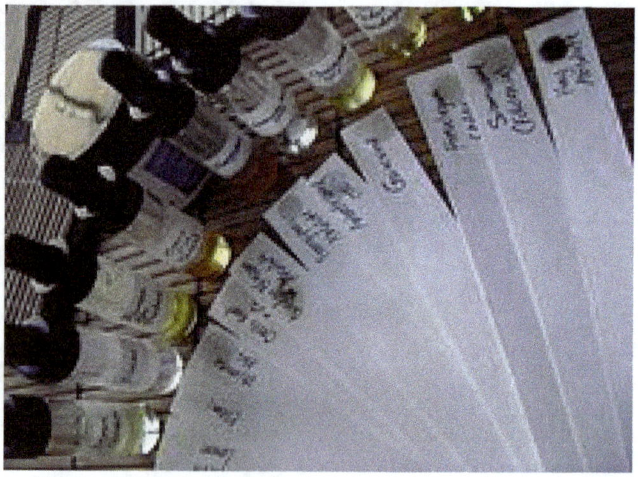

Paper blotters (fr:*mouillettes*) are commonly used by perfumers to sample and smell perfumes and odorants.

Although there is no single "correct" technique for the formulation of a perfume, there are general guidelines as to how a perfume can be constructed from a concept. Although many ingredients do not contribute to the smell of a perfume, many perfumes include colorants and anti-oxidants to improve the marketability and shelf life of the perfume, respectively.

Basic Framework

Perfume oils usually contain tens to hundreds of ingredients and these are typically organized in a perfume for the specific role they will play. These ingredients can be roughly grouped into four groups:

- *Primary scents* (Heart): Can consist of one or a few main ingredients for a certain concept, such as "rose". Alternatively, multiple ingredients can be used together to create an "abstract" primary scent that does not bear a resemblance to a natural ingredient. For instance, jasmine and rose scents are commonly blends for abstract floral fragrances. Cola flavourant is a good example of an abstract primary scent.
- *Modifiers*: These ingredients alter the primary scent to give the perfume a certain desired character: for instance, fruit esters may be included in a floral primary to create a fruity floral; calone and citrus scents can be added to create a "fresher" floral. The cherry scent in cherry cola can be considered a modifier.
- *Blenders*: A large group of ingredients that smooth out the transitions of a perfume between different "layers" or bases. These themselves can be used as a major component of the primary scent. Common blending ingredients include linalool and hydroxycitronellal.
- *Fixatives*: Used to support the primary scent by bolstering it. Many resins, wood scents, and amber bases are used as fixatives.

The top, middle, and base notes of a fragrance may have separate primary scents and supporting ingredients. The perfume's fragrance oils are then blended with ethyl alcohol and water, aged in tanks for several weeks and filtered through processing equipment to, respectively, allow the perfume ingredients in the mixture to stabilize and to remove any sediment and particles before the solution can be filled into the perfume bottles.

Fragrance Bases

Instead of building a perfume from "ground up", many modern perfumes and colognes are made using *fragrance bases* or simply bases. Each base is essentially modular perfume that is blended from essential oils and aromatic chemicals, and formulated with a simple concept such as "fresh cut grass" or "juicy sour apple". Many of Guerlain's *Aqua Allegoria* line, with their simple fragrance concepts, are good examples of what perfume fragrance bases are like.

The effort used in developing bases by fragrance companies or individual perfumers may equal that of a marketed perfume, since they are useful in that they are reusable. On top of its reusability, the benefit in using bases for construction are quite numerous:

1. Ingredients with "difficult" or "overpowering" scents that are tailored into a blended base may be more easily incorporated into a work of perfume
2. A base may be better scent approximations of a certain thing than the extract of the thing itself. For example, a base made to embody the scent for "fresh dewy rose" might be a better approximation for the scent concept of a rose after rain than plain rose oil. Flowers whose scents cannot be extracted, such as gardenia or hyacinth, are composed as bases from data derived from headspace technology.
3. A perfumer can quickly rough out a concept from a brief by combining multiple bases, then present it feedback. Smoothing out the "edges" of the perfume can be done after a positive response.

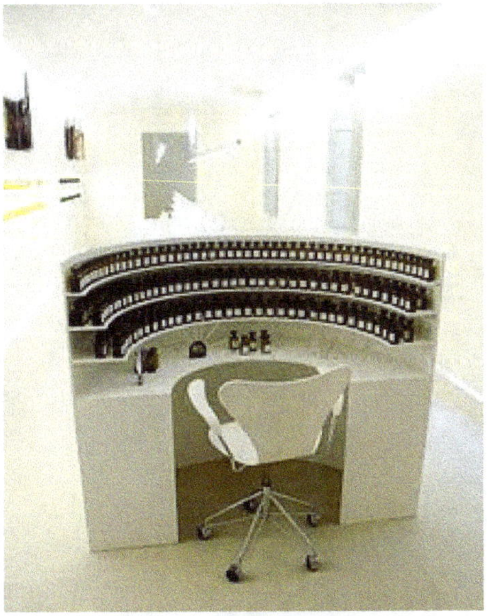

A "perfume organ", where perfumers play around with hundreds of essences, in Grasse

Reverse Engineering

Creating perfumes through reverse engineering with analytical techniques such as Gas chromatography–mass spectrometry (GC/MS) can reveal the "general" formula for any particular perfume. The difficulty of GC/MS analysis arises due to the complexity of a perfume's ingredients. This is particularly due to the presence of natural essential oils and other ingredients consisting of complex chemical mixtures. However, "anyone armed with good GC/MS equipment and experienced in using this equipment can today, within days, find out a great deal about the formulation of any perfume... customers and competitors can analyze most perfumes more or less precisely."

Antique or badly preserved perfumes undergoing this analysis can also be difficult due to the numerous degradation by-products and impurities that may have resulted from breakdown of the odorous compounds. Ingredients and compounds can usually be ruled out or identified using gas chromatograph (GC) smellers, which allow individual chemical components to be identified both through their physical properties and their scent. Reverse engineering of best-selling perfumes in the market is a very common practice in the fragrance industry due to the relative simplicity of operating GC equipment, the pressure to produce marketable fragrances, and the highly lucrative nature of the perfume market.

Chapter 3

Makeup for Face

Face base is mainly applied on the face and the neck area to hide scars and pimples and to create a uniform skin tone. It is mainly classified in different shades, such as warm, cool or neutral. Foundation can be applied by using either one's fingers or sponges and brushes. The topics discussed in this section focus on the methods and techniques used by Asian women for applying foundations and face powder.

How to Determine your Skin Type

Determining your skin type is easy, and the information will help you when buying moisturizers, cosmetics and facial cleansers.

Instructions

- STEP 1: Wash your face with a skin cleanser, then rinse and pat dry.
- STEP 2: Wait one hour.
- STEP 3: Note whether your skin feels "tight."
- STEP 4: Press a separate piece of tissue onto each area of your face: chin, center of cheeks, outer cheeks, center of forehead, outer forehead and nose.
- STEP 5: Examine each tissue and look for oily residue or flaky skin residue.
- STEP 6: Interpret the results. Oil on each tissue indicates an oily skin type, while oil on only some tissues (specifically those on the T-zone, which is the center of forehead, nose, chin and center of cheeks) indicates a combination skin type.

Flaky skin residue on all tissues - without oily residue - or a tight feeling in the skin indicates a dry skin type. No oil and no flaky residue on any parts of the tissue indicates a normal skin type.

Tips & Warnings

- Pore size is another indication of skin type; small pores generally indicate dry skin, while large pores mean oily skin.
- Remember that there are many factors that affect your skin type, such as weather, emotions, hormones and stress, and this will cause your skin type to be in a constant state of fluctuation.
- "Combination skin" products that claim to serve different functions on different parts of the face are suspicious. You're better off using different products on different areas.

- Overall Things You'll Need
- Mild Facial Cleansers
- Hand Or Wash Towels
- Oil-free Moisturizers
- Oil-free Facial Cleansers

Foundation

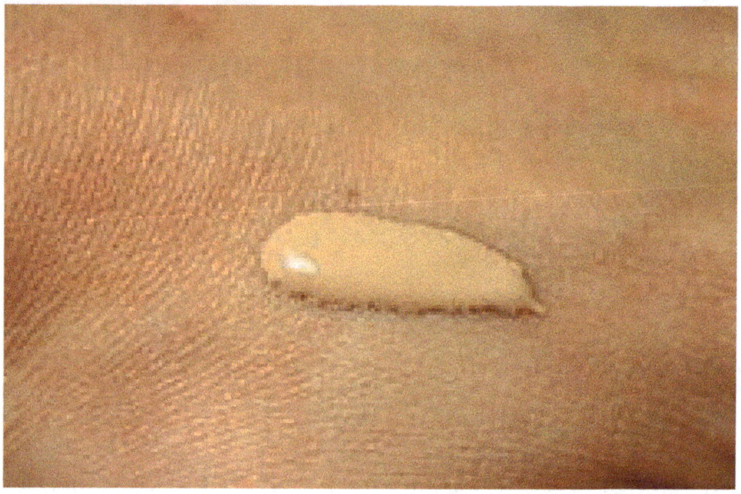

Thick, unblended foundation on skin

Foundation is a skin coloured makeup applied to the face to create an even, uniform colour to the complexion, to cover flaws and, sometimes, to change the natural skintone. Some foundations also function as a moisturizer, sunscreen, astringent or base layer for more complex cosmetics. Foundation applied to the body is generally referred to as "body painting."

Pan-Cake

The first commercially available foundation was Max Factor's *Pan-Cake*. Originally developed for use in film, actresses were so taken with the results that Max Factor was overwhelmed with demand for the product for their personal use. The breakthrough in his formula was the first "foundation and powder in one"; traditionally, an actor was made up with an oil/emollient-based make-up, which was then set with powder to reduce the reflection and ensure it would not fade or smudge. Pan-Cake used talc—rather than oil or wax—as the base, and, applied directly to the skin with a wet sponge, it offered enough coverage (it could be layered without caking on the skin) to eliminate the need for a foundation underneath. This was considered significantly more lightweight and natural-looking on the skin than the standard method, hence people's eagerness to wear the item in public. Although foundation make-up was widely available and used within the film industry, the use of cosmetics in general was still somewhat disreputable, and no one had tried to market foundation (although lipstick, blush and nail polish were popular for daily use) as an everyday item. Factor had the product patented in 1937, and, despite the economic turmoil of the era, Pan-Cake became one of the most successful cosmetic launches of all time. By 1940, it was estimated that one in three North American women owned and wore Pan-Cake. As of February 2009, Procter and Gamble, the brand's current owner, confirmed that the original formula Factor developed and used himself is still sold today.

Modern Formulations

Colour

Colour may be identified by a name, number, letter, or any combination of the three. However, unlike the Pantone or Munsell systems used in the art and fashion industries, commercial cosmetic product names are not standardised. If a make-up artist requests a "Medium Beige" foundation, the result can vary drastically from brand to brand, and sometimes, within one brand across different formulas. Cosmetic companies can also edit and adjust their formulations at any time, resulting in the 'Medium Beige' foundation a consumer has been wearing for years becoming a slightly different shade or color without prior notice.

Colour Classification

Many companies classify their shades as Warm, Neutral, or Cool. Adding to the confusion is the different color wheels used between the art and beauty industry. The traditional artist's palette places the line dividing Cool and Warm across Primary Blue, whereas the cosmetic palette places the line across Primary Red. Thus, on the artists' color wheel, Yellow is always Cool, Red is always Warm, and Blue can be Neutral (Primary), Warm (Violet), or Cool (Green). In contrast, the cosmetic palette classifies Yellow as always Warm, Blue as always Cool, and Red as either Neutral (Primary), Warm (Orange) or Cool (Blue-Red). The cosmetic palette is never used outside of make-up, and is very common in the industry – though a handful of professional lines, such as William Tuttle, Ben Nye, Visiora, M.A.C. and even Max Factor all use the conventional artist's palette. Thus, a Warm Beige foundation may either have a yellow tint or a pink tint, depending on the palette the company's creative director uses. Note that the artist's palette is designed to be used on canvas (which is white) compared to the make-up palette – which is used on flesh (an ivory to brown tone).

Selection

Although most artists differ over the significance of selecting an exact match to the wearer's skin tone, intentionally using a mismatch can achieve a desired result. An excessively red complexion can be minimised by using a clear (meaning neither yellow nor pink) beige toned foundation. A sallow or dull complexion can be brightened with a rose to red tint, mature skin that has lost its color and appears pale and dull can be brightened with a tint of clear pink, and olive or ashy skin can be brightened with a shot of peach. A crucial point in selecting a foundation shade is to recognise that the appearance of the shade in the container may not accurately gauge the colour impact on the skin – a foundation that appears very yellow in the bottle may go on much less yellow, or not appear yellow at all.

Coverage

Coverage refers to the opacity of the makeup, or how much it will conceal on the skin.

- Sheer is the most transparent and contains the least amount of pigment. It will not hide discolorations on the skin but it can minimise the contrast between the discoloration and the rest of the skin tone. Although pigment technology has evolved dramatically since 2004, the traditional protocol for sheer foundations called for pigment to comprise 8–13% of the finished formula.
- Light can cover unevenness and slight blotchiness, but is not opaque enough to cover freckles. It contains 13–18% pigment.
- Medium coverage can, when set with a tinted (instead of translucent) powder, cover freckles, discolorations, blotchiness, and red marks left by pimples. It contains 18–23% pigment.
- Full coverage is very opaque, and used to cover birthmarks, vitiligo, hyperpigmentation and scars. It is sometimes referred to as "corrective" or "camouflage" make-up. In general it contains up to 35% pigment, though professional brands, designed for use on stage, can contain up to 50% pigment.

Application Tools

There are various tools that can be used to apply foundation including your fingers, a sponge, and several varieties of foundation brushes, each providing a different finish. Before applying foundation always start with clean, moisturized skin. Any dry, flaky skin patches will be highlighted when makeup is applied so users should exfoliate their skin first if required.

- Fingers: Using your fingers is great for creating a natural look. The natural body heat in your fingers helps the foundation to melt into your skin and it's easy to blend in a sheer layer of makeup. Using your fingers isn't recommended for applying full cover makeup though as streaks and finger marks can occur.
- Sponge: Using a sponge to apply foundation is great for creating a sheer to medium cover look. A triangular sponge is good for blending in liquid foundation and concealer, whilst a rounded sponge is best for powder foundations. Wet a clean sponge with water first: the moisture will help prevent the sponge from absorbing the makeup, but make sure to squeeze out excess water. The sponge will also assist in blending. Try to find sponges with pointed tips for superb blending of the eye area. Also, note that reusing sponges can be unhygienic, so sponges should be washed and dried thoroughly after every use.
- Brush: For liquid foundation, a brush with a synthetic bristle is recommended as the brush won't soak up too much of the liquid. Alternatively, a natural bristle which is more porous works best for powder foundations such as mineral makeup. A densely bristled brush is best for foundation as it is less likely to leave tell-tale streaky brush marks. As with all tools used to apply makeup to the face, brushes should be soft and gentle, as anything too stiff will scratch and irritate the skin.
- Airbrush: Liquid foundation is applied with an air stream. The airbrush mixes the founda-

tion with a controllable stream of compressed air. It adheres with the skin as millions of tiny droplets of foundation. This technique can create an even, sheer, natural appearance to the skin that, if applied properly for a natural look, can appear natural and non-heavy like traditional makeup. Airbrush makeup application is also frequently used in special effects makeup.

Formulation

The formula refers to the ingredients blended together, and how the makeup is formulated.

- Oil and emollient-based are the oldest type of make-up. An oil (usually mineral oil) or emollient (such as petrolatum, beeswax, or lanolin) is used as the main ingredient, with pigment added to it. The texture and application is extremely thick and dense, most closely resembling modern lip balms or lipsticks. The extremely emollient nature stays moist and will not cake, is moderately waterproof, and provides the most opaque coverage; but it can smudge, fade, and change colour (darkening or oxidising) during wear. Since the 1970s, synthetic wax has also been used, which is less greasy and more reliable than other emollients. Used professionally, it is sometimes referred to as Greasepaint. Examples: Pan-Stik (Max Factor's follow-up to his Pan-Cake make-up), Elizabeth Arden Sponge-On Cream, Mehron, Dermablend.

- Oil-based shakers are different from traditional oil-and-emollient-based makeup in that they were liquid foundations developed before emulsifiers and binding agent were available, and thus separate in the bottle, like the alcohol-based formulas mentioned below. Once shaken, this is akin to applying coloured oil to the skin, with a smooth texture than can provide medium coverage with a moist finish. Liquid foundation is applied using a damp makeup sponge and is especially effective around the eye. It was a marked improvement in application, stability and finish over the tradition oil bases, but improvements since then have rendered these nearly extinct. Examples: Alexandra de Markoff Countess Isserlyn, Frances Denney Incandescent.

- Alcohol based uses a blend of water and denatured alcohol as the base, with pigment added to it. Developed by Erno Laszlo for problematic skin, it eliminated emollient and binding agent that could clog pores, and needs to be shaken before use. Alcohol-based foundations have the most lightweight, "nothing on my face" feel, and nearly impossible to clog pores, but provide only the sheerest coverage and can be tricky to apply and blend. They work better with cotton balls or pads, instead of latex or sea sponges. Examples: Erno Laszlo Normalizer Shake-It, Clinique Pore Minimizer.

- Powder-based began with Max Factors' Pan Cake, using powder — usually talc — as the main ingredient. Pigment is added, along emollients, skin adhesion agents and binding agents to the formula before it is pressed into pans. The difference between this type of foundation and pressed powder is that this provides more coverage (due to more pigment), and contains more skin adhesion agents (to help it stick to the skin – because pressed powder is lighter weight, it requires less). Some formulas — such as Pan Cake — also contain wax, and can only be applied with a wet sponge; others, such as M.A.C. StudioFix contain no emollient, and can only be used dry; the last group, such as Lançome Dual Finish, contain a smaller amount of oil and can be used either way. This provide a "finished" look and can blend from sheer to nearly full coverage, but can look too floury and dry, especially around the eyes, or on drier/mature skin. They can also flake and trickle down as they are applied and blended.

- Mineral makeup most commonly refers to a foundation in loose powder format. The most common minerals used as the base are mica, bismuth oxychloride, titanium dioxide or zinc oxide. However, talc is also a mineral, so a talc-based powder could be considered a "mineral makeup" — although most mineral make-up sold makes a point of being talc-free. A "mineral make-up" may be all mineral, part mineral — or contain less than 1% mineral as part of the finished formula. Using this logic, practically all make-up could be considered mineral.

- Water-based make-up appeared after the end of World War II, with emulsifiers that could successfully keep a water-and-oil blended emulsion stable being the key to their development. This creamy liquid provided medium coverage with a far more natural feel and appearance than oil, powder or emollient bases of the time, and became popular with women since then. Examples include: Cover Girl Clean Makeup, Estee Lauder Country Mist. Since then, variations on the formula have expanded the category significantly:

    - Water-based cream make-up has a rich, creamy texture that can be sheer to full coverage with a moist, satiny finish. It usually comes in a jar or tube, and is much more comfortable and realistic looking on the skin than the oil or emollient-based predecessors. Examples: Elizabeth Arden Hydro-Light, Guerlain Issima.

    - Water-based oil-free eliminates oil altogether, but substitutes an emollient ester or fatty alcohol in the base, and adds a mattifying agent — usually clay — to dry to a flat, non-reflective ("matte") finish. Oil-free liquids are quite thick and heavy, and the earliest versions took time to pour out of the bottle. They provide solid medium coverage but dry quickly, and can thus set before blended is complete. The result is streaking, which is then difficult to smooth out without starting over from scratch. The usual recommendation is to divide the face into quarter sections, and to apply and blend the makeup over one section (rather than the entire face) at a time. Blending over moisturised skin with a wet sponge can also help compensate for the lack of slip. However, they will last a long time and resist smudging, even on very oily skin. Examples: Estee Lauder Fresh Air.

    - Water-based transfer-resistant follows the same formulation as oil-free, but uses a film former or polymer instead of (or in addition to) the clay to achieve a matte finish that resists being rubbed off. Transfer-resistant make-up was launched in 1993 by Revlon-owned Ultima II with *Lipsexxxy*, the first lip-colour that included film former to prevent rubbing off. By 1996, *WonderWear* foundation and Revlon *Colorstay* had been launched, using the same technology as the lipsticks. Transfer-resistant (sometimes called *transfer-proof*) makeup will last on very oily skin, skin that perspires heavily, or in humid climates longer than any other type of foundation, though it is even more difficult to apply than oil-free makeup. The thick texture dries almost instantly, and requires a fair amount of experimentation to master. The most modern versions (such as *Revlon Colorstay SoftFlex*) have made marked improvements over predecessors in that regard.

- Silicone-based make-up uses a silicone — or a blend of water and silicone — as the main ingredient. The most typical silicones used are dimethicone, polysiloxane and volatile silicones such as cyclomethicone and phenyl trimethicone. The silicone provides lubrication and viscosity (what some artists refer to as "slip") at a level equal to, or often, even better than oil allowing a product to apply and blend over the skin smoothly and evenly. Silicones have a lighter weight and are thus more comfortable on the skin, as well as resisting filling in lines or large pores on the face. Conventional silicones stay supple and smooth, even in dry climates, whereas volatile silicones last long enough to blend over the face, then evaporate (like alcohol), leaving little to no feel behind. Silicone-based makeups are less likely to oxidise or change colour during wear. One of the biggest challenges facing silicone bases is the tendency for the product to break and/or ball up on the skin, something unique to silicones and out of control of the user. Ionizing the silicones (electrically charging the silicone positive) helps it adhere to (negatively charged) skin, although this technology is in its infancy and thus rather expensive. Examples: Maybelline Dream Matte Mousse.

How to Make Liquid Foundation

Liquid foundation offers a beautiful, full coverage base for your makeup look. It can cover up any blemishes or imperfections, and make your skin look flawless. If liquid foundation has become a staple in your beauty routine, it can be a nightmare if you go to apply your makeup only to discover your trusty bottle is empty. Don't freak out – there are a few different ways to make your own, homemade liquid foundation.

Method 1

Creating Homemade Lotion and Color

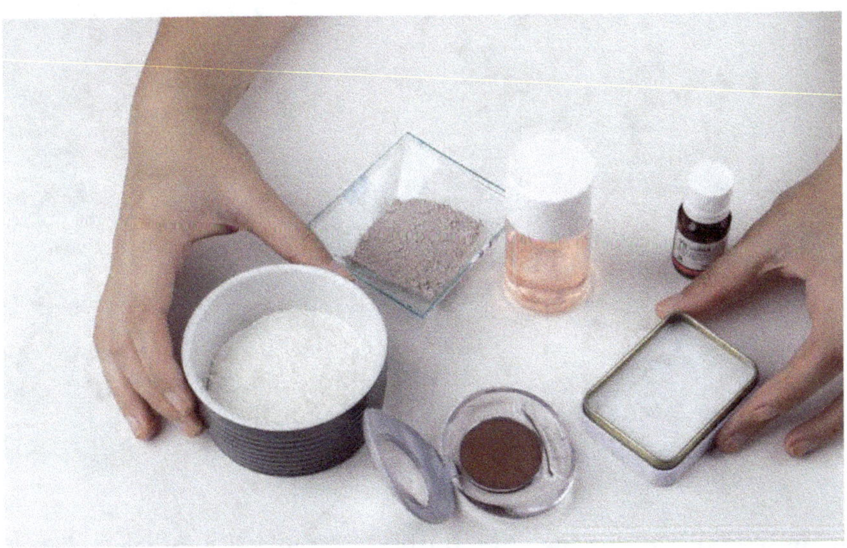

1. Gather the ingredients. If you want to truly create your liquid foundation from scratch, you'll need about five ingredients to create your base and four to create your custom color. For your base lotion, you'll need shea butter, emulsifying wax, argan oil, aloe, and witch hazel. For coverage and color, you'll need zinc oxide, cosmetic clay, mica powder, and cocoa powder.

- You can find shea butter, argan oil, aloe, and witch hazel – an astringent – at your local pharmacy or beauty supply store. You may need to search a bit harder for the emulsifying wax, but can certainly order it from Amazon if you can't find it locally.
- You can find zinc oxide at your local pharmacy. You'll find cosmetic clays at natural beauty supply stores – a quick Google search will bring up several options. The easiest place to find mica powder is online. Cocoa powder can be found in any grocery store.

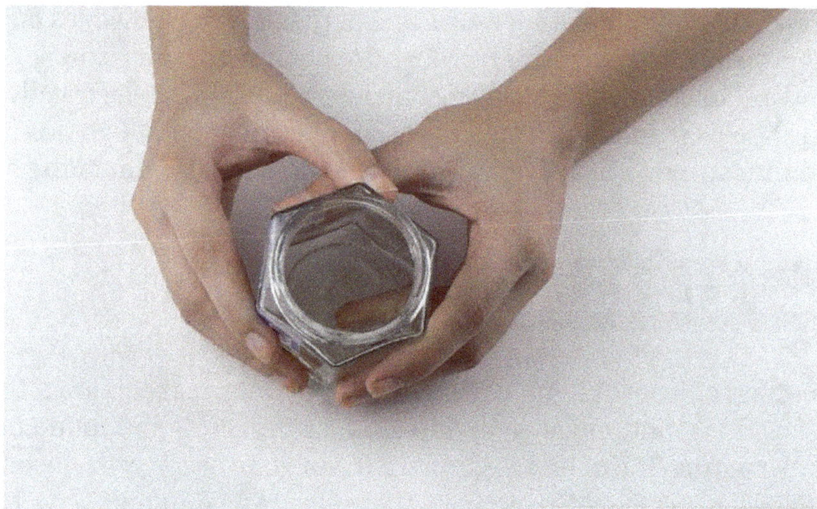

2. Melt shea butter in a small pan. If you have one, a double boiler also works great for this step. Add one teaspoon (4.93 mL) of shea butter into the pan, and set your stovetop to low heat. This shouldn't take long at all, so don't step away. Continue stirring the shea butter as it begins to melt.

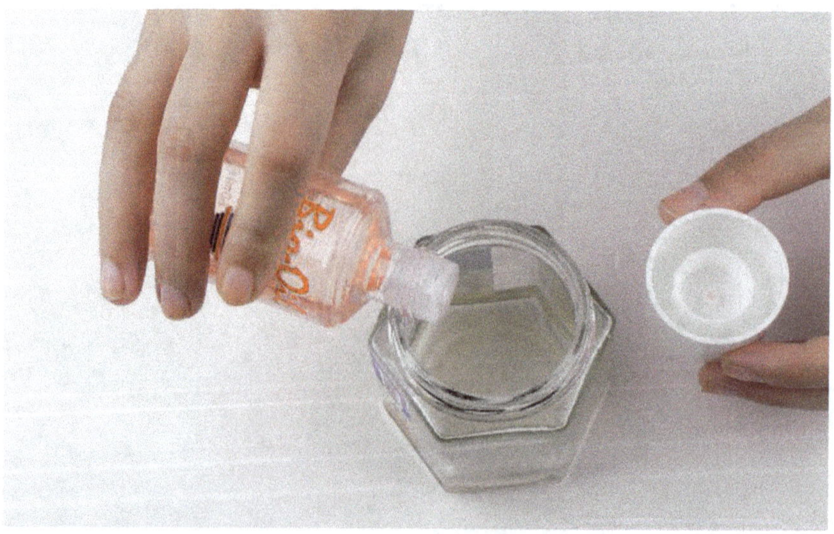

3. Add your other ingredients. Once the shea butter has melted, you'll need to throw in two tea-

spoons (9.86 mL) of argan oil and half a teaspoon (2.46 mL) of wax. Continuously stir your mixture as it warms and melts together. Once those have melted, add one tablespoon (14.79 mL) of the aloe and one teaspoon (4.93 mL) of the witch hazel.

- Mix until everything is thoroughly blended, and remove from heat.

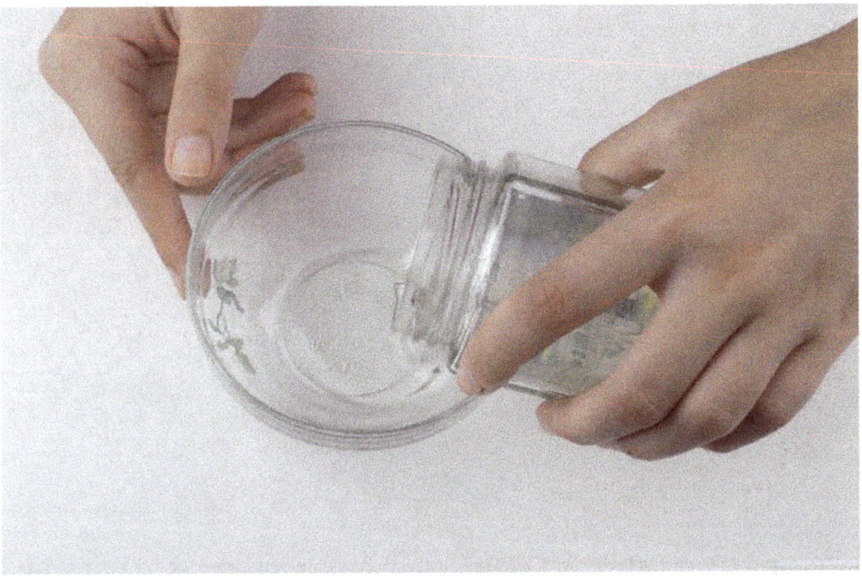

4. Put your lotion into a bowl or small container. You'll be adding the color ingredients next, so make sure there is plenty of room for mixing in this container. You may want to create your foundation in whatever container you'll use for storage, like a small makeup container or cup. Just make sure that whatever container you use has a lid.

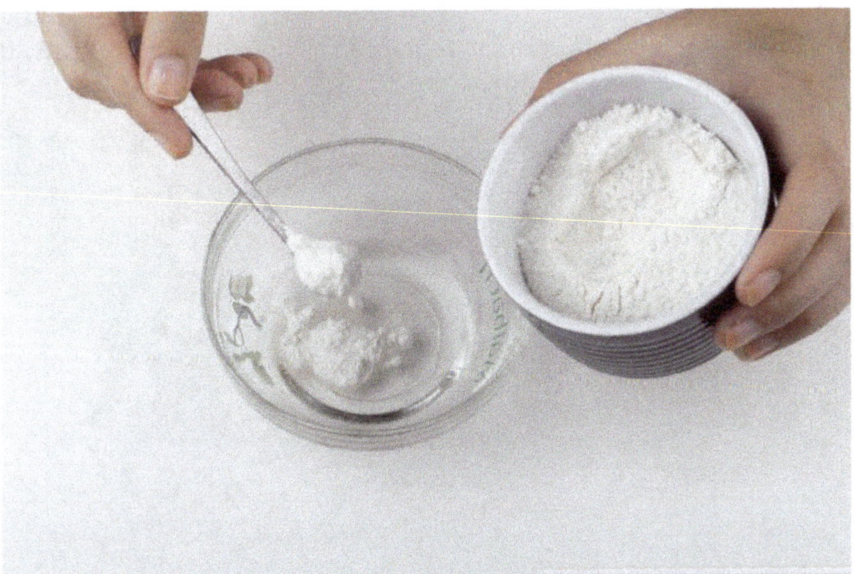

5. Add zinc oxide to your moisturizer. Zinc oxide will add sun protection to your liquid foundation, which will help keep your skin healthy and wrinkle-free. Because the zinc is a pretty thick

substance, it will ensure your liquid foundation provides the coverage you desire, concealing any blemishes. It will make your skin appear smooth and soft.

- You may need to experiment a bit to find out how much zinc oxide you like in your recipe. Typically, it requires anywhere from one teaspoon (4.93 mL) to four teaspoons (19.72 mL).

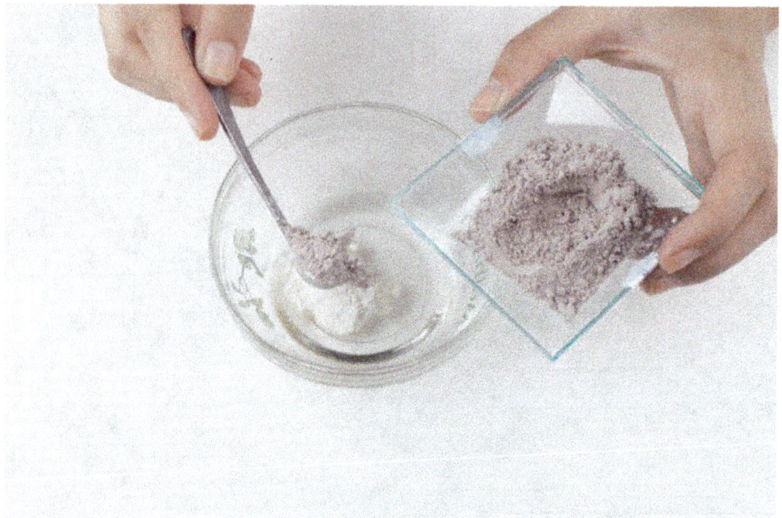

6. Mix clay in your foundation. While the word "clay" probably brings to mind images of modeling clay you used back in art class, there is actually powder cosmetic clay to use for recipes like these. However, this is an optional ingredient, and you don't need much – about half a teaspoon (2.46 mL) will do the trick.

- These clays contain minerals that are healthy for your skin and absorb excess oil so they're a great addition to your liquid foundation.
- Bentonite clay is the most popular clay to use, so as a beginner, you can start with that!

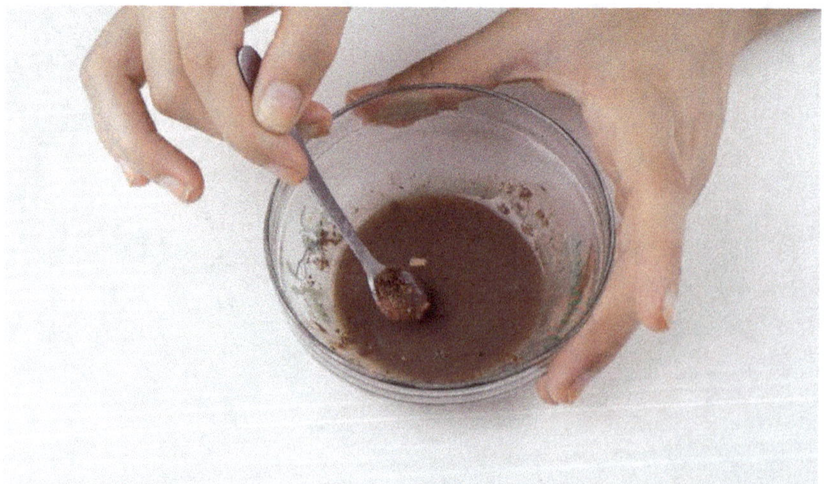

7. Add mica powder and cocoa powder. These powders will provide the color and bronzing to your liquid foundation. This is where you can really customize your foundation to match your skin tone,

so do this step slowly and carefully. Sprinkle in a bit of mica powder, then a bit of cocoa powder, stir, and test the color. Tweak as needed, and continue mixing until you've created a shade that matches your skin tone.

- Choose mica powder in gold and bronze to match your skin tone and create a beautiful glow.

Method 2

Using Store Bought Cosmetics to Create Foundation

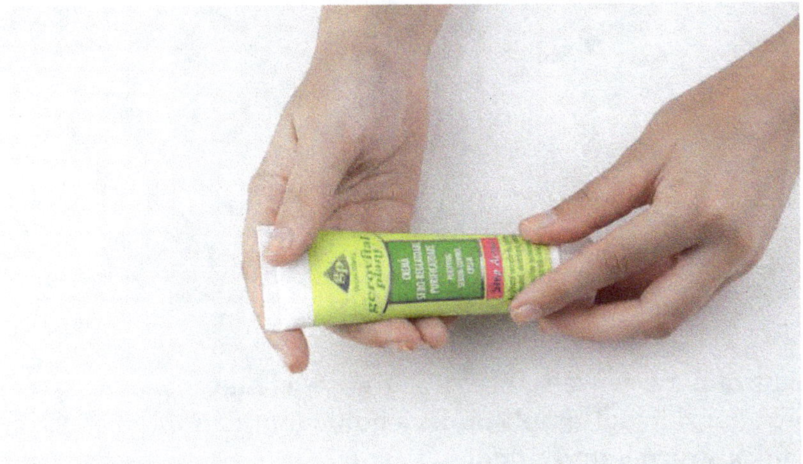

1. Purchase a moisturizer. If you aren't interested, or don't have the time, to make your own lotion, you can simply buy some. If you have a great facial lotion that you use religiously, stick with that one. It's great to use one that you know won't make you break out or cause any unfortunate side effects. If you don't have a trusted moisturizer, head to your local pharmacy or beauty supply store to pick one up. A lotion with shea butter is great for your skin, and works well to make liquid foundation.

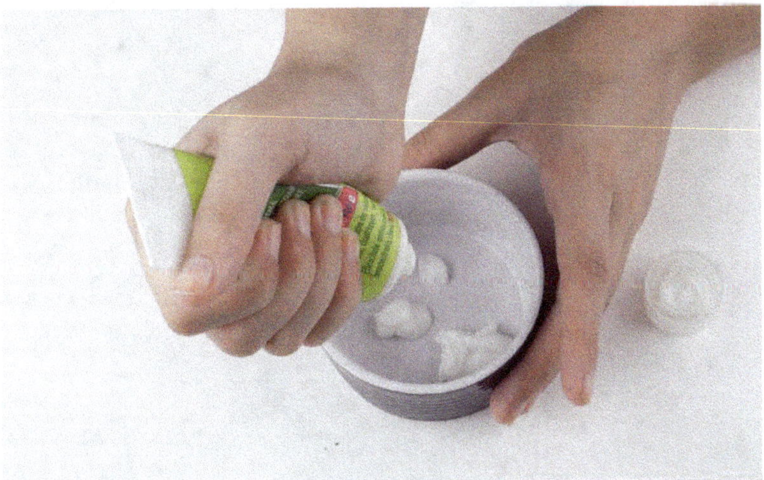

- If you aren't sure which lotion to choose, make sure you buy the smallest available bottle. That way, you won't waste money (or lotion) if you discover you don't like it.

2. Squirt your lotion into a container. It's simple to put it into whatever container you'll be storing your foundation in, so put it in anything with a tight lid. Make sure there is adequate room for mixing as well. Decide how much liquid foundation you want to make, and add that much lotion to the container. Just remember that if you add a lot of lotion, you'll need a lot of powder foundation as well.

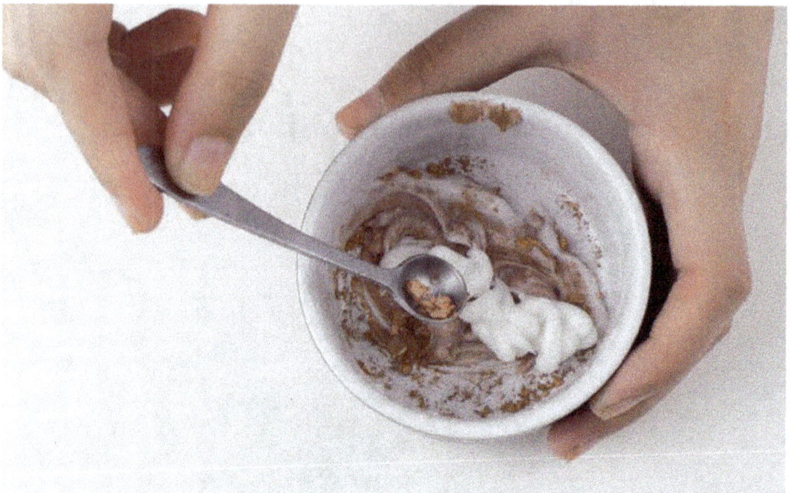

3. Use a store-bought mineral powder. Feel free to use whatever powder you like. If you have a powder that matches your skin but simply prefer a liquid foundation, go ahead and combine it with the moisturizer to quickly turn it into a liquid.

- Picking the perfect powder for your skin tone can be tricky. If you've never purchased powder before, it might be smart to head to a cosmetic store or a beauty counter in a department store and ask a professional for help finding your shade.

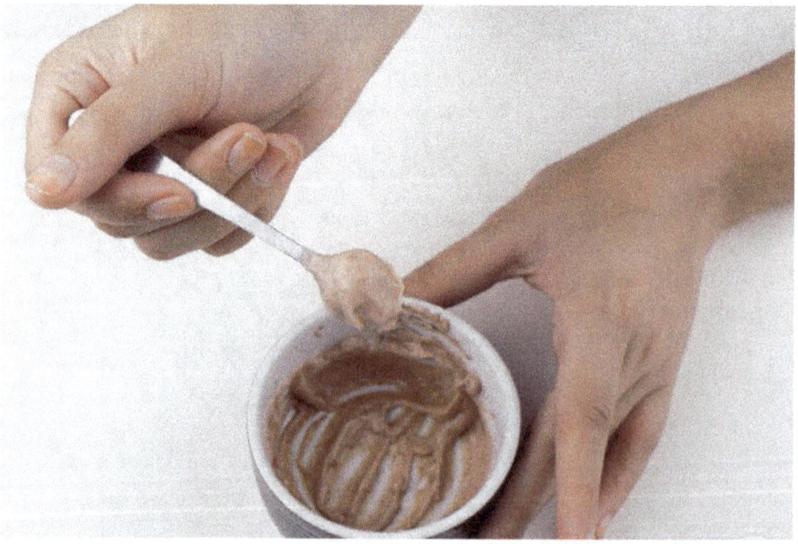

- If there is no one to ask for help, make sure you test the powder before buying it. The right shade should blend naturally on your jawline. Make sure that you check the color on yourself in natural light, because the bright lights of stores can be deceiving.

4. Stir until satisfied with the consistency. Add one teaspoon (4.93 mL) and stir, another another, stir, and so on. Continue doing this until you've reached a color and consistency that you like for your liquid foundation. When the color and consistency look good to you, test it on your forehead to ensure you like the product you've created. The great thing about making your own product is that you can always tweak the ratios, make new batches, and find the recipe that works best for you.

How to Apply Foundation

To quote makeup artist Nam Vo, "If someone compliments you on your foundation, you're doing something wrong." If you struggle with applying your foundation for a natural look, don't worry - it's a common problem. Look out for the perfect shade, take your time to apply it the right way, then set your foundation for the best of makeup circumstances. Soon enough, you'll be praised for the quality of your skin rather than the talent of your makeup application.

Part 1

Getting Started

1. Know your skin type. It is important to know whether you have dry, oily, normal or combination skin before applying foundation. This will determine what foundation is right for you. Some foundations are specially designed for different skin types. A mousse foundation is light and great for oily skin, whereas, a liquid foundation with a built in moisturising element is perfect for dry skin.

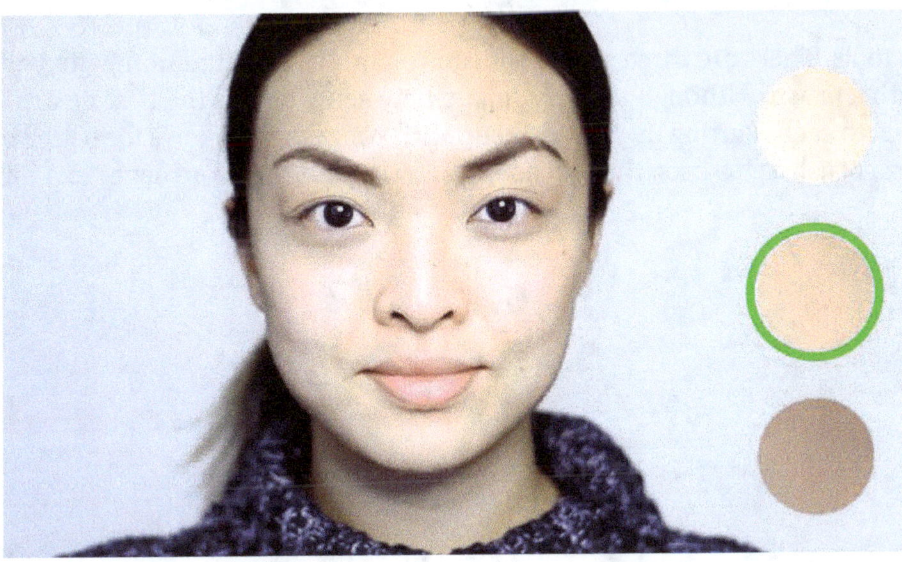

2. Choose the right foundation color. As the name implies, your foundation is the basis for the rest of your makeup. To make sure that it acts as a blank canvas, choose a foundation that identically matches your skin tone. Try multiple shades of foundation on your face (rather than your hand or your neck), and stick with the color that matches your skin tone without blending.

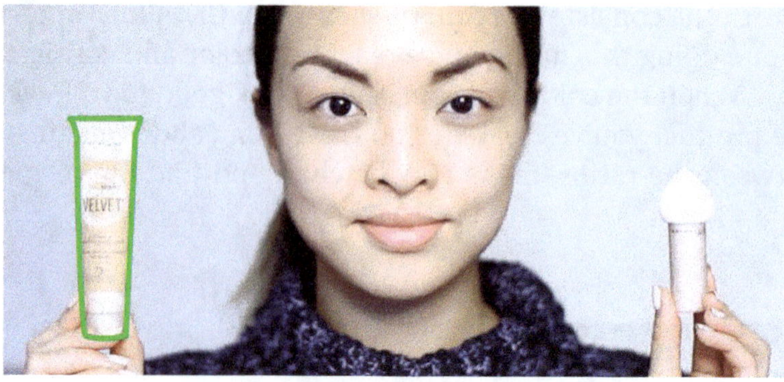

3. Decide on a medium. Foundation comes in a varieties of mediums and textures, including loose powders, compact powders, creams, liquids, and aerosols. All the variety can seem daunting, but really doesn't change much except for the application of the makeup. Visit the makeup counter at a local department store and try on versions on each to determine which feels the most comfortable and looks the most realistic on your skin.

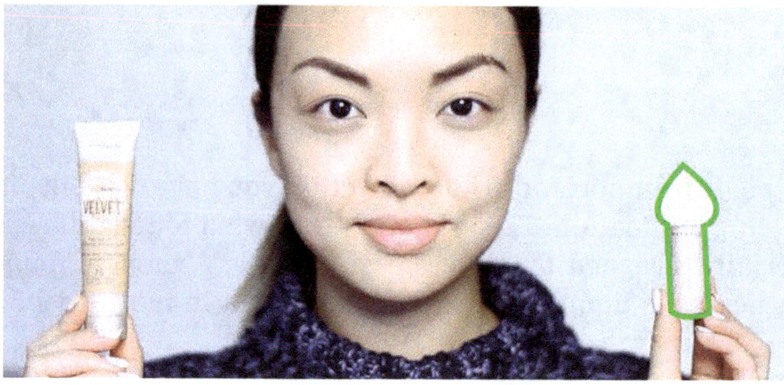

4. Get the right tools. There are three primary means of applying foundation: with your fingers, with a sponge, or with a brush. Although there is debate between which is the best means of application, there are benefits to each. Putting on your makeup with your fingers allows for better blending, while applying it with a brush helps keep the spread of bacteria (and therefore acne) to a minimum.

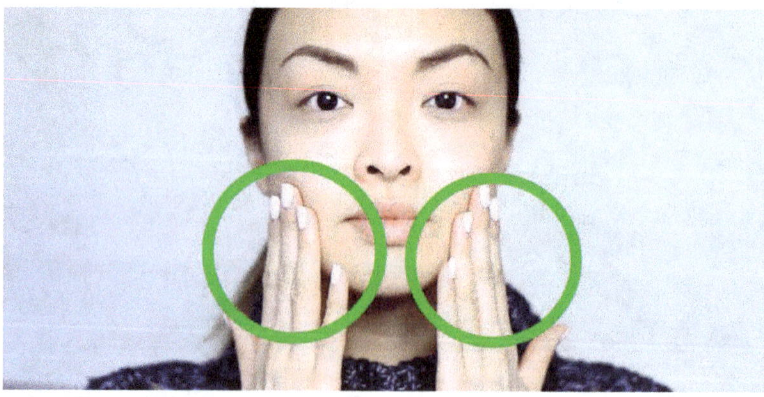

5. Prep your face. Foundation glides on most smoothly with a clean, well moisturized face. Wash your face with a gentle face cleanser, and follow up with a facial moisturizer. Wait five minutes for the lotion to set before applying your foundation.

Part 2

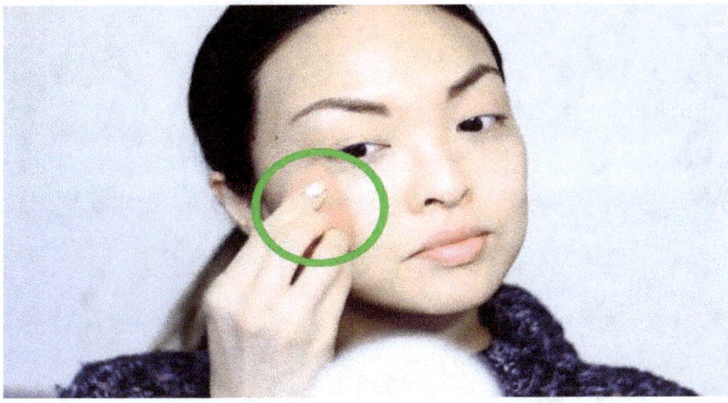

1. Put on your pre-foundation makeup. A slight misnomer, foundation isn't actually the first make-up you apply. Add a primer to your face, which is a clear gel that work to smooth out your skin and seal in imperfections. Some people also choose to apply their concealer prior to putting on their foundation, although this can be applied afterwards as well.

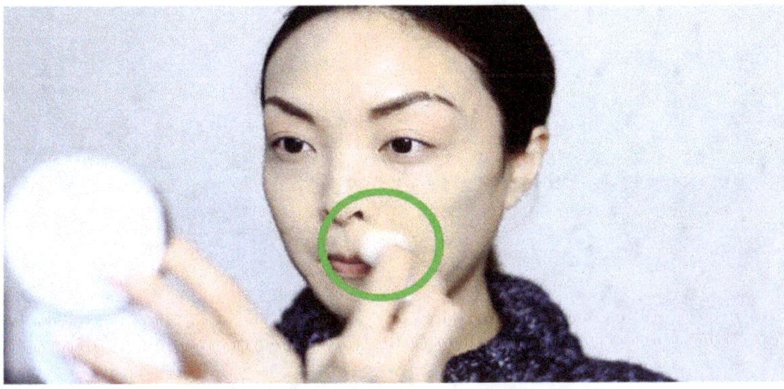

2. Put on your foundation. Regardless of whether your foundation is a liquid, cream, or powder, it should be applied first in the center of your face. Add a few dabs to either cheek near your nose, your chin, and a bit on your forehead.

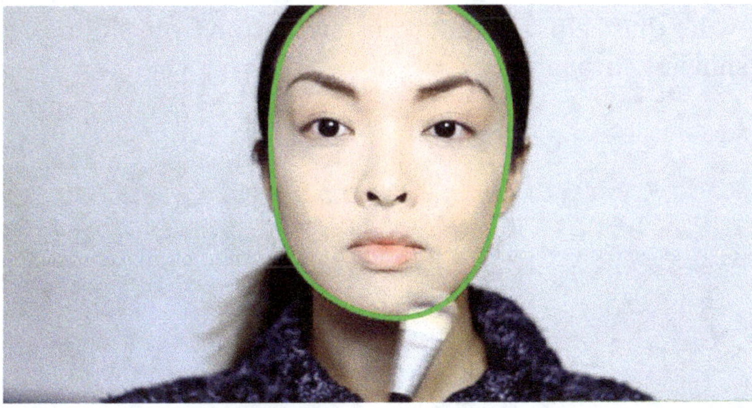

3. Blend your foundation with your selected tool. Use your tool of choice to blend your foundation around your face. There shouldn't be any noticeable lines where your foundation starts or ends; it

should blend smoothly into your neck and hairline. Prevent your foundation from being too thick by spreading it out. Otherwise, your face will look cakey and fake, rather than airbrushed and lustrous.

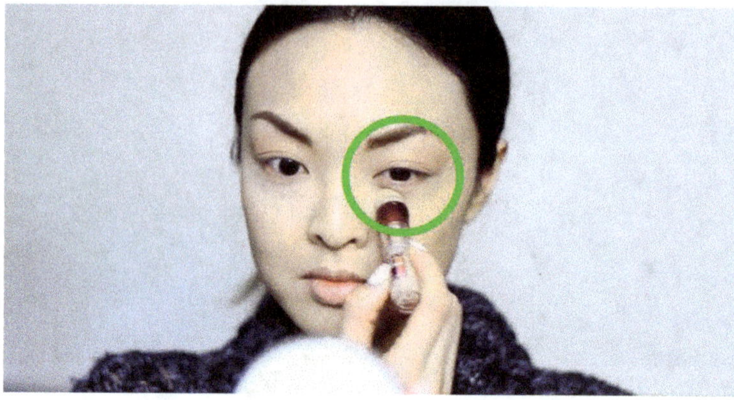

4. Touch up on difficult areas. If you do have particularly uneven skin in certain areas, acne, dark spots, or under-eye circles, use your foundation to touch up on these areas. Use a concealer brush to apply foundation more heavily on these spots. Make sure to blend it in well to prevent dark or orange dots on your face.

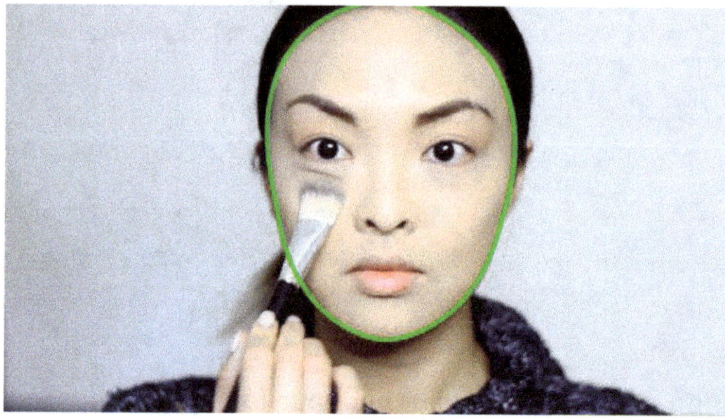

5. Finish up on your foundation. If you haven't yet already, apply concealer to troubled areas on your face. Finish up your entire face by applying your foundation with setting powder. This is a translucent, matte powder that helps prevent your foundation from sliding around while preventing oil buildup from showing through.

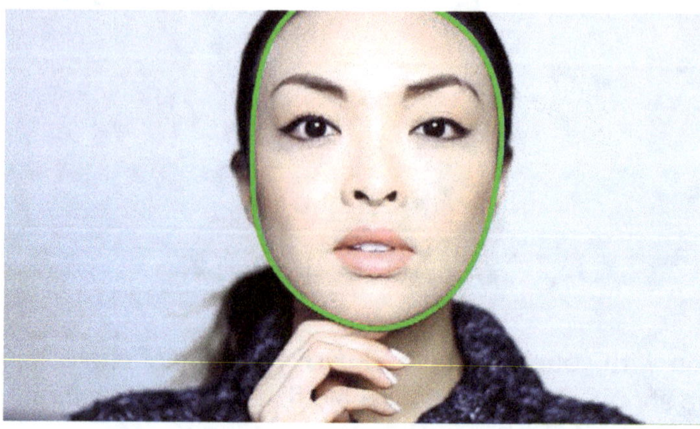

How to Apply Blush

Bring radiance and glow to your face with a little sweep of blush. The application is quick and the results gratifying.

Instructions

- STEP 1: Select a color of blush that resembles the natural glow of your cheeks after you exercise. Consider having a lighter color for day, and a darker tone for a more dramatic evening look. Keep your blush in the same color family as your lipstick.
- STEP 2: Consider the type of blush best suited to your skin type. Cream blush works very well for drier skin, as it can help to keep skin hydrated. Powder blush is better suited to oily skin.
- STEP 3: Complete the application of foundation, powder and all eye makeup before applying blush.
- STEP 4: Use a full, round brush for the application of your powder blush, as it will make for a softer and more professional look than the brush that comes with the blush. This should not be the same brush you use to apply your loose powder.

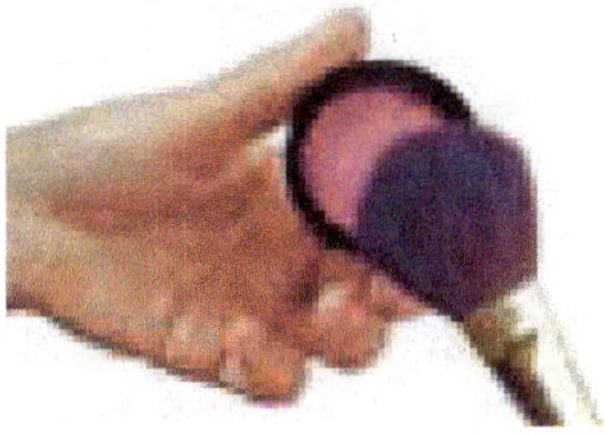

- STEP 5: Place a small amount of blush on the brush and gently tap off any excess. Or, place a small amount of cream on your middle finger.

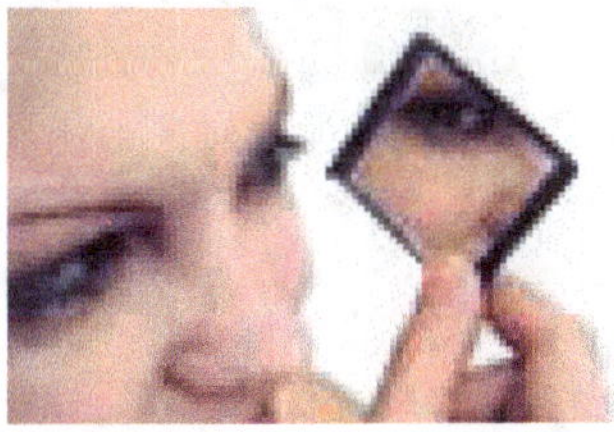

- STEP 6: Look in the mirror and smile.

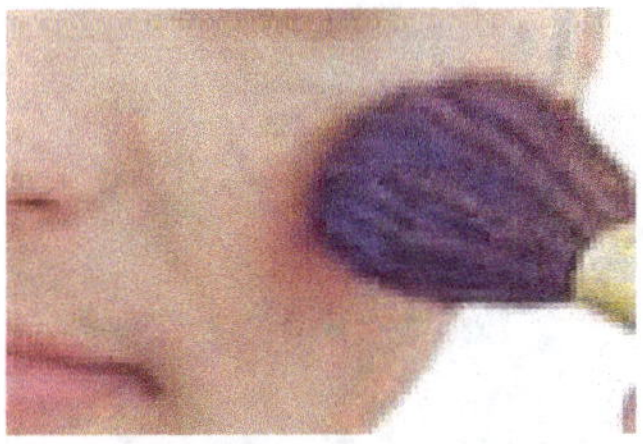

- STEP 7: Place powder blush on the apple of your cheek and gently brush up your cheekbone toward your hairline. Dot cream blush beginning at the apple, and gently blend up the cheekbone toward the hairline.

- STEP 8: Focus your blush at the outside of your face near your hairline if you have a fuller face. For high cheekbones, concentrate blush in the center of your face to accentuate your bones.
- STEP 9: Blend a little blush down your cheek for a little more natural, less dramatic look.

Tips & Warnings

- For rosier cheeks, consider gel or liquid tints. Wash your hands after use, as these products may stain the hands.
- Remember that the lighter your skin tone, the lighter your blush color should be.
- Wash brushes regularly with a makeup remover or nonsoap cleanser.
- Avoid following the underside of your cheekbones, which makes for an artificial and unbecoming look.

Overall Things You'll Need

- Blush Brush
- Blush
- Mirrors

Face Powder

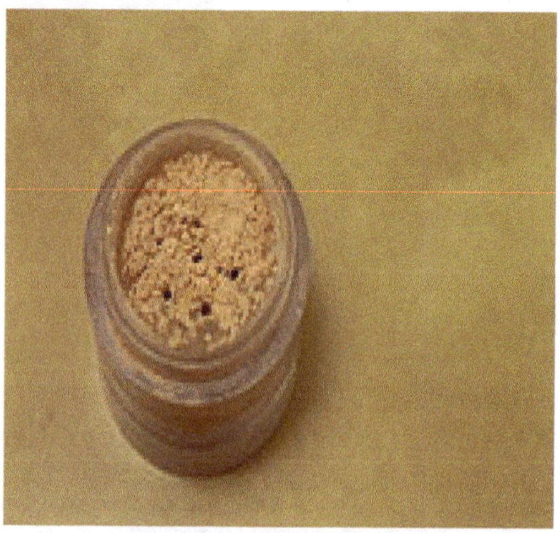

Loose mineral powder

Face powder is a cosmetic powder applied to the face to set a foundation after application. It can also be reapplied throughout the day to minimize shininess caused by oily skin. There is translucent sheer powder, and there is pigmented powder. Certain types of pigmented facial powders are meant be worn alone with no base foundation. Powder tones the face and gives an even appearance. Besides toning the face, some powders with sunscreen can also reduce skin damage from sunlight and environmental stress. It comes packaged either as a compact or as loose powder. It can be applied with a sponge, brush, or powder puff. Uniform distribution over the face is achieved more easily when a loose powder is applied.

Because of the wide variation among human skin tones, there is a corresponding variety of colors of face powder. There are also several types of powder. A common powder used in beauty products is talc (or baby powder), which is absorbent and provides toning to the skin.

It can also be applied generously to the higher points of the face to brighten, colour correct and highlight, through a technique termed baking (a.k.a. cooking). This technique also helps to increase the coverage of the make-up whilst helping the makeup stay in place for longer.

Application

Face powder should be carefully chosen to match the skin tone in order to show the best results.

Ingredients

- talcum powder.
- cornstarch

How to Choose a Powder Color

A good powder sets your makeup, creating a smooth, shine-free and even complexion. For a natural and flawless finish, select colors that match your skin tone or foundation as closely as possible.

Instructions

- STEP 1: Make sure your foundation, if you wear any, disappears as you blend it into your skin. Powder can either complement the perfect foundation color or serve to neutralize any slight color imbalance.
- STEP 2: Head to a department store counter and talk to a veteran beauty consultant. Bring your foundation along, or go with freshly applied foundation so you can test powder colors over your everyday makeup.
- STEP 3: Start with colors that match your skin tone. You may be inundated with pink, yellow, green and purple shades all designed to make your skin look its best. Stick to what you feel comfortable with and what you can see makes your skin look good.
- STEP 4: Check the colors you test in good lighting, or step outside to consider your options

in natural light. You're looking for a color that blends with your skin, rather than sitting on top of it.

- STEP 5: Remember that translucent powder still has color in it. Some may advise that this is the most natural option, but it may render you pale or pasty.

Tips & Warnings

- Loose powder sets your makeup in the morning; pressed powder is for daily touchups. Pressed powder may seem darker because it's packed more densely. Test all colors before buying.
- Bring a trusted companion along for an honest second opinion.

Overall Things You'll Need

- Foundation
- Makeup Brushes
- Mirrors
- Face Powder

How to Apply Foundation and Powder

Applying foundation and powder together sounds simple enough. It can leave you with a smooth finish, but only if done right. If done wrong, your skin might look too shiny or too dry. This article will show you the proper way to apply different types of foundation. It will also give you tips on what brushes, foundation, and powder you should use.

Part 1

Applying Foundation

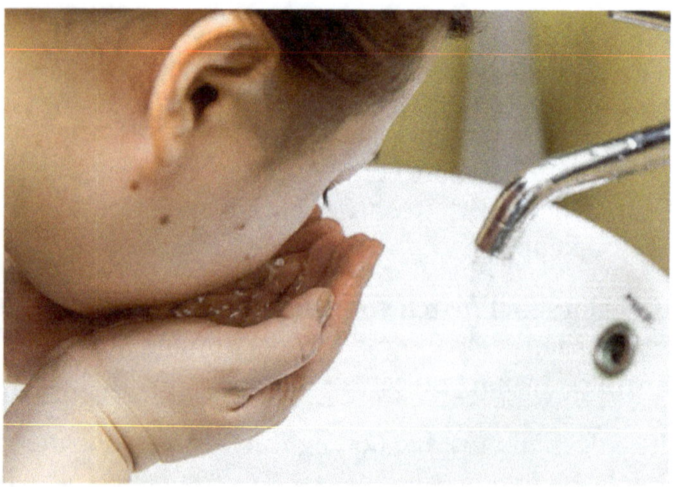

1. Start with a clean face, then apply some toner and moisturizer. Apply the toner first using a cotton ball, and the moisturizer using your fingers. The toner will help balance the pH of your skin. It will also help tighten pores and make them less noticeable. The moisturizer will help keep your skin feeling smooth and soft. It will also help prevent foundation (especially powder-based ones) from looking flaky.

- If you have very sensitive skin, try using a rosewater-based toner or an alcohol-free toner. This will make it sting less.
- If you have oily skin, consider using a lightweight or an oil-free moisturizer.

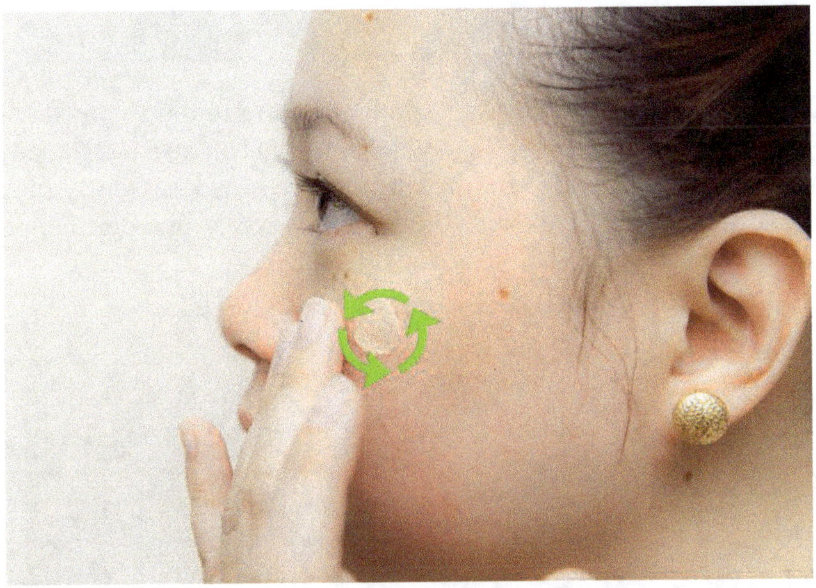

2. Consider applying some primer to your face. You don't need a lot; a little bit goes a long way. Primer will help fill in large pores and fine lines. This will make your skin appear smoother. It will also make the foundation easier to apply and blend in.

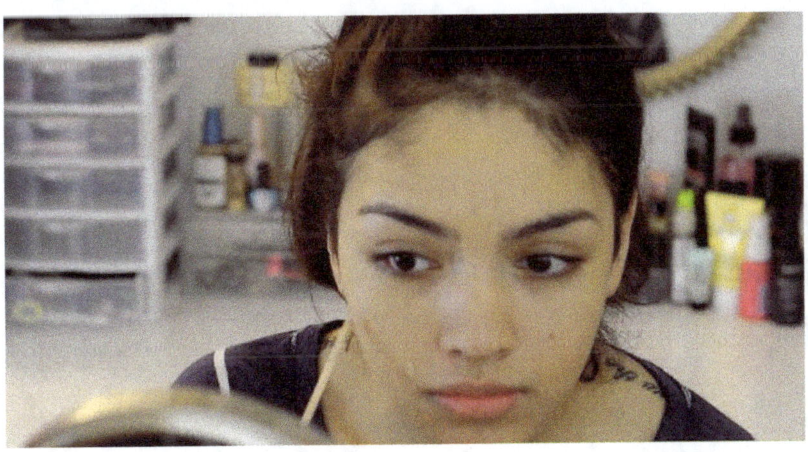

3. Apply concealer now if you are using a cream-to-powder type of foundation. This will help prevent any blending issues. Keep in mind, however, that the foundation may also wipe away the concealer. If you are using any other type of foundation, hold off on the concealer for now.

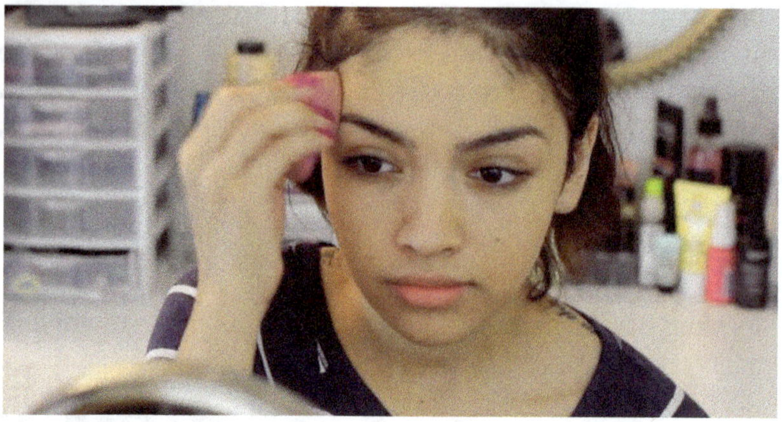

4. Get out a powder brush or a foam makeup sponge if you are using powder foundation. If the foundation is pressed, sweep a makeup sponge across it. You can also swirl a powder brush across it. If the foundation is loose, lightly dip the brush into the powder. Gently blow on the brush or tap the handle against the counter. This will shake off any excess powder. Do not use the makeup sponge to apply loose powder.

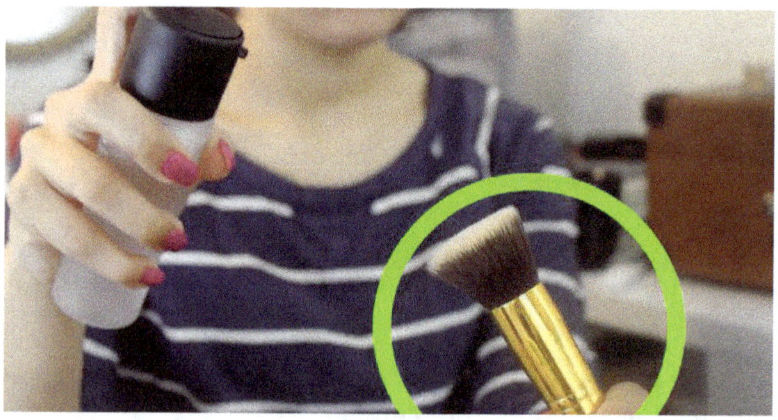

5. Get out a foam makeup sponge or a foundation brush if you are using liquid foundation. Shake the bottle first. This will help mix up the pigments inside the foundation. Then, pour out some foundation onto the back of your hand or onto a little dish. This will help prevent you from accidentally picking up too much foundation.

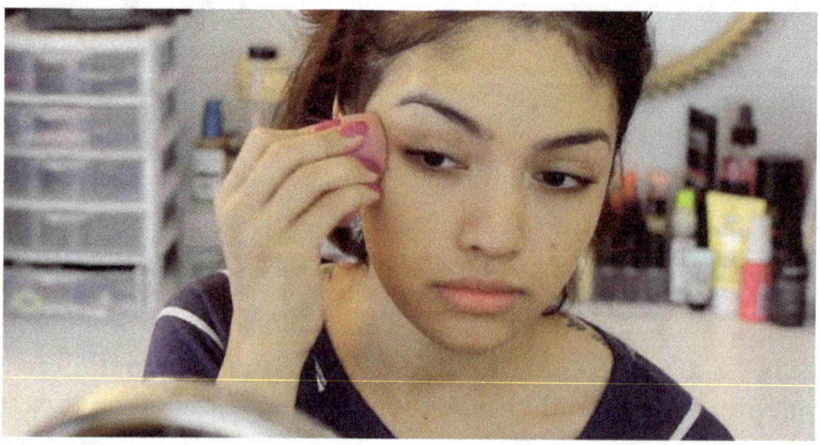

- If you are using a makeup sponge, consider soaking the sponge in water first and then squeezing it to get rid of the excess water. This will keep the sponge from soaking up too much foundation and wasting it.
- Avoid using a powder brush with soft bristles. Try to get a foundation brush. It will have stiffer bristles that can hold the weight of the liquid foundation.
- You can also apply liquid foundation if you are in hurry. Keep in mind that this may not give you the smoothest result.

6. Get out a foam makeup sponge or a foundation brush if you are going to apply cream foundation. Cream foundation usually comes in a compact case. It may also come in a tube, sort of like lipstick. Simply swipe the sponge or brush across the surface of the foundation. If your foundation comes in a stick, you can roll the stick over your forehead, nose, cheeks, and chin. Use your fingers or a foam sponge to blend it in.

- Don't use a powder brush to apply cream foundation. The bristles will only stick together. Use a foundation brush. Its stiffer bristles will hold up to the weight of the cream foundation.

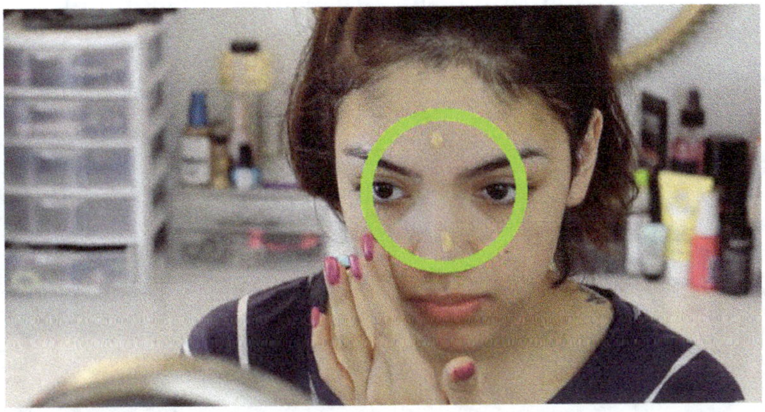

7. Start applying the foundation to the center of your face. No matter what type of foundation you are using, or what type of tool you are using to apply it, it is always a good idea to start from the center if your face. Simply brush the foundation down the center of your face.

- If you are using your fingers, consider creating little dots instead. Blend these dots in with your fingers or a foam makeup sponge.

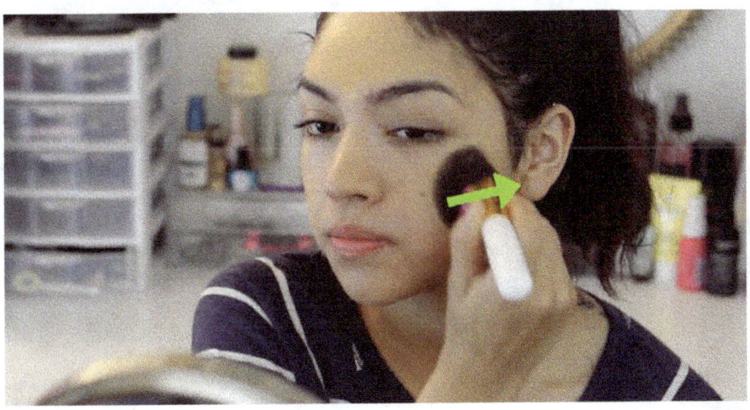

8. Smooth the foundation down the sides of your nose and towards the sides of your face. You want the foundation to get thinner as you get closer to the sides of your face. If it gets too thin on your cheeks and you want more coverage, dab more foundation onto your cheekbones and blend it outwards.

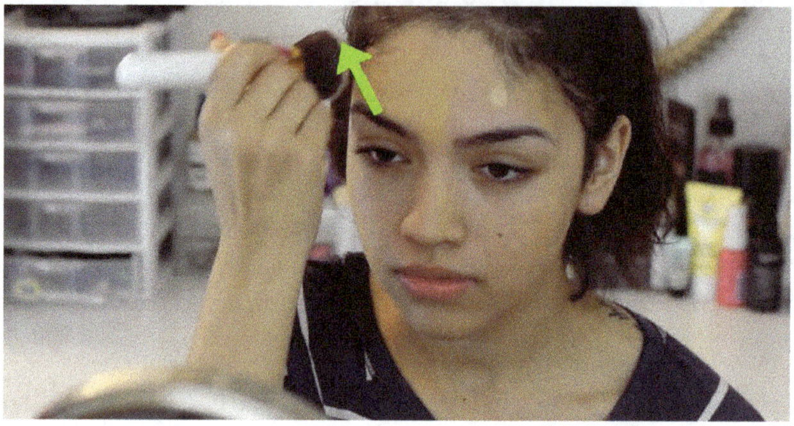

9. Spread the foundation across your forehead. Brush the foundation up towards your hairline. Then, brush it to the left and right above your eyebrows.

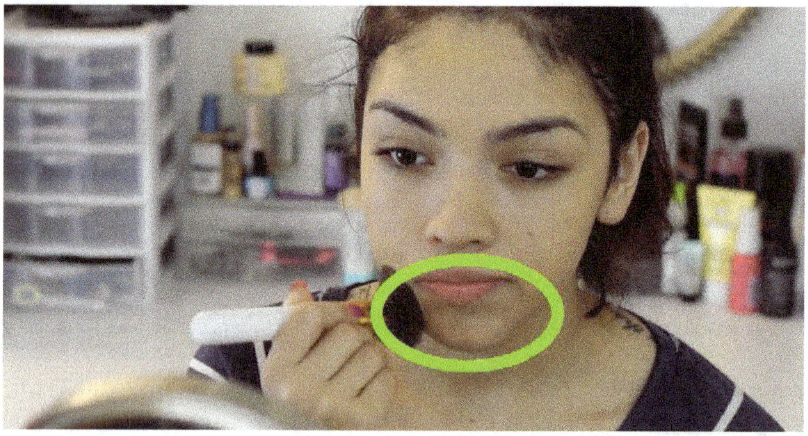

10. Spread the foundation down your chin and along your jaw line. Use your brush, fingers, or sponge to pull the foundation down towards your chin. Then, spread it sideways along your jaw.

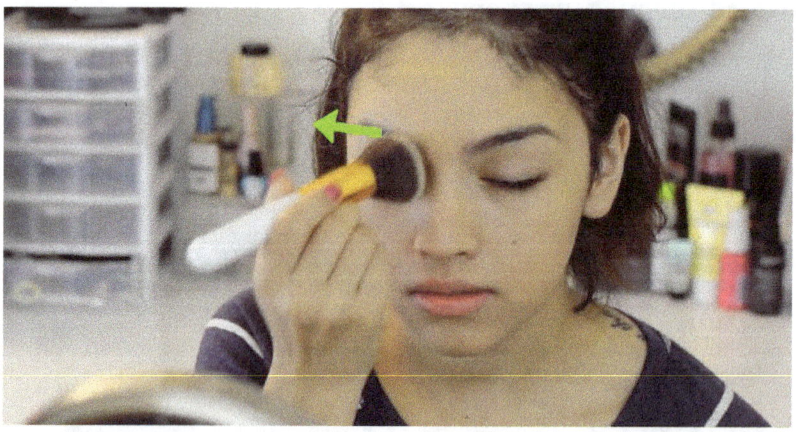

11. Blend the foundation using a foam sponge or a brush. Always blend from the center outward. You want the foundation to fade the closer it gets to your hairline and the sides of your face. This will create the smoothest transition and prevent any harsh lines.

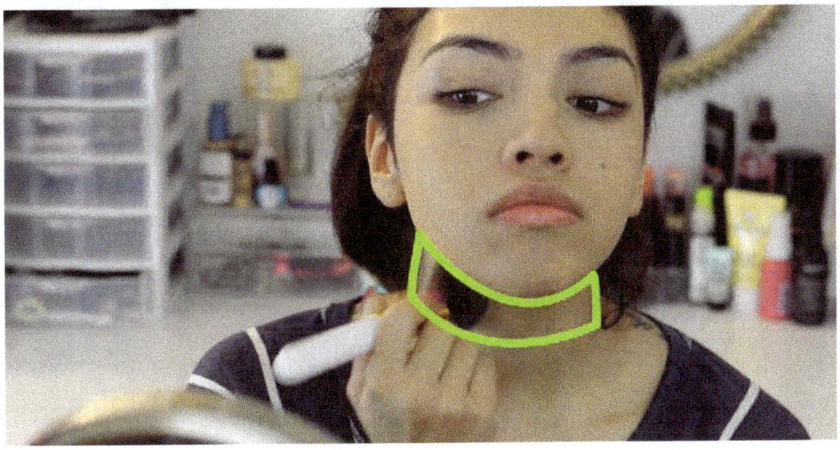

12. Consider applying foundation to your neck. This is great for those who have dull or grayish skin on their necks.

Part 2

Applying Concealer and Powder

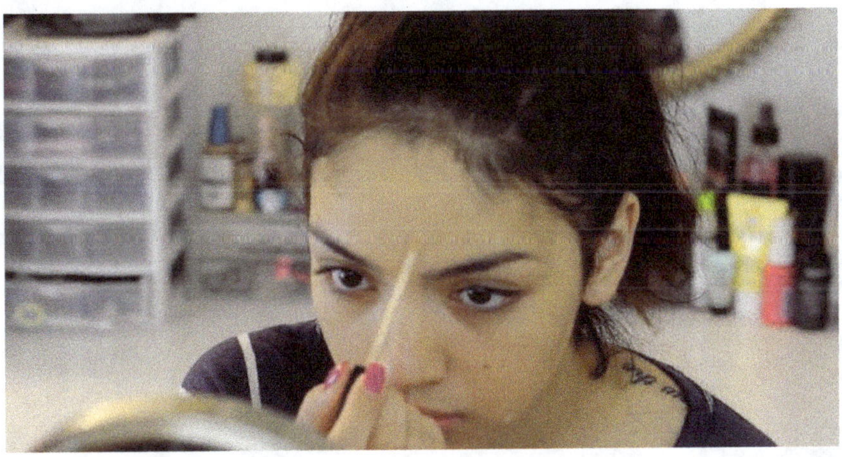

1. Apply some concealer. Use a brush or your fingers to tap it onto the area that needs to be concealed. Then, blend it into the foundation using light, feathery strokes. Always blend outward, away from the center of the concealer spot.

- If you are applying concealer under your eyes, use your ring finger. This is the weakest finger on your hand, and thus the gentlest.
- Applying concealer after foundation makes it easier to blend in. It also lessens the chances of the foundation getting wiped off.

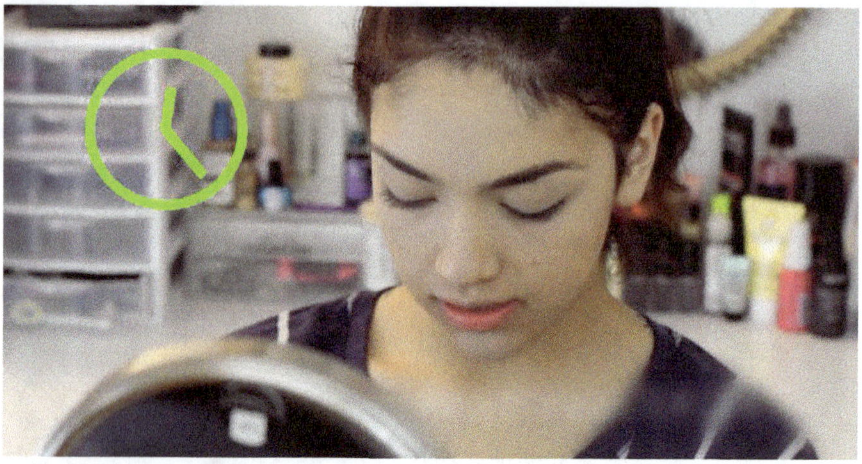

2. Let the foundation dry. This can take anywhere from 1 to 5 minutes. Some foundations, such as cream, are oil-based and will never fully dry. Other foundations, such as powder, are already dry to begin with.

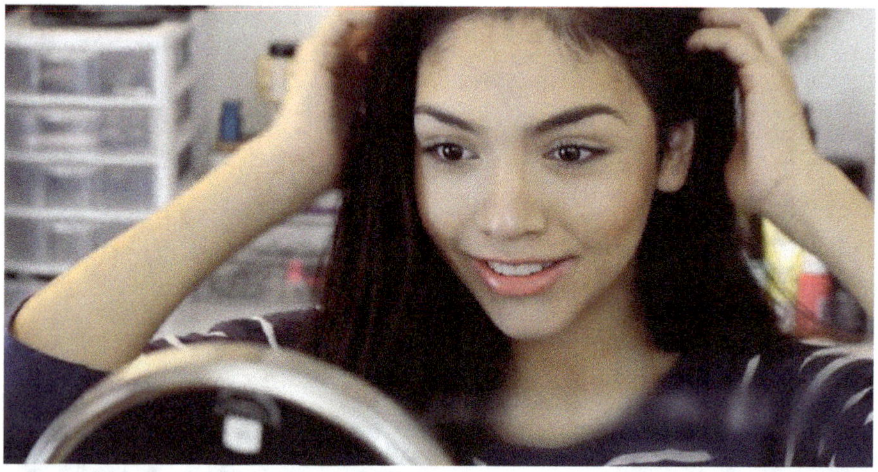

3. Consider doing the rest of your makeup. At the point, you can apply the rest of your makeup, including your lipstick, blush, and eye makeup.

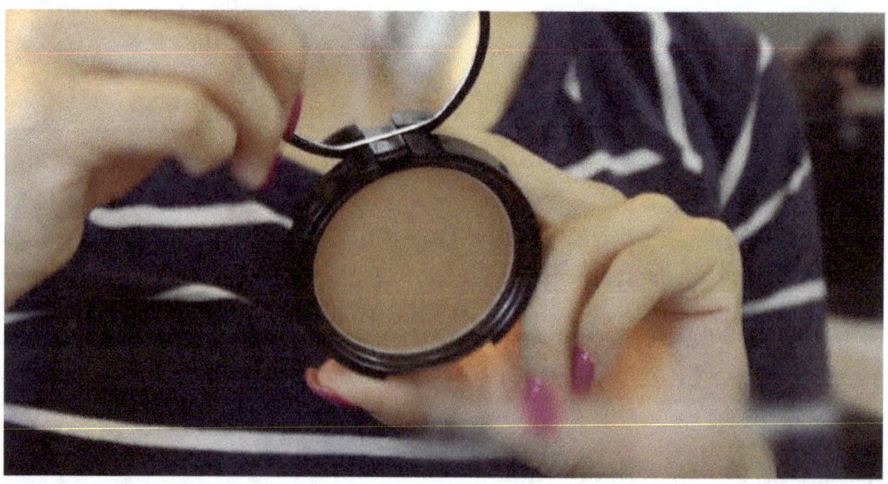

4. Open up your powder case. You can use a powder foundation or a setting powder. Both will help give your skin a smoother finish and get rid of shine. They will also help soak up any excess oils.

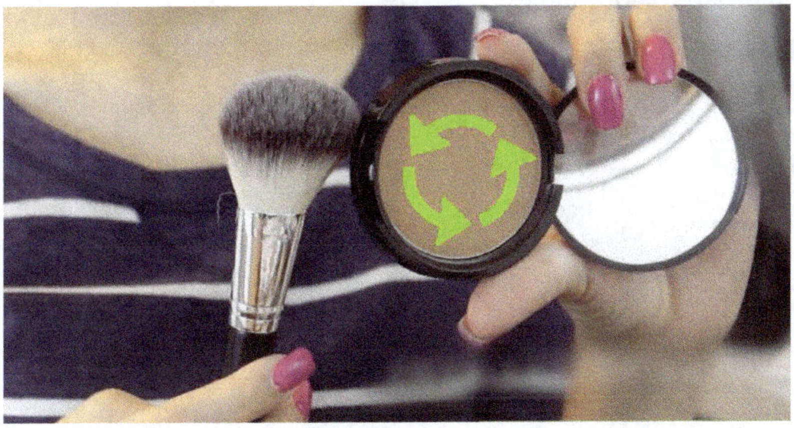

5. Swirl a powder brush into the powder. Most powder will be compact or pressed. If you are using a loose powder, simply dip the brush into the powder.

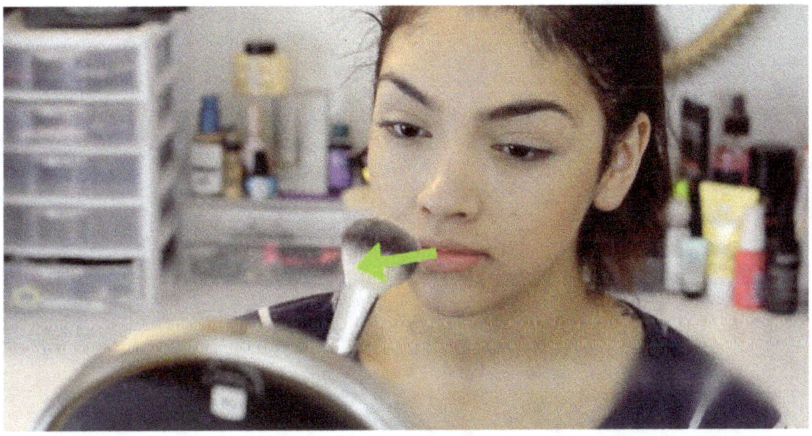

6. Gently puff on the brush to get rid of any excess powder. You can also tap the brush handle against the counter edge. This will keep you from applying too much powder at one time, which can result in a cake-y look. You can always apply more powder later.

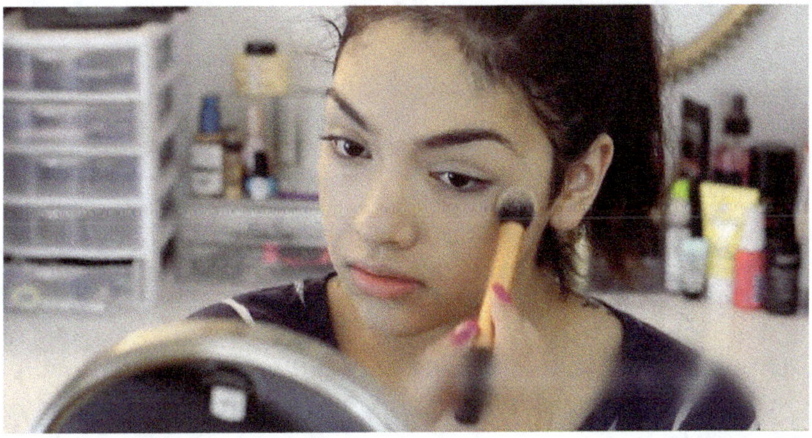

7. Dust the powder onto your face. Start from the middle or your face and brush outward. If needed, dip your brush into the powder and keep dusting your face. Always tap off the excess powder before you touch the brush to your face.

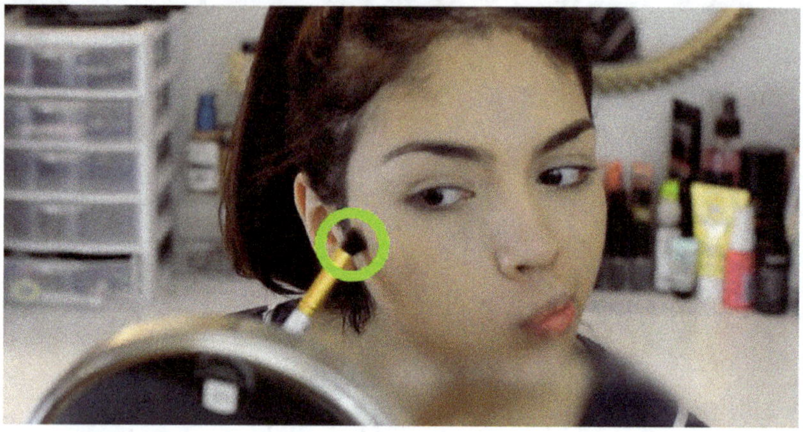

8. Use a clean brush to dust off any excess powder. Look carefully into the mirror. If you see any excess powder, take a clean brush and lightly dust it off.

Part 3

Choosing Your Foundation, Powder, and Tools

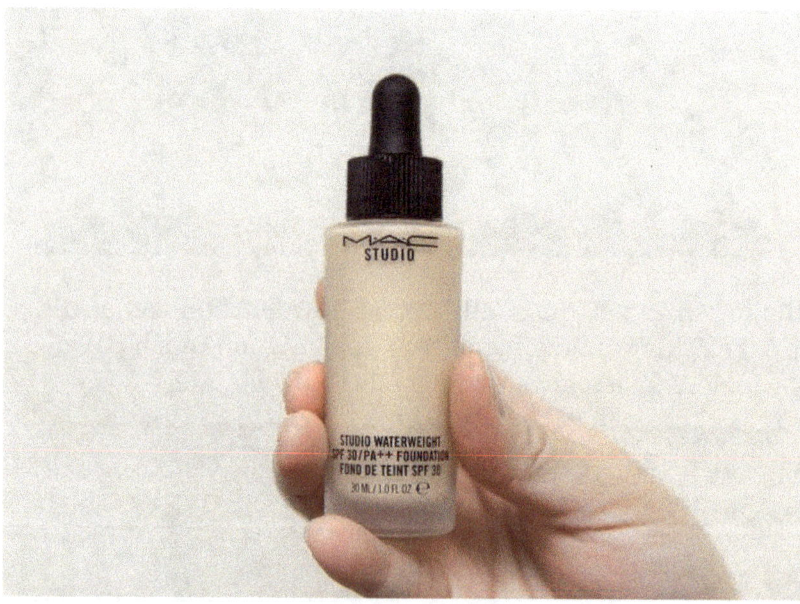

1. Choose a foundation. There are many different types of foundation. Some are better for certain skin types than others. The main three are: powder, liquid, and cream. Here's what you need to know based on your skin type:

- If you have dry skin, go for a moisturizing liquid or cream foundation. Avoid using powder foundation. It will make your skin appear even more dry. If you must use a powder foundation, choose a hydrating one.

- If you have oily skin, choose a lightweight, oil-free liquid or powder foundation. You can also use mineral-based powder foundation; it will absorb the oil better. Don't use cream foundation. It will be too heavy and oily for your skin.
- If you have normal skin, you can use any type of foundation you want: powder, liquid, or cream.
- If you have combination skin, consider using a powder foundation. Use more on the oily parts, and less on the dry parts.

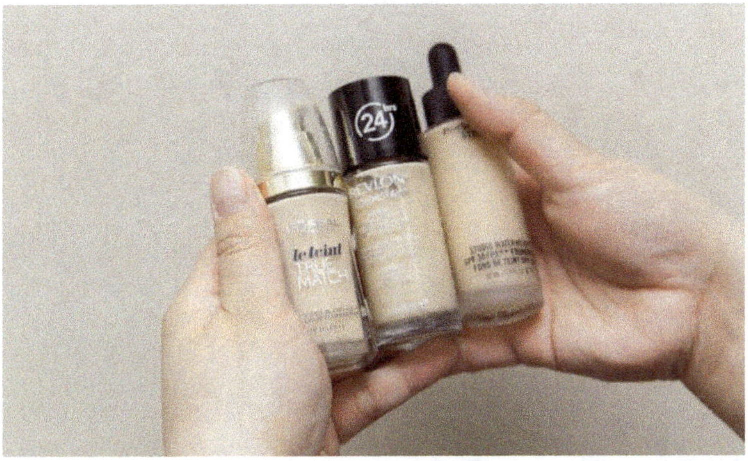

2. Choose your foundation finish. There are also different types of foundation finishes. Some are more sheer while others are more matte. Here's what you need to know:

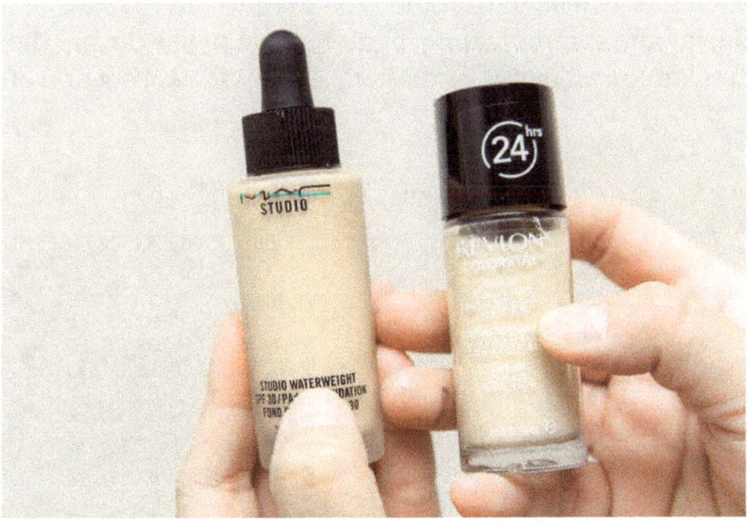

- Use a semi-matte foundation if you want a natural look. Most foundations are semi-matte.
- Use a dewy or illuminizing finish if you want to give your skin a healthy glow. This is great for the cold, winter months.
- Use a matte or flat finish if you want your face to look smooth. This is great for pictures. It will also get rid of shine.

3. Choose your foundation coverage. Some foundations are sheer and light, while others are thick and heavy. Use a sheer foundation if you want to just even out your skin tone, but still let your natural features (such as freckles and beauty marks) show. Use a full coverage foundation if you want to cover freckles, dark spots, and other blemishes. Keep in mind that for things like pimples, you might also need to use a concealer.

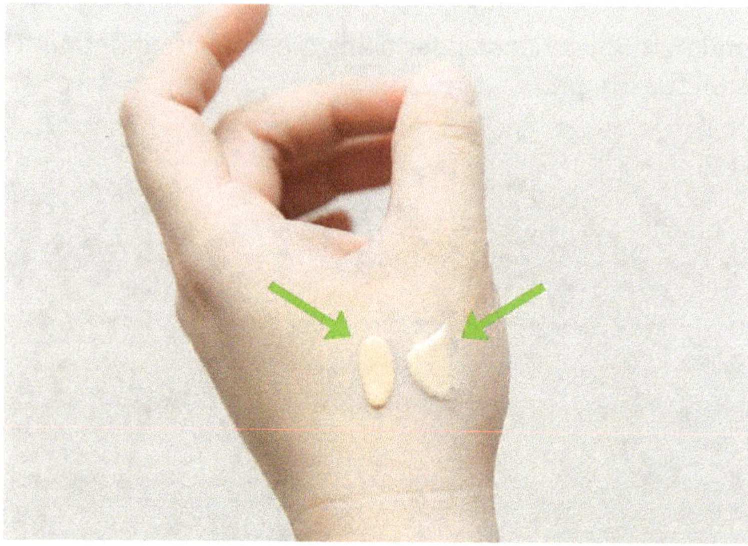

4. Plan on having at least two different shades. You skin will be lighter during the winter months when there is less sunlight. It will be darker in the summer when the sun is brighter. As such, the foundation you use in the winter may be too light for your skin during the summer, and the foundation you use in the summer will be too dark for you in the winter. To avoid these problems, get a darker shade to use during the summer, and a lighter shade to use during the winter. You can mix the two shades as your skin tone lightens or darkens during the spring and fall.

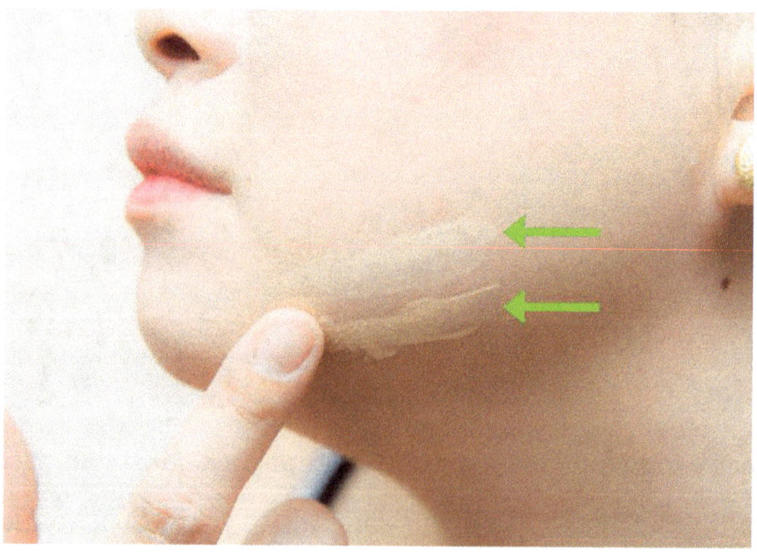

5. Know that foundation oxidizes as it dries. When shopping for foundation, choose a few shades that you think match your skin tone. Apply each one along your cheek. Wait one to two minutes before looking at the foundation again. Choose the color that blends into your skin the best.

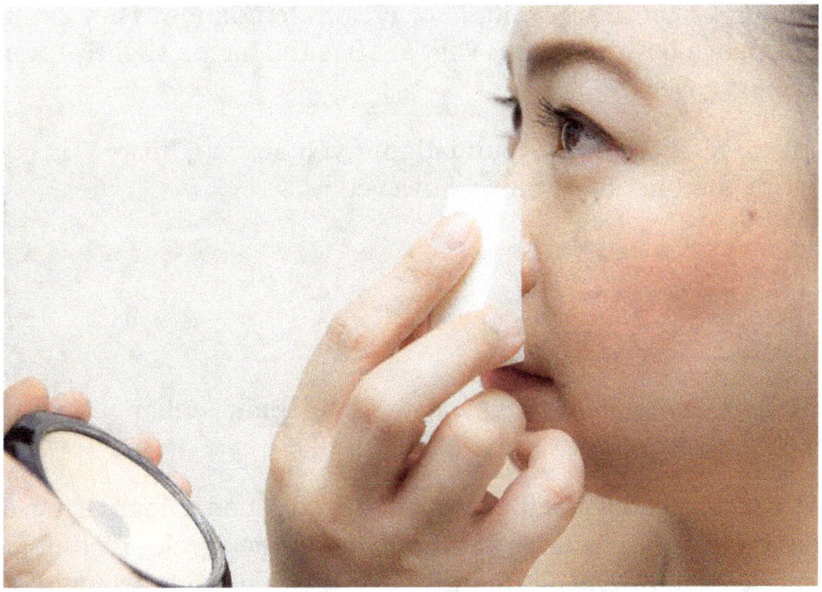

6. Choose your powder. You can use powder foundation to soak up any excess oil or shin. You can also use a setting powder to set your makeup and keep it from moving around.

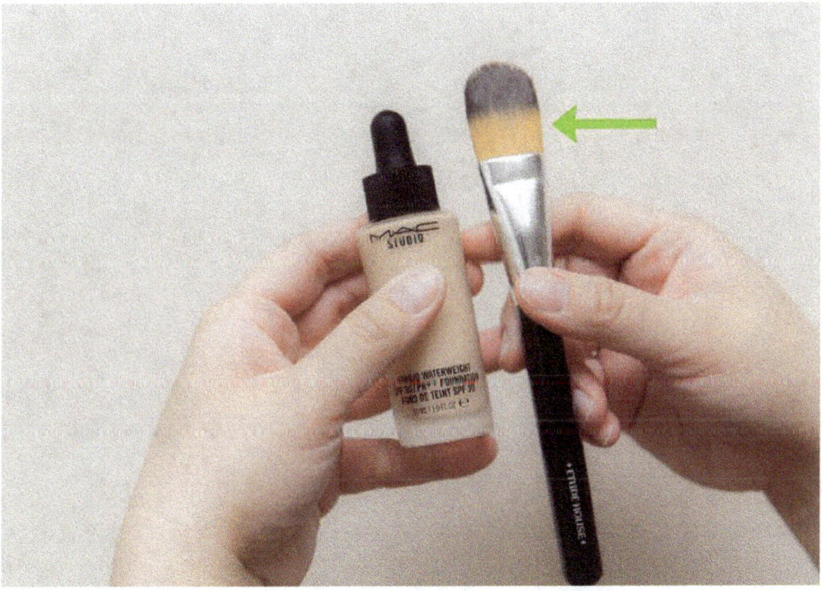

7. Choose your tools based on your foundation type and desired coverage. The type of foundation you use will determine what you use to apply it. Here is what you need to know:

- Use a fluffy powder brush to apply powder foundation. This will work on both pressed and loose powder. You can also use this brush to apply setting powder when you are done doing your makeup.
- Use a foam makeup sponge to apply *pressed* powder foundation, liquid foundation, or cream foundation. They are usually white, and come in wedge or disk shapes. They will give you the smoothest, most even coverage.

- Use a foundation brush to apply liquid or cream foundation. They are made with slightly stiffer bristles than a powder brush. They are flat and have a slightly rounded tip. They will give you the most coverage.
- Use your fingers to apply liquid foundation if you are in a hurry. This won't give you the best coverage or the smoothest finish, however.

Contouring

Contouring is a makeup technique that uses cosmetics to define, enhance and sculpt the structure of the face or other body parts, such as breasts.

Contouring is usually produced by placing a warm or cool toned colour that is one or two shades darker than the skin color in areas such as in the hollows of the cheeks, on the side of the nose, and on the temples to give a shadow and slimming effect. It can be complemented with a highlighter that is one or two shades lighter than the skin color on areas of the face that is more prominent such as on the apples on the cheeks and the tip of the nose or the t-zone.

Chapter 4

Lip Care and Makeup

Lipsticks are applied on the lips to color them and to protect them from drying. Lipsticks have different shades, ranging from dark red to a nude shade. Matte, shimmery and normal lipsticks are distinctive types of lipsticks that are worn by women as per their taste. The following chapter explains to the readers the various kinds of lip makeup and how to apply it.

How to Get Natural Red Lips

Are you tired of getting red lipstick on everything your lips touch? If you want lips that look red without the mess, start by conditioning your lips to bring out their natural color. Using a subtle lip stain made with berry or beet juice adds is a great natural trick to have up your sleeve for days when your lips need a colorful boost. To keep your lips looking their best, use sunscreen and moisturizer so they'll always look bright and supple instead of flaky and dull.

Method 1

Prepping Your Lips

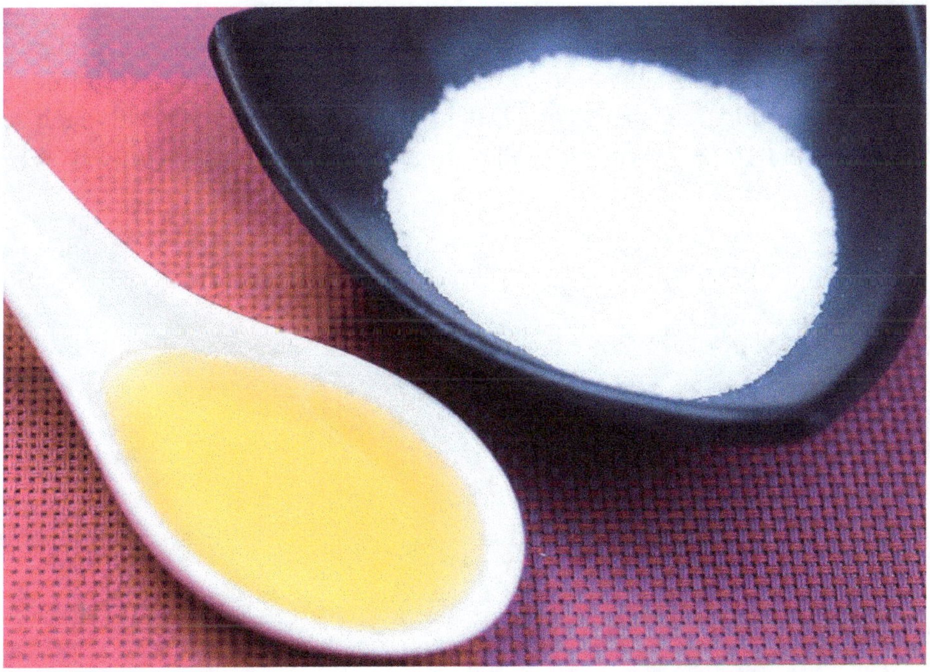

1. Use a sugar scrub. Dry, dead skin that builds up on your lips can cause them to look paler than they otherwise would. To bring out your natural reddish hue, you need to exfoliate your lips to uncover the fresh skin underneath. An easy way to do this is by mixing up a homemade lip scrub with ingredients you probably already have on hand. Here's how to do it:

- Mix a teaspoon of sugar and a teaspoon of honey (or olive oil, if you don't have honey available).
- Scrub the mixture over your lips using a circular motion.
- Rinse and repeat until your lips are dry-skin free.

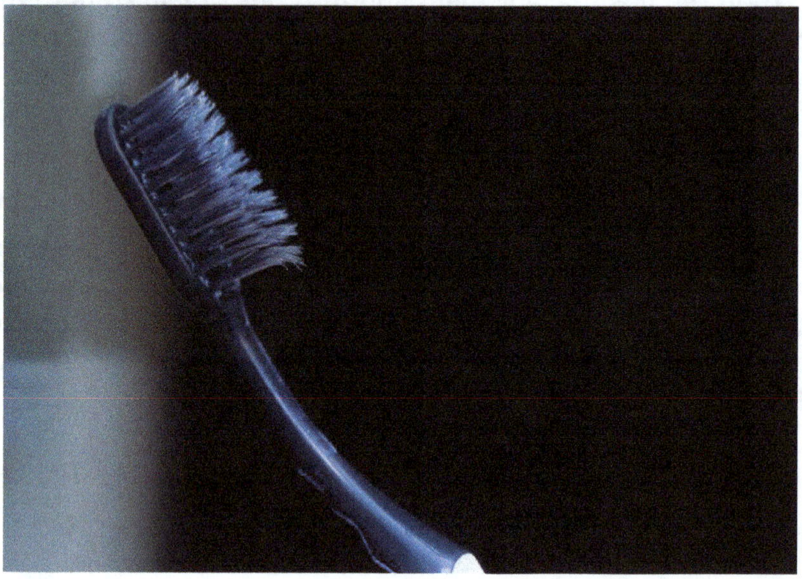

2. Brush your lips with a toothbrush. If your lips are too flaky for a simple scrub to get through the skin, try brushing them with a soft-bristled toothbrush. Cover your lips in baseline, wet the toothbrush with warm water, and then scrub your lips in a circular motion. Scrub each section of your lips for 20 to 30 seconds before moving on to the next. Your lips will be good as new when you're finished.

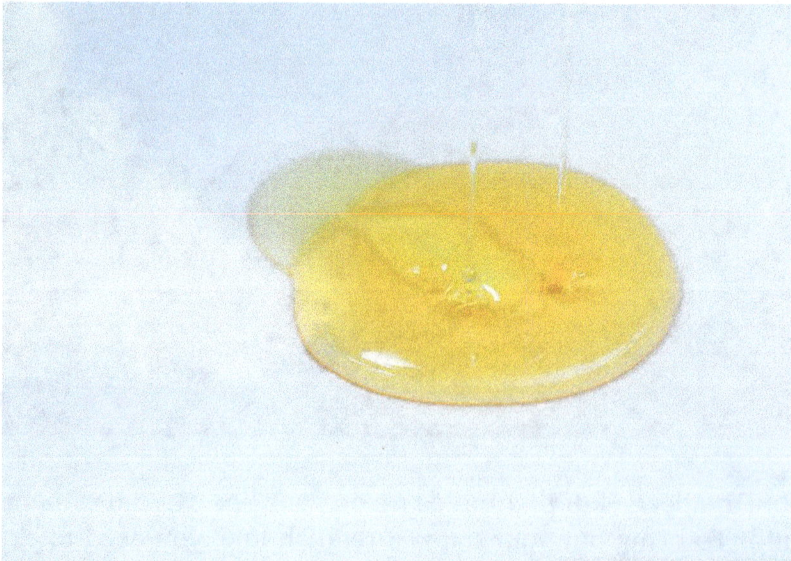

3. Condition your lips with serum. Now that you've uncovered your natural reddish color, condition your lips with a layer of lip serum to keep them in good shape. Applying a serum overnight will

give you even better results; you'll wake up with soft, pink-hued lips. Try using one of the following oils as a natural lip serum:

- Coconut oil
- Almond oil
- Olive oil
- Jojoba oil

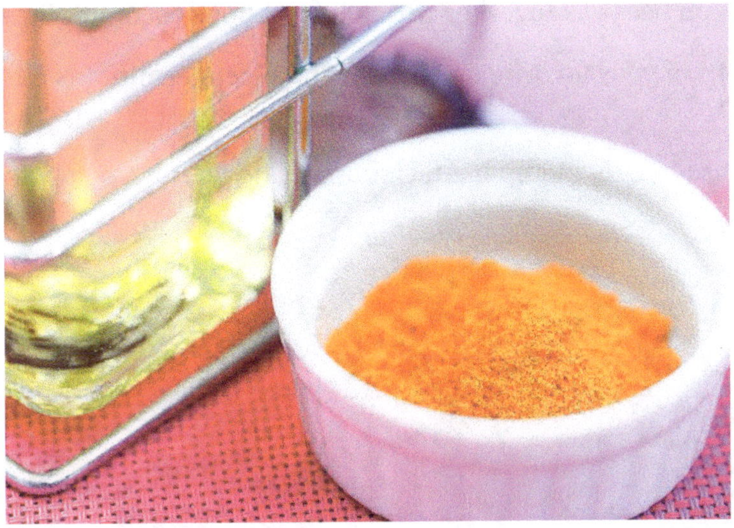

4. Plump your lips to add natural color. Just as pinching your cheeks makes them look rosy, increasing circulation in your lips brings up their natural red color and causes them to look pleasantly plump. You can buy a lip plumper from the store, but it's just as effective to make one yourself. Try one of these natural lip plumpers:

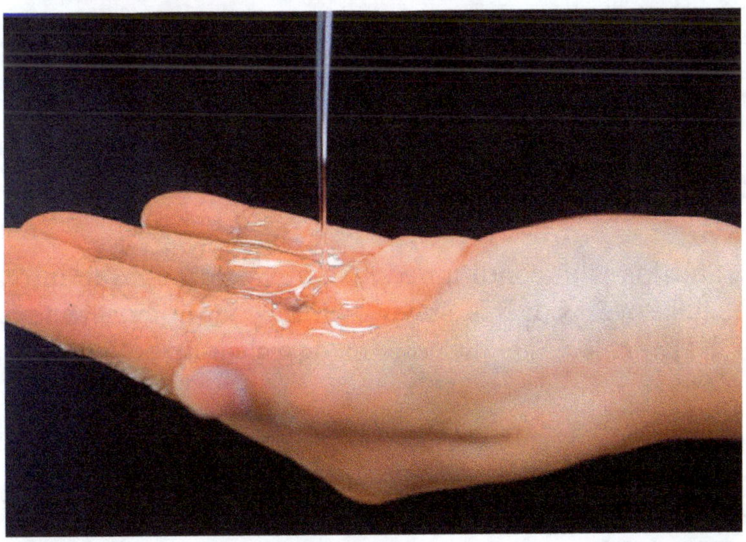

- Mix 1/4 teaspoon cinnamon or cayenne pepper with enough olive oil to make a paste. Apply to your lips for five minutes, then rinse.

- Mix 5 drops of peppermint extract with 1/2 teaspoon olive oil. Apply to your lips for five minutes, then rinse.
- Cut a small piece of fresh ginger, or cut a jalapeno pepper in half. Rub the cut part on your lips for five minutes.

5. Moisturize your lips. Keeping your lips moisturized is essential to having good natural color. If your lips get dry, they'll start looking pale and dull again. Use a good natural lip balm to ensure your lips never dry out. You can make your own lip balm using the following method:

- Melt 1 tablespoon beeswax together with 3 tablespoons coconut oil.
- Add a few drops of your favorite essential oil, like peppermint (as a bonus, it'll also plump your lips).
- Pour the mixture into an old lip balm container and let it harden before use.

Method 2

Adding Natural Color

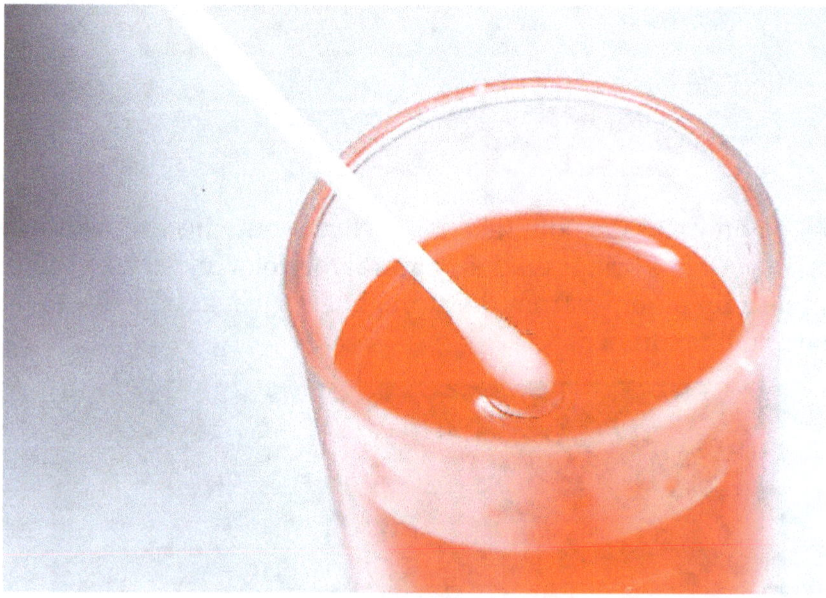

1. Use red fruit juice. Starting with conditioned lips, dip a cotton swab into a small container of red fruit juice. Rub the juice over your lips, staying within your lip lines, and allow the juice to dry. Apply more layers for deeper color. Seal the color using a clear lip balm. Any of the following types of juice will work:

- Cherry juice
- Cranberry juice
- Pomegranate juice
- Strawberry juice (for a pinker hue)

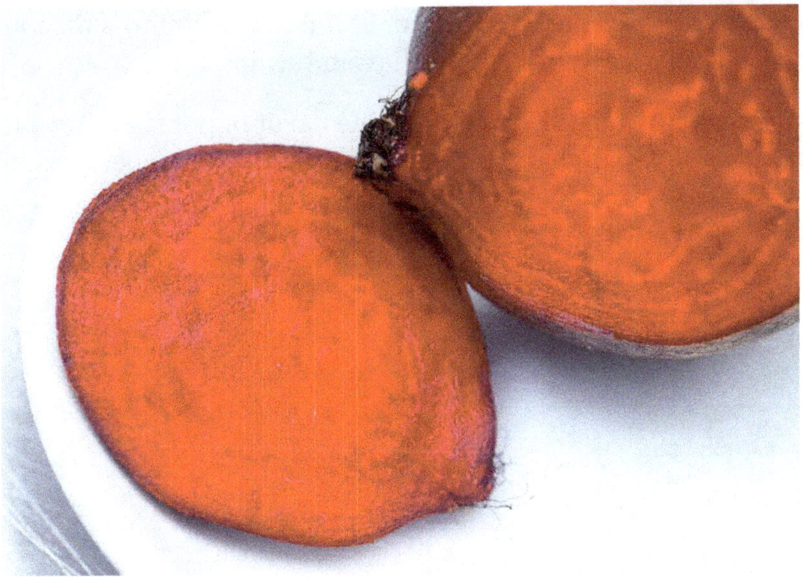

2. Try a slice of beet. Cut off a slice of fresh beet, making sure the interior flesh is bright red. Rub the slice over your lips, squeezing gently as you go to release the juice. Let the juice dry, then apply more layer for deeper color. Seal it using a clear lip balm.

- Beet root powder is also an effective lip stain. Mix a little powder with enough olive oil to make a paste. Apply to your lips, and let the paste dry completely. Wipe off the excess paste, then seal the color with clear lip balm.
- You can also use canned beets, although the pigment won't be as strong.

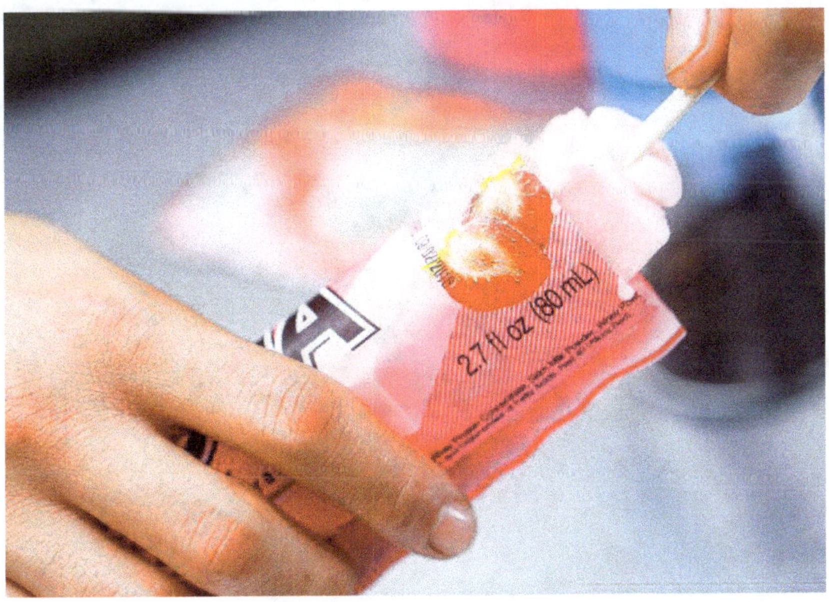

3. Eat a red popsicle. Red popsicles contain just the right amount of food coloring to make your lips look naturally red. Choose a cherry or raspberry popsicle and eat it slowly, making sure the melted popsicle coats your lips. By the time you're finished eating the popsicle, your lips will have a bright red hue.

- For a more precise application, you can melt the popsicle into a dish and apply it using a cotton swab. This also prevents your teeth from turning red.
- Make a custom color by mixing more than one flavor of popsicle. Try mixing a grape and a cherry to make a rich red plum color, or an orange and a raspberry for a pretty coral hue.

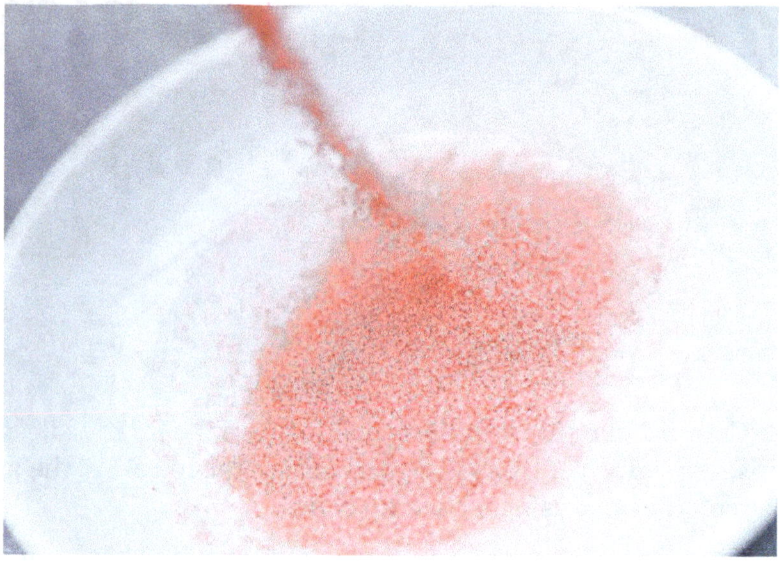

4. Use Kool-Aid powder. Red Kool-Aid powder has been used as a lip stain since the 1950s. Who knew this simple drink mix would make the perfect addition to your cosmetic bag? Grab a cherry or strawberry-flavored packet of Kool-Aid powder. Mix it with enough olive oil to make a paste, and rub it on your lips. Let it sit for five minutes, then wipe off the excess paste.

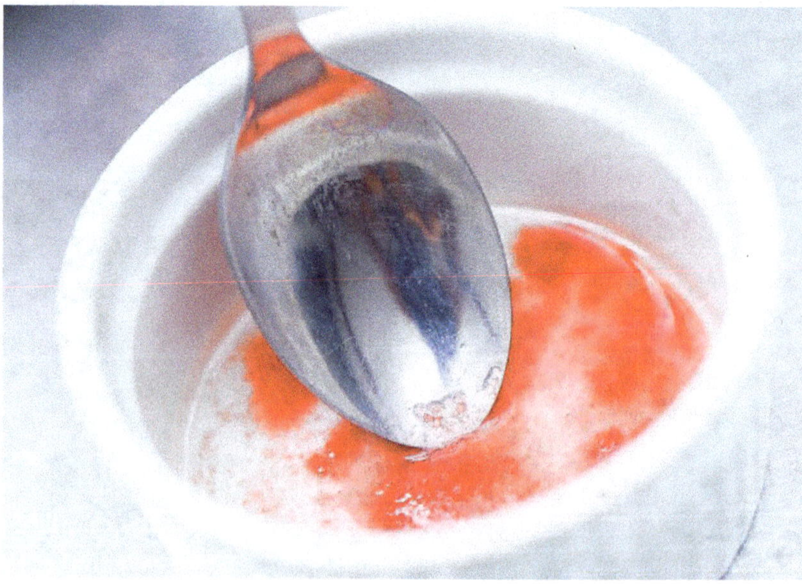

5. Make your own portable lip stain. If you want to have a stain handy to use whenever your lips need a lift, it's easy to make your own using either beet root powder or Kool-Aid powder. Mixing the powder with coconut oil will make a stain that absorbs into your lips, so you don't have to wipe it off. Here's how to do it:

- Melt 1 tablespoon coconut oil.
- Mix in 1 tablespoon Kool-Aid powder or beet root powder.
- Pour the mixture into a small jar with a tight-fitting lid.
- Apply it with your finger or a cotton swab. The stain will melt at warm temperatures.

Method 3

Keeping Your Lips Healthy and Bright

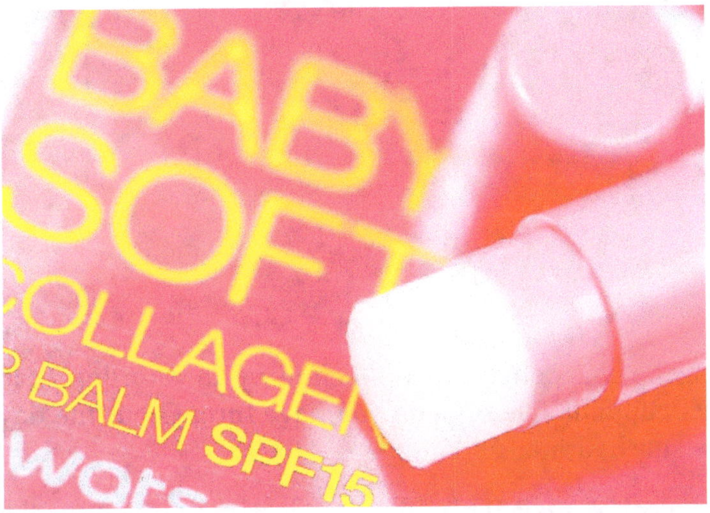

1. Protect them from the sun. Too much sun exposure can cause lip discoloration, including dark spots. Keep your natural lip color safe by protecting your lips with lip balm that has at least SPF 15. It's best to use sunscreen all year long, even in the winter when the sun isn't as strong.

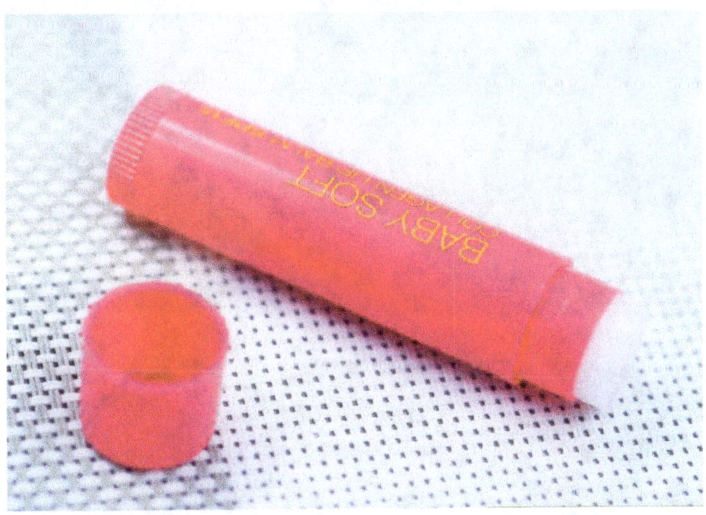

2. Keep them moisturized. Moisturizing your lips helps them look bright and fresh, preventing cracks and flaking. It's especially important when the air is dry and cold. To keep your lips moisturized, do the following:

- After exfoliating your lips, always apply a good nourishing lip balm to keep extra moisture from escaping.
- If you have trouble with flaky lips, try sleeping with a humidifier.

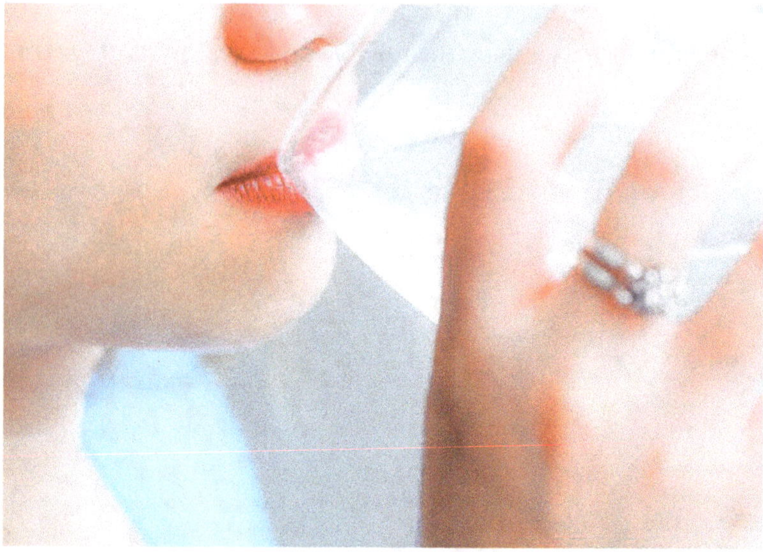

3. Stay hydrated. If your body is dehydrated, it'll show up in your lips. Start each day with a full glass of water. For each cup of coffee or soda you have throughout the day, drink a full glass of water to make sure you stay hydrated.

- When you have alcohol, make sure to follow it with plenty of water. That way you won't wake up with dry lips.
- Avoid extremely salty foods, since they can dry out your lips.

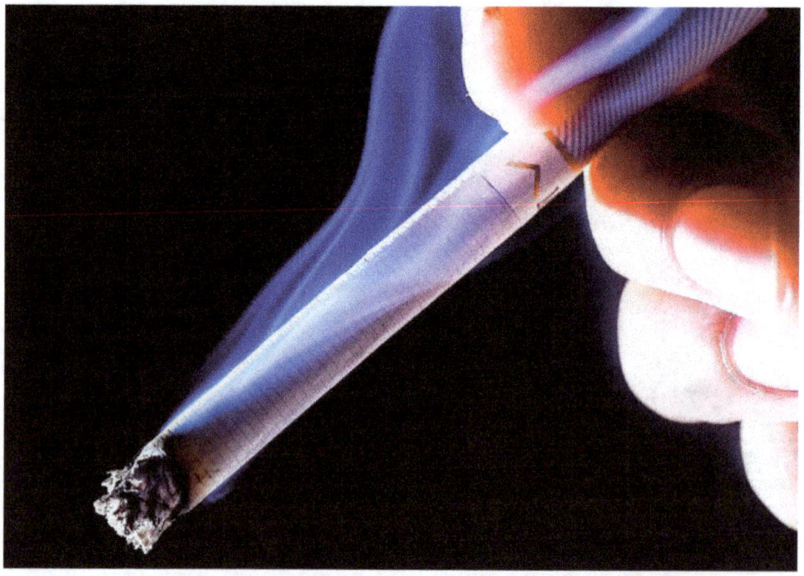

4. Avoid smoking. Smoking tobacco products can lead to lip discoloration. It also causes lip wrinkles and thinning. When you're going for a natural red color, it's best to avoid smoking altogether.

How to Get Red Lips without Lipstick

If you're looking for a good alternative to wearing lipstick, there are many ways to make your lips red without it. Several fruits and foods with red dye will stain your lips red for several hours, so you can get the look you want without having to buy cosmetic products. Try using fruit, red popsicles, or Kool-Aid powder to get pretty red lips.

Method 1

Using Kool-Aid Powder

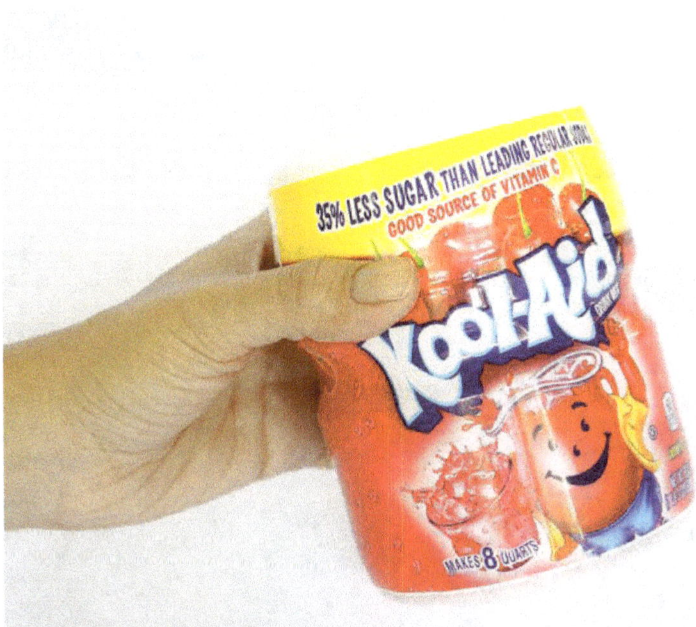

1. Buy red Kool-Aid powder. Look for a bright red shade that you like. Cherry, cranberry or strawberry-flavored powder will result in a pretty red stain.

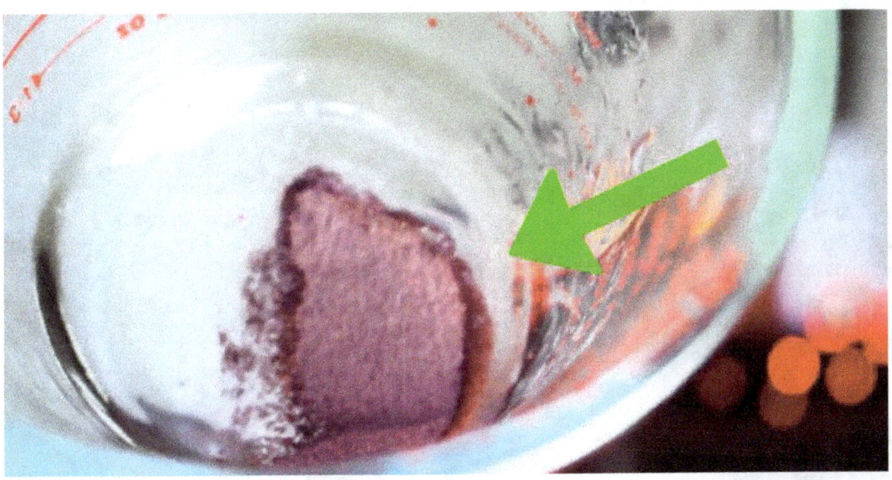

2. Pour the powder into a bowl. Any bowl or cup works just fine.

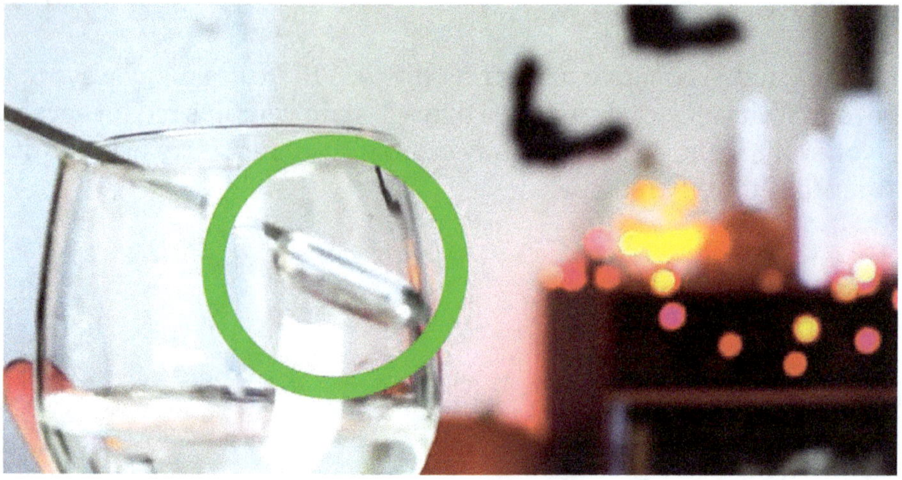

3. Add enough water to make a paste. Just add a few drops at a time. Stir in the water until you have a thick, spreadable paste.

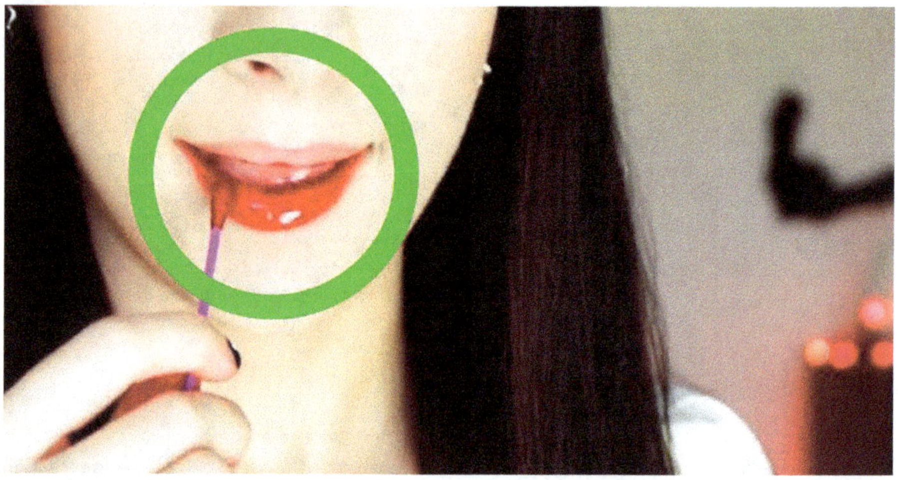

4. Apply the paste to your lips with a cotton swab. Dip a cotton swab in the paste and apply it neatly to your lips, making sure to stay within your lip lines.

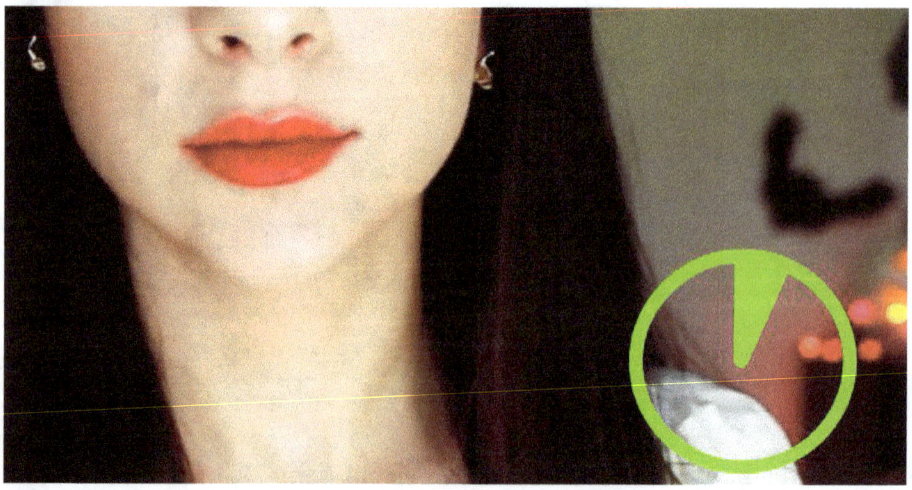

5. Let the paste dry for three minutes. This will give it time to stain your lips. When three minutes are up, rinse the paste away and check out your new lip stain.

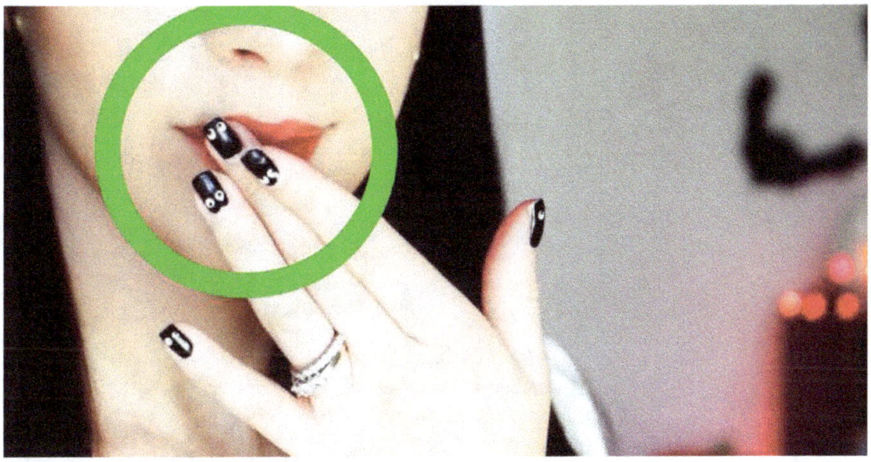

6. Apply more layers for a deeper color. Repeat the process as many times as you'd like until your lips are stained just the right bright red color.

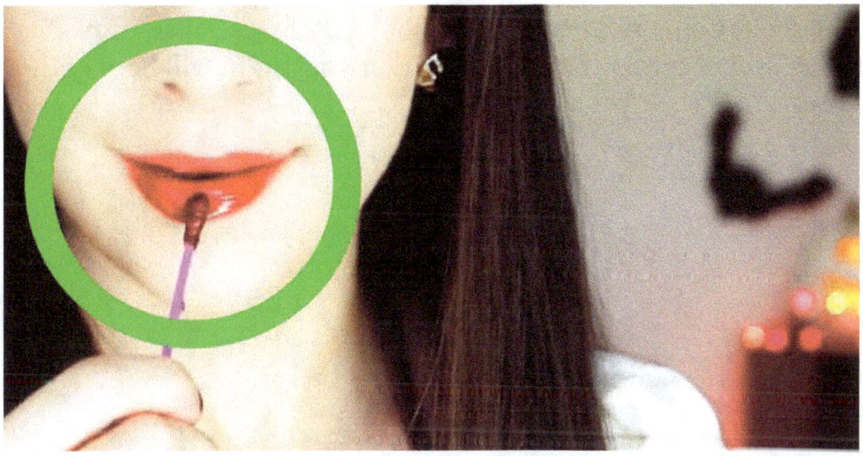

7. Seal the stain with clear lip gloss. This will keep your color in place for several hours and make your lips look bright and shiny.

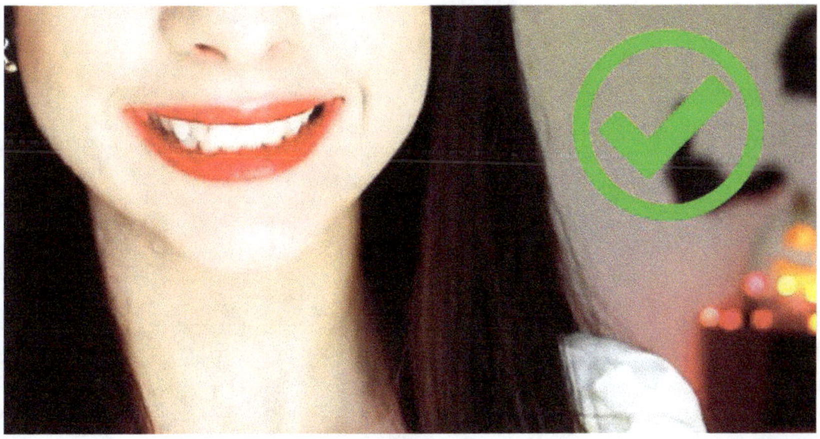

Method 2

Using Fruit

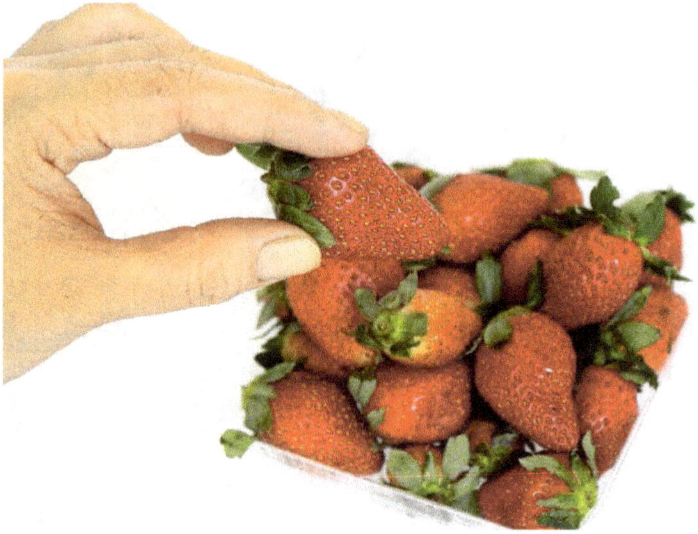

1. Choose bright red fruit. Using red fruit to give your lips a natural stain results in a pretty deep pink or red color. The deeper the fruit color, the darker your stain will be. Try the following different types of fruit to create the perfect stain:

- Cherries
- Cranberries
- Raspberries
- Pomegranate seeds
- Strawberries
- Beets (not technically fruit, but they work just as well)

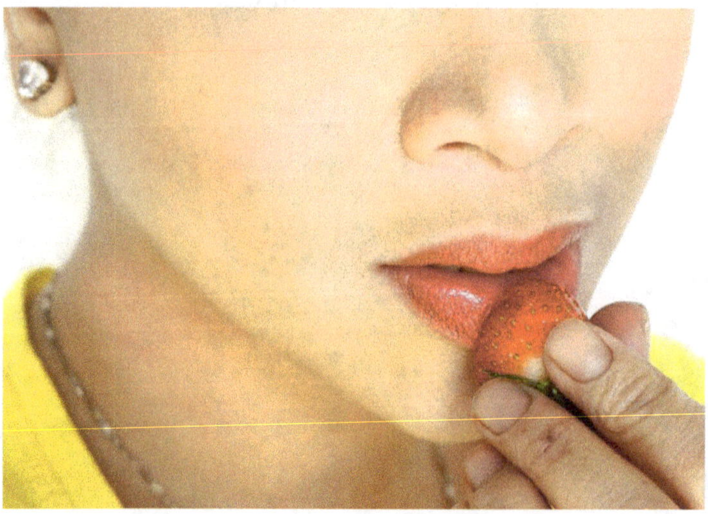

2. Rub the fruit on your lips. Just as you would if applying lipstick, rub the fruit over your lips. Try to stay within your lip lines instead of letting fruit juice get above or below your lips. Keep rubbing until your lips are completely coated in juice.

- Squeeze the fruit as you rub to release the red juice.
- If you're working with a large piece of fruit, it might help to cut it into smaller slices for a more precise application.
- You could also squeeze out the juice into a bowl and apply it using a cotton swab.

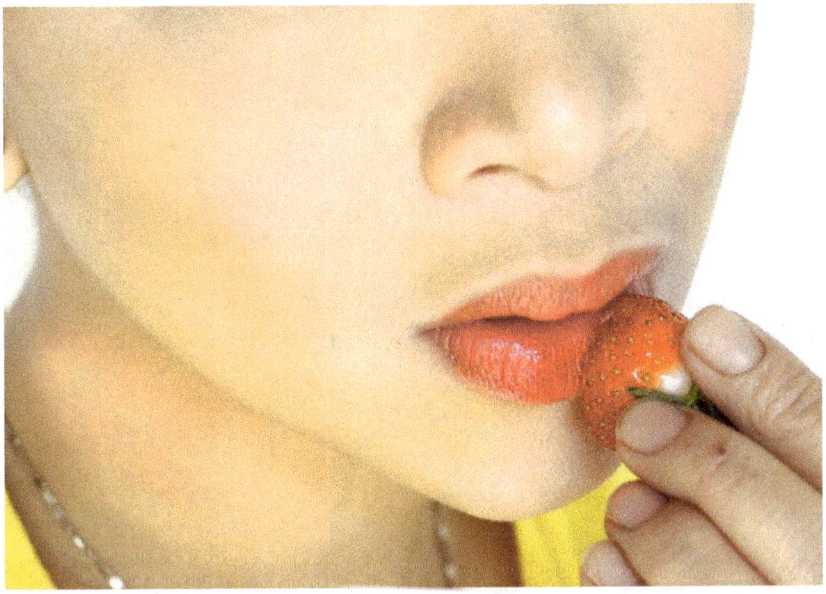

3. Apply additional layers of color. Once the first layer of juice dries, you might decide you want a darker, more vibrant red. The more layers of fruit juice you add, the more red your lips will look. Let each layer dry for a minute before adding the next.

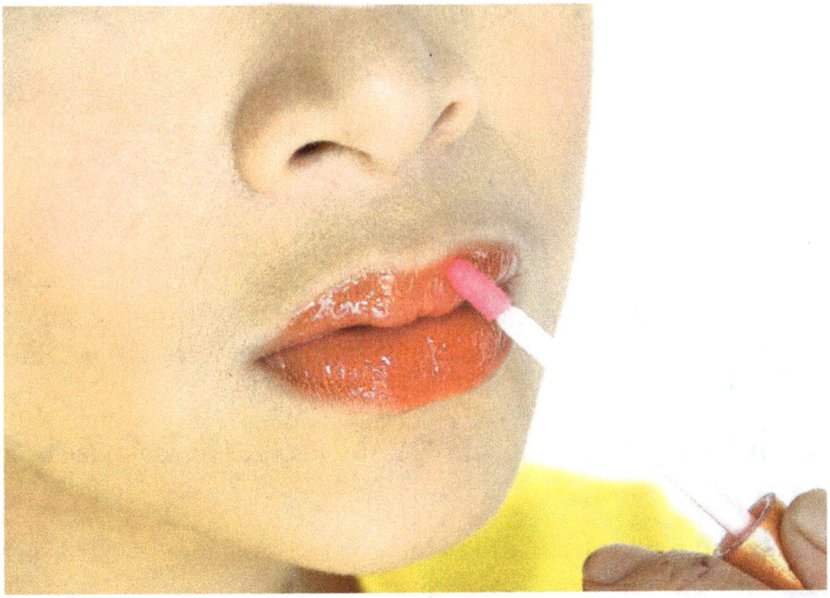

4. Seal the stain with clear lip gloss. This will help keep the fruit juice from rubbing off too quickly. A clear lip gloss will also add shine to make your lips look brighter and more vibrant.

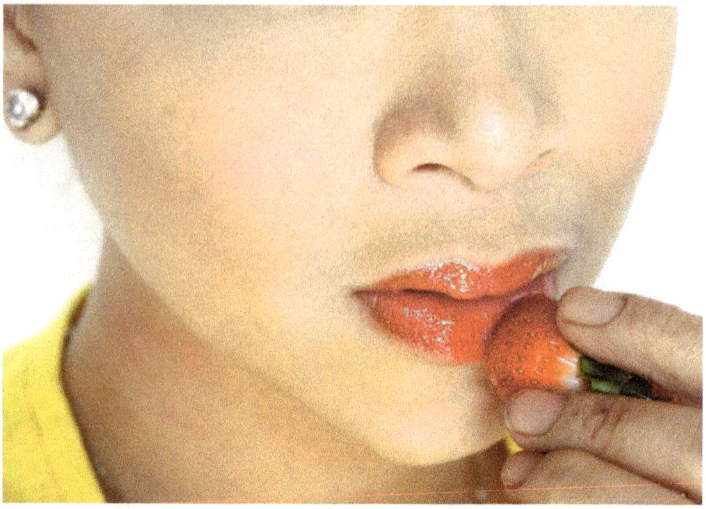

5. Reapply throughout the day. A natural fruit stain will fade away within a few hours. If you want to keep your lips red all day, keep some fruit with you so you can reapply color as necessary.

Method 3

Using Popsicles

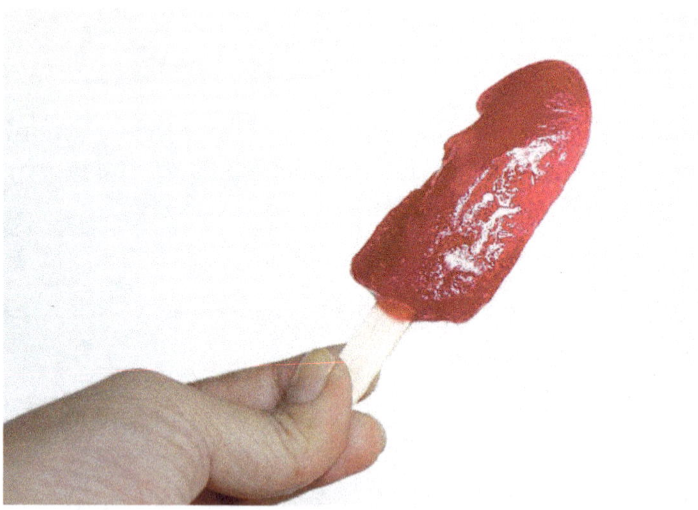

1. Buy red popsicles. Red popsicles contain artificial food coloring that will stain your lips red, just like lipstick. Choose the brightest red popsicles you can find. Look for flavors like cherry, red raspberry or strawberry.

- You can use any food product with red dye. If you don't have popsicles available, look for red soda.
- You can also use red food coloring, the kind used in baked goods. This is highly pigmented and will stain your lips for hours, so be careful.

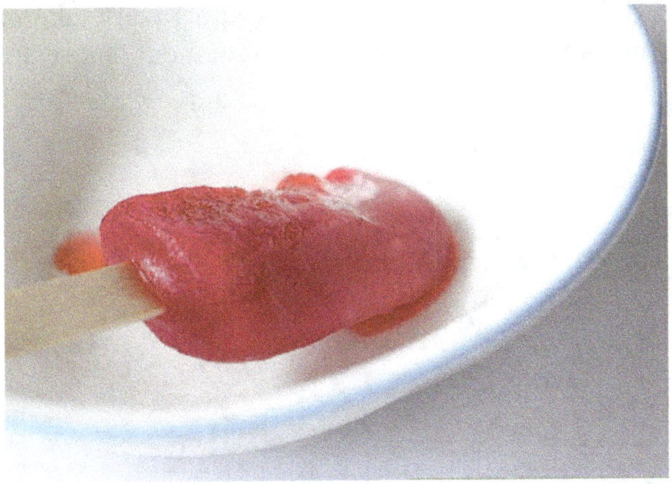

2. Melt a popsicle into a bowl. You'll apply the melted popsicle to your lips just like you would fruit juice. If you'd prefer, you can eat the popsicle and let it stain your lips red, but it may end up looking a little messy.

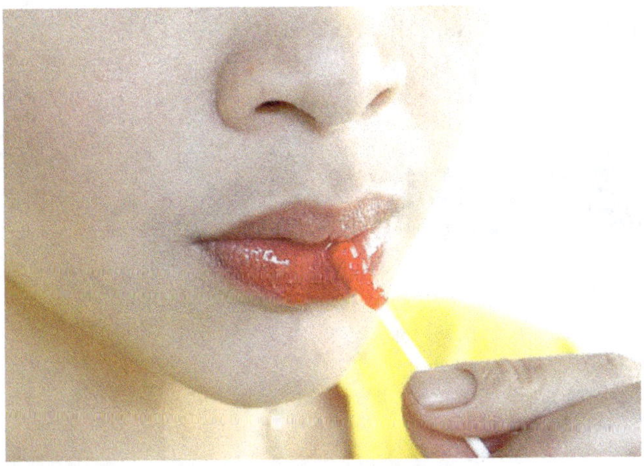

3. Use a cotton swab to apply the melted popsicle to your lips. Rub it over your lips to coat them, making sure to stay within your lip lines. Let the liquid dry on your lips.

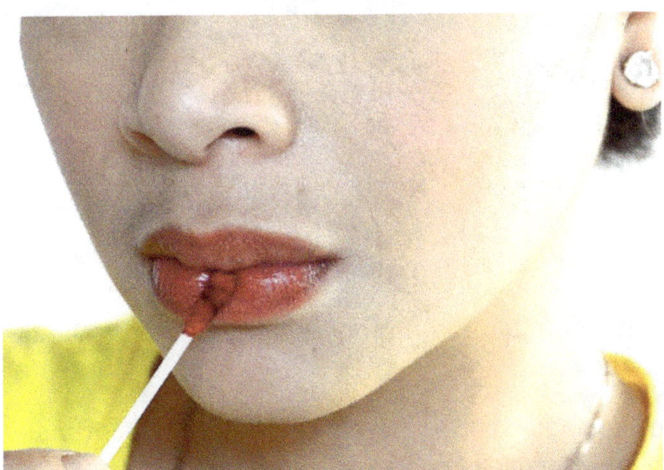

4. Add more layers for a deeper color. Every layer you apply will make your lips look redder, so apply as many coats as you want. Let each one dry for a moment before applying the next.

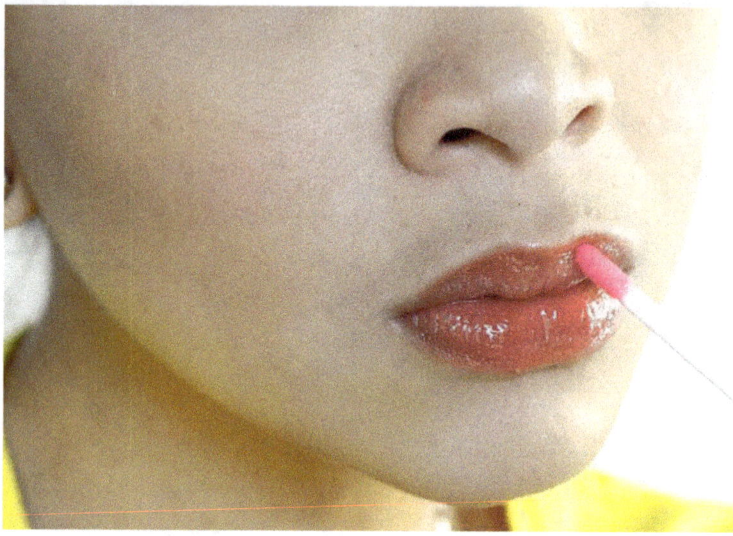

5. Seal the stain with clear lip gloss. This will prevent your stain from rubbing off and give your lips a pretty shine.

Lipstick

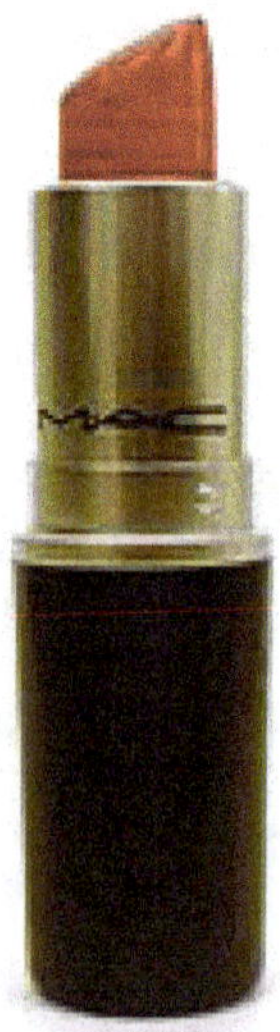

A tube of lipstick

Lipstick is a cosmetic product containing pigments, oils, waxes, and emollients that apply color, texture, and protection to the lips.

Many colors and types of lipstick exist. As with most other types of makeup, lipstick is typically, but not exclusively, worn by women. Some lipsticks are also lip balms, to add color and hydration.

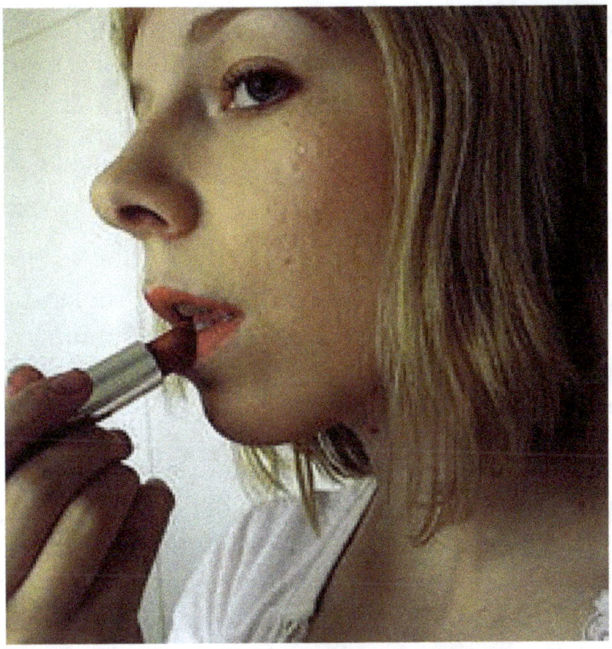

A woman applying lipstick

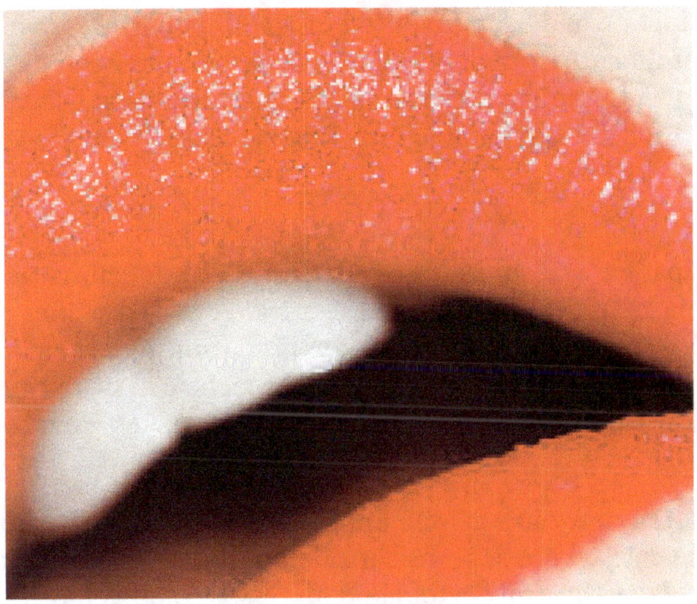

Closeup of red lipstick.

Ancient Sumerian men and women were possibly the first to invent and wear lipstick, about 5,000 years ago. They crushed gemstones and used them to decorate their faces, mainly on the lips and around the eyes. Also Egyptians like Cleopatra crushed bugs to create a colour of red on their lips. Also around 3000 BC to 1500 BC, women in the ancient Indus Valley Civilization applied red tinted lipstick to their lips for face decoration. Ancient Egyptians wore lip-stick to show social status rather than gender. They extracted the red dye from fucus-algin, 0.01% iodine, and some bromine mannite, but this dye resulted in serious illness. Lipsticks with shim-mering effects were initially made using a pearlescent substance found in fish scales.

During the Islamic Golden Age the notable Andalusian cosmetologist Abu al-Qasim al-Zahrawi (Abulcasis) invented solid lipsticks, which were perfumed sticks rolled and pressed in special molds, and he described them in his *Al-Tasrif*.

In Australia, Aboriginal girls would paint their mouths red with ocher for puberty rituals.

United Kingdom

Lip colouring started to gain some popularity in 16th-century England. During the time of Queen Elizabeth I bright red lips and a stark white face became fashionable. At that time, lipstick was made from a blend of beeswax and red stains from plants. Only upper class women and male actors wore makeup.

Throughout most of the 19th century the obvious use of cosmetics was not considered acceptable in Britain for respectable women, and it was associated with marginalized groups such as actors and prostitutes. It was considered brazen and uncouth to wear makeup. In the 1850s, reports were being published warning women of the dangers of using lead and vermilion in cosmetics applied to the face. By the end of the 19th century, Guerlain, a French cosmetic company, began to manufacture lipstick.

The first commercial lipstick had been invented in 1884, by perfumers in Paris, France. It was covered in silk paper and made from deer tallow, castor oil, and beeswax. Prior to this, lipstick had been created at home. Complete acceptance of the undisguised use of cosmetics in England appears to have arrived for the fashionable Londoner at least by 1921.

United States

In the 19th century, lipstick was colored with carmine dye. Carmine dye was extracted from cochineal, scale insects native to Mexico and Central America which live on cactus plants. Cochineal insects produce carminic acid to deter predation by other insects. Carminic acid, which forms 17% to 24% of the weight of the dried insects, can be extracted from the insect's body and eggs. Mixed with aluminum or calcium salts it makes carmine dye (also known as cochineal).

This lipstick did not come in a tube; it was applied with a brush. Carmine dye was expensive and the look of carmine colored lipstick was considered unnatural and theatrical, so lipstick was frowned upon for everyday wear. Only actors and actresses could get away with wearing lipstick. In 1880, few stage actresses wore lipstick in public.

The famous actress, Sarah Bernhardt, began wearing lipstick and rouge in public. Before the late 19th century, women only applied makeup at home. Bernhardt often applied carmine dye to her lips in public.

In the early 1890s, Carmine was mixed with an oil and wax base. The mixture gave a natural look and it was more acceptable among women. At that time, lipstick was not sold in screw up metal tube; it was sold in paper tubes, tinted papers, or in small pots. The Sears Roebuck catalog first offered rouge for lips and cheeks by the late 1890s.

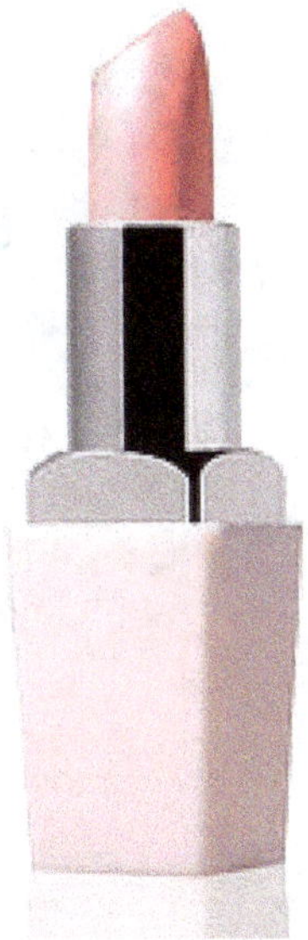

A tube of lipstick

By 1912 fashionable American women had come to consider lipstick acceptable, though an article in the *New York Times* advised on the need to apply it cautiously.

By 1915, lipstick was sold in cylinder metal containers, which had been invented by Maurice Levy. Women had to slide a tiny lever at the side of the tube with the edge of their fingernail to move the lipstick up to the top of the case, although lipsticks in push-up metal containers had been available in Europe since 1911. In 1923, the first swivel-up tube was patented by James Bruce Mason Jr. in Nashville, Tennessee. As women started to wear lipstick for photographs, photography made lipstick acceptable among women. Elizabeth Arden and Estee Lauder began selling lipstick in their salons.

During the Second World War, metal lipstick tubes were replaced by plastic and paper tubes. Lipstick was scarce during that time because some of the essential ingredients of lipstick, petroleum and castor oil, were unavailable. World War II allowed women to work in engineering and scientific research, and in the late 1940s, Hazel Bishop, an organic chemist in New York and New Jersey, created the first long lasting lipstick, called No-Smear lipstick. With the help of Raymond Specter, an advertiser, Bishop's lipstick business thrived.

Another form of lip color, a wax-free, semi-permanent liquid formula, was invented in the 1990s by the Lip-Ink International company. Other companies have imitated the idea, putting out their own versions of long-lasting "lip stain" or "liquid lip colour."

Lipstick Trends

Throughout the early 20th century, lipstick came in a limited number of shades.

Dark red was one of the most popular shade throughout the 19th and 20th century. Dark red lipstick was popular in the 1920s. Flappers wore lipstick to symbolize their independence. Lipstick was worn around the lips to form a "Cupid's bow," inspired by actress Clara Bow. At that time, it was acceptable to apply lipstick in public and during lunch, but never at dinner.

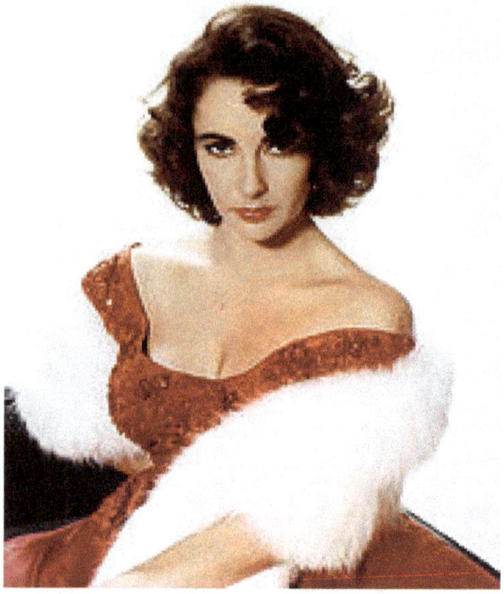

Elizabeth Taylor helped to popularize red lipstick.

In the early 1930s, Elizabeth Arden began to introduce different lipstick colors. She inspired other companies to create a variety of lipstick shades. In the 1930s, lipstick was seen as symbol of adult sexuality. Teenage girls believed that lipstick was a symbol of womanhood. Adults saw it as an act of rebellion. Many Americans, especially immigrants, did not accept teenage girls wearing lipstick. A study in 1937 survey revealed that over 50% of teenage girls fought with their parents over lipstick.

In the mid-1940s, several teen books and magazines stressed that men prefer a natural look over a made-up look. Books and magazines also warned girls that wearing cosmetics could ruin their chances of popularity and a career. The implication of these articles was that lipstick and rouge were for teen girls who acted very provocatively with men. Despite the increased use of cosmetics, it was still associated with prostitution. Teen girls were discouraged from wearing cosmetics for fear that they would be mistaken for "loose" girls or prostitutes.

By the 1950s, movie actresses Marilyn Monroe and Elizabeth Taylor helped bring back dark red lips. A 1951 survey revealed that two-thirds of teenage girls wore lipstick.

In 1950 chemist Hazel Bishop formed a company, Hazel Bishop Inc., to promote her invention of long-lasting, non-smearing 'kissproof' lipstick ("stays on you... not on him"), which quickly gained acceptance. At the end of the 1950s, a cosmetic company named Gala introduced pale shimmery lipstick. Later, Max Factor created a popular lipstick color called Strawberry Meringue. Lipstick manufacturers began creating lipsticks in lavender, pale pink, white, and peach. Since parents generally frowned on teen girls wearing red lipstick, some teen girls began wearing pink and peach lipsticks, which became a trend. White or nearly white lipstick was popular in the 1960s. Rock groups such as the Ronettes and the Shirelles popularized white lipstick. Girls would apply white lipstick over pink lipstick or place under-eye concealer on their lips. During that time, many lipsticks were either matte, sheer, or slightly shiny. In the 1960s, lipstick was associated with femininity. Women who did not wear lipstick were suspected of mental illness or lesbianism.

In the 1970s, a number of cosmetic companies introduced lipsticks in more unusual colors such as iridescent light blue (Kanebo), frosted lime green (*Conga Lime* by Revlon), and silver sparkled navy blue (*Metallic Grandma* by Biba). M•A•C cosmetics continues to release limited edition and highly collectible lipsticks in a wide range of colors and finishes, including unusual hues of violets, blues, and greens.

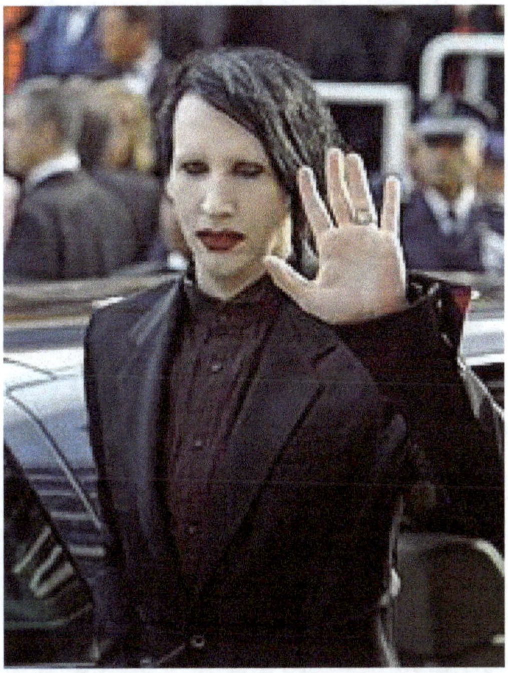

Rocker Marilyn Manson helped popularize dark lipsticks in alternative subcultures.

Black lipstick became popular in the late 1970s and into the 1990s. In the 1950s, black lipstick had been worn by actresses starring in horror films. It became popular again due in part to punk and goth subcultures.

In the mid-1980s, so-called mood lipstick were sold to adults by mainstream cosmetic companies. This type of lipstick changes colors after it is applied, based on changes in skin's pH that supposedly reflect the wearer's mood. Previously these had been available as little girls' play makeup. They had another resurgence in the very early 21st century, offered by inexpensive as well as more exclusive cosmetic lines, and color changing chemicals also appeared in lip gloss, such as Smashbox O-Gloss, and blush, such as Stila Custom Color Blush.

In the 1990s, lipstick colors became semi-matte. Shades of brown were very popular. These shades were inspired by several shows such as "Friends". In the late 1990s and into the 21st century, pearl shades became very popular. Lipsticks were no longer matte or semi-matte, they were shiny and contained several interference pearls.

In 2012, bright bold lip colors became trendy again with saturated colors such as hot pink, neon, and orange.

In 2014 and early 2015 nude lipsticks were coming up to be incredibly popular. These lipsticks follow the general trend where "less is more". Examples of celebrities promoting this trend are Paris Hilton and Gigi Gorgeous.

In late 2015 and 2016 liquid lipstick, which applies like a gloss but dries matte, became popularized with brands such as Anastasia Beverly Hills. Its most common form comes in a tube, applied with an applicator wand.

Lipstick also has many variations including lip balms, glosses, crayons, pencils, liners, and stains. Balms and glosses tend to be clear and not as dark or vibrant.

Ingredients

Lipstick contains wax, oils, antioxidants and emollients. Wax provides the structure to the solid lipstick. Lipsticks may be made from several waxes such as beeswax, ozokerite and candelilla wax. Because of its high melting point, Carnauba wax is a key ingredient in terms of strengthening the lipstick. Various oils and fats are used in lipsticks, such as olive oil, mineral oil, cocoa butter, lanolin, and petrolatum.

Lead and other trace metals are also found in many lipsticks. It is impossible to know whether these metals are in the lipstick by looking at the ingredient list because they are not an intentional ingredient added, but rather, an unintentional contaminant. These trace metals are naturally occurring and accidentally get taken up with other chemicals that are used in lipstick production. Lead and other trace metals will not be listed in the ingredients section of different lipsticks. Look for lead acetate, chromium, thimerosal, hydrogenated cotton seed oil, sodium hexametaphosphate on the ingredients list of lipsticks. These chemicals contain trace amounts of naturally occurring metals, such as lead.

Lipsticks get their colors from a variety of pigments and lake dyes including, but not limited to bromo acid, D&C Red No. 21, Calcium Lake such as D&C Red 7 and D&C Red 34, and D&C Orange No. 17. Pink lipsticks are made by mixing white titanium dioxide and red shades. Both organic and inorganic pigments are employed.

Matte lipsticks contain more filling agents like silica but do not have many emollients. Creme lipsticks contain more waxes than oils. Sheer and long lasting lipsticks contain more oil, while long lasting lipsticks also contain silicone oil, which seals the colors to the wearer's lips. Glossy lipstick contain more oil to give a shiny finish to the lips.

Shimmery or frost lipstick may contain mica, silica, and synthetic pearl particles, such as bismuth oxychloride, to give them a glittery or shimmering shine.

Lipstick is made from grinding and heating ingredients. Then heated waxes are added to the mix for texture. Oils and lanolin are added for specific formula requirements. Afterwards, the hot liquid is poured onto a metal mold. The mixture is then chilled. Once they have hardened, they are heated in flame for half a second to create a shiny finish and to remove imperfections.

How to Choose the Right Lipstick for You

With its endless palette of lipsticks, glosses, and stains, the makeup counter can be pretty overwhelming. This article will teach you how to choose the right lip color to match your skin tone, outfit, and the occasion.

Part 1

Determining your Skin Tone

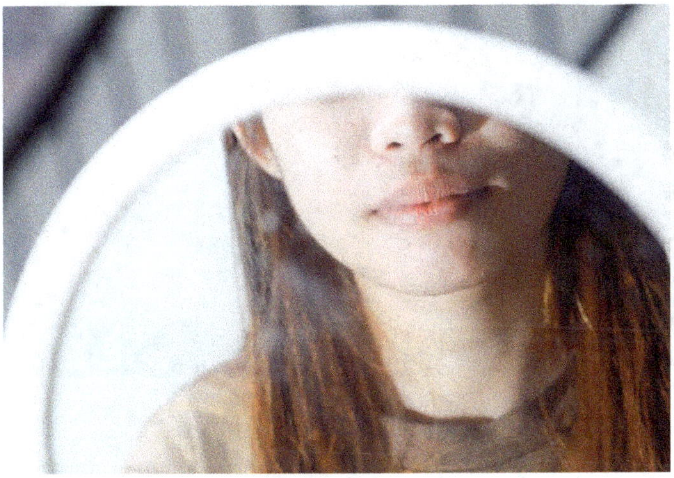

1. Examine your skin in natural lighting to determine your complexion: fair, light, medium, tan, deep. Concentrate on the skin around your jaw line.

- Fair skin: your skin is very pale or translucent and you burn very easily. You may have freckles and some redness.
- Light skin: your skin is pale. When you are in the sun, you burn and then may possibly tan.
- Medium: you tan easily and generally don't burn or have sensitive skin.
- Tan: your skin is tan or olive. You rarely burn and look tanned even in the winter.
- Deep: your skin is dark and you never get sunburned. Your hair is possibly black or dark brown.

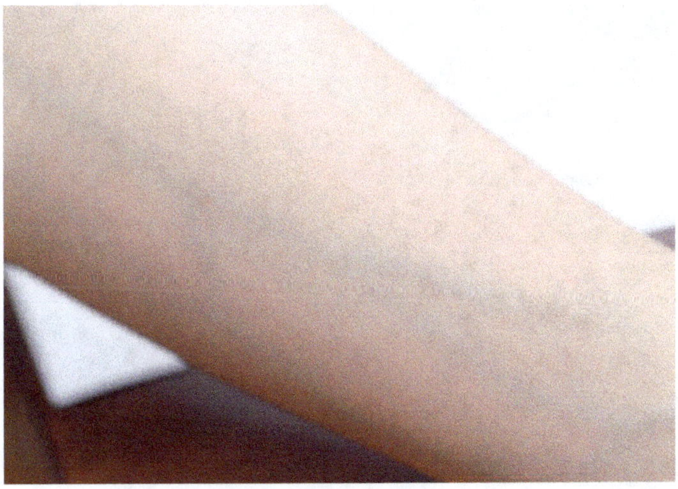

2. Look at the color of the veins on the inside of your wrist. This is a quick way to figure out if you have a warm, neutral, or cool skin tone.

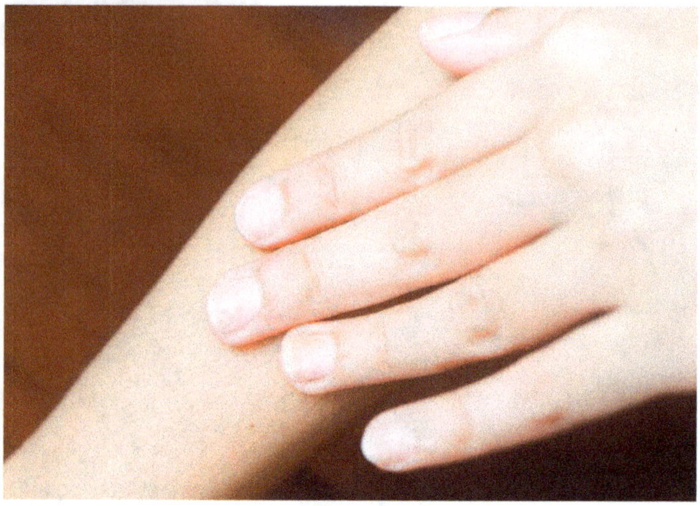

- Blue or purple veins indicate you have a cool skin tone.
- Green veins mean you have a warm skin tone.
- If you have difficulty deciding if your veins are blue or green, you likely have a neutral skin tone and can choose colors from both the cool and warm spectrum. People with olive skin usually have neutral undertones.

3. Notice how your skin reacts to the sun: do you tan or burn easily?
   - Skin that tans easily has more melanin indicates a warm skin tone. Most women of African-American and Indian descent fall into this category.
   - If you burn before you tan (and maybe can't tan at all), then your skin has less melanin and you have a blue skin tone. If you have deep ebony skin, you may actually fall into this category.

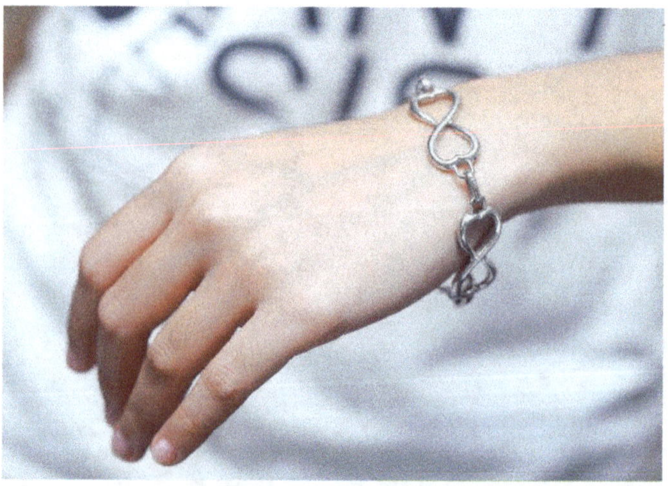

4. Try on gold and silver jewelry. Which looks better?
   - Gold jewelry looks best with warm skin tones.

- Silver jewelry looks best on cool skin tones.
- Both look good on a more neutral skin tone.
- This can be a good "tie breaker" if you don't clearly meet the criteria listed already.

Part 2

Choosing an Everyday Color

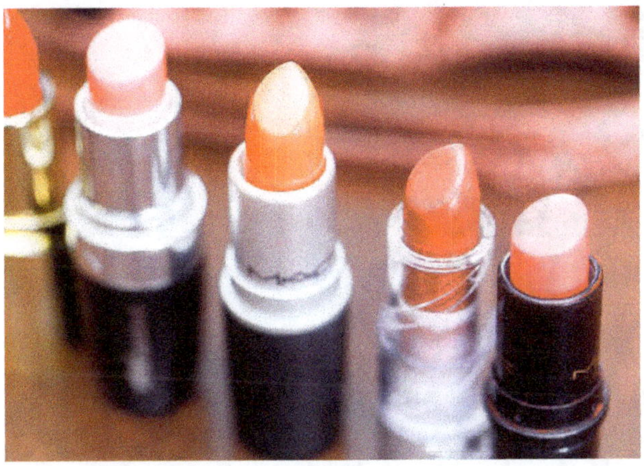

1. Find a color that is one to two shades deeper than your natural lip color.

    - To test how close the shade is to your natural color, apply the lipstick only to your lower lip. Compare that shade to the your upper lip. If the shades are drastically different, you need to keep looking.

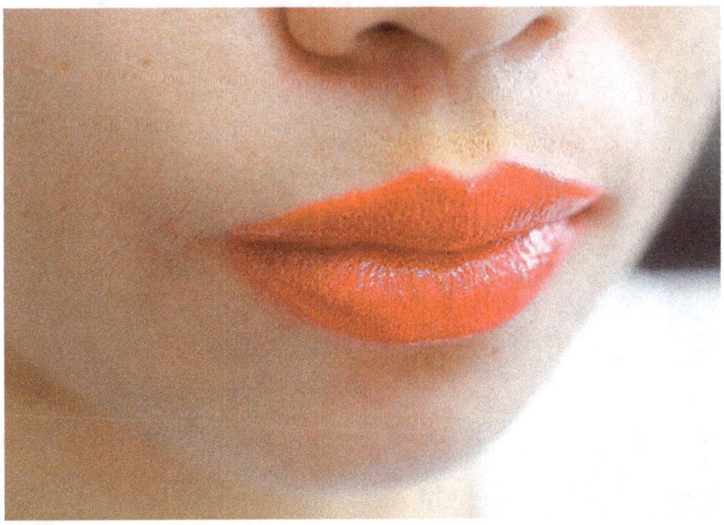

2. Decide if you want your lips to look smaller or larger. Dark shades will actually make your lips look smaller, while lighter shades can add plumpness.

    - Lipstick with a matte finish can also cause lips to look thinner, while glosses and shimmery shades can make them look fuller.

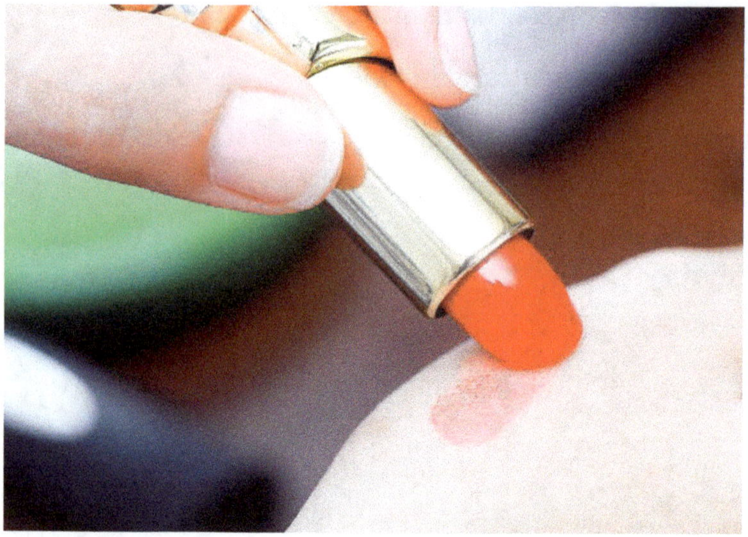

3. Determine your undertone and complexion.

    - Remember that your undertone and complexion will help guide you, but they aren't the be-all-end-all of choosing a lipstick color. It is important to try on different shades and, ultimately, choose what *you* feel looks best.

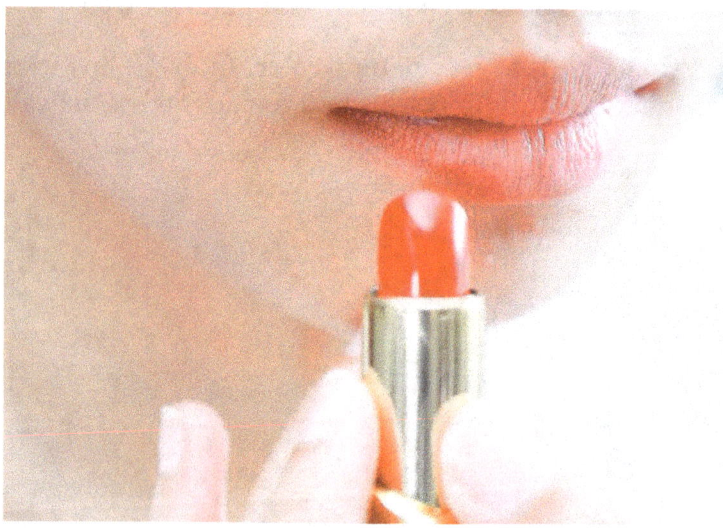

4. Experiment with shades that experts recommend for your complexion and skin tone.

    - If you have fair or light skin, try light pink, coral, peach, nudes, or beige. If you have cool undertones, try a soft mocha and nude. Warm undertones, try pale pinks or a nude with a little peach.
    - If you have medium skin, try rose, mauve, or berry shades. Cool undertones: try shades of pink or cranberry. Warm undertones: experiment with copper or bronze.

- If you have tan skin, try to avoid browns and purples and go for colors with an orange undertone. Most other colors will look great. Try coral, or deep pink.
- If you have a deep complexion, try browns or purples like walnut, caramel, plum, or wine. Cool undertones should look for ruby and wine-colored reds. Warm undertones: try copper or bronze.

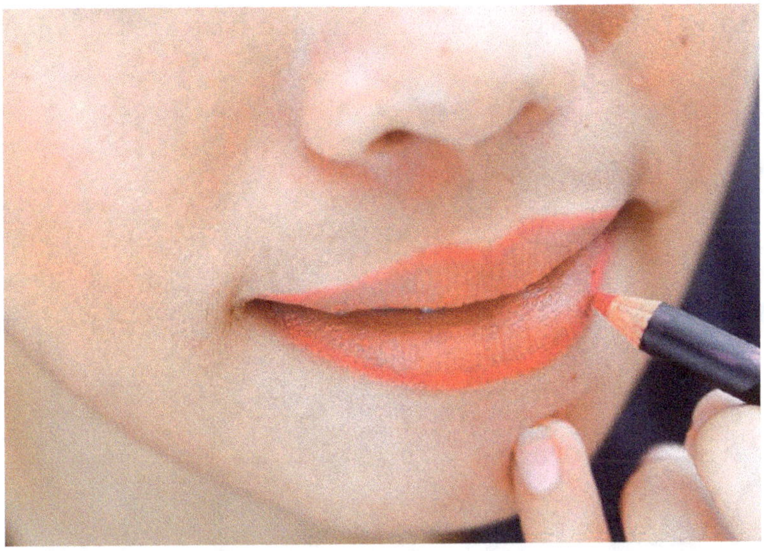

5. Keep it subtle. Unless you're feeling like making a statement with bold lips (which is totally fine!), apply strong shades to your lower lip only. Press your lips together, then use your finger to even out the color.

Part 3

Choosing the Right Red

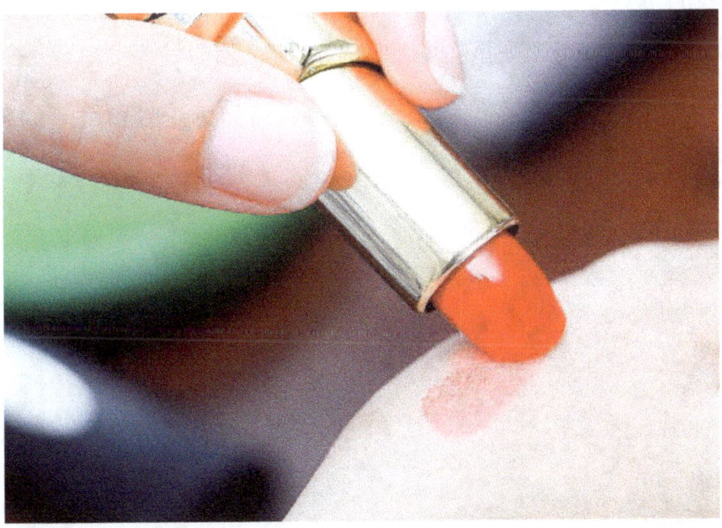

1. Find the right color for your skin tone. Again, use your skin tone and complexion as a guide--if you find a color you love that breaks the "rules"--go for it!

- Fair or light skin should look for dusty, pinkish red or coral. Cool undertones: raspberry. Warm tones: try reds with a blue undertone or coral.
- Tan or medium skin should look for bright red cherry red, or true red with no undertone (if you have a neutral undertone). Warm undertones: orangey-red or tangerine. Cool undertones: wine.
- Deep skin with warm undertones should try blue-based red. Cool: Metallic ruby red or deep wine.

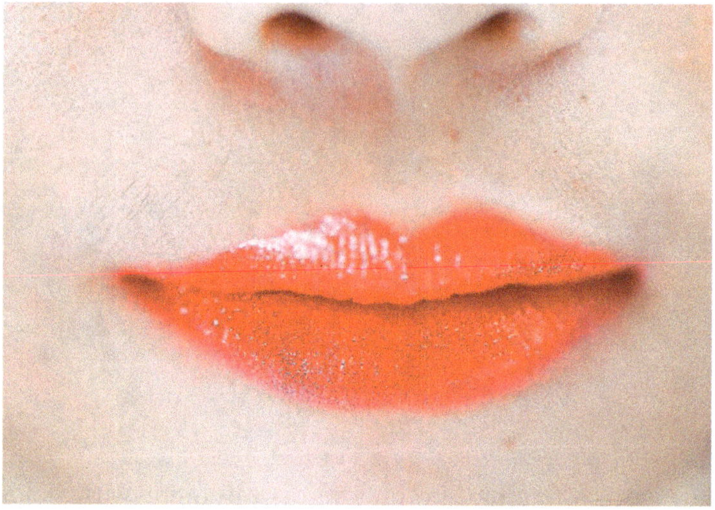

2. Wear red with pride. This is a classic look that any woman can pull off, regardless of age, skin, hair, eye, or lip color. Own it!

Part 4

How to Shop for Lipstick

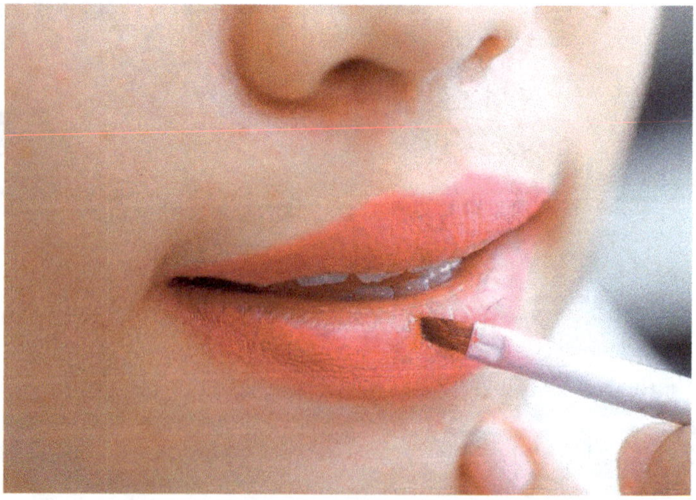

1. Try the lipstick on before you buy it. Clean the tester with a little alcohol (the store should provide this in a spray bottle) and use a test brush or a cotton swab to apply the color to your lips.

- If you don't want to apply the tester lipstick to your mouth, test it on the pads of your fingertips. Your fingertips are closer to your lip color than your wrist or the side of your hand.

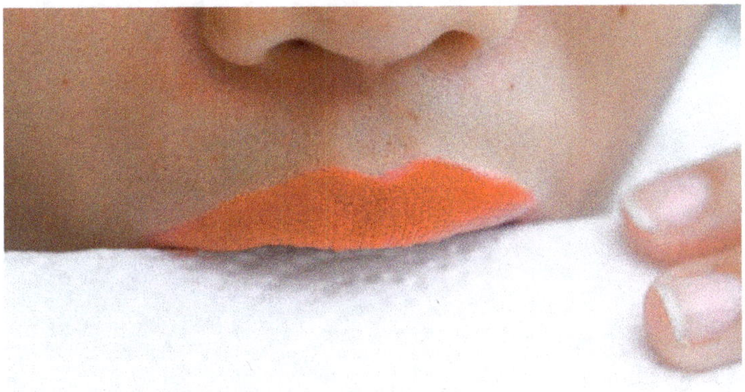

2. Remove one lip color completely before trying on the next. Otherwise, you will be mixing multiple colors together. Ask a sales rep for makeup remover or lotion.

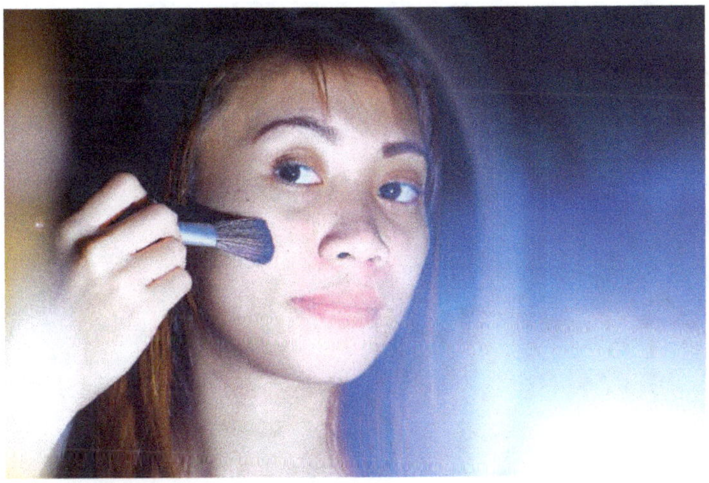

3. Make sure you are in a well-lit area.

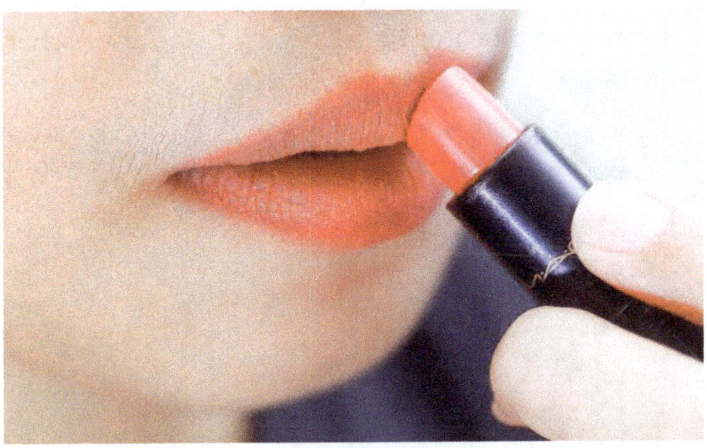

4. Try on lipstick with little or no other makeup on your face. Look for a shade that, worn with no other make up, brightens your face and makes other makeup unnecessary.

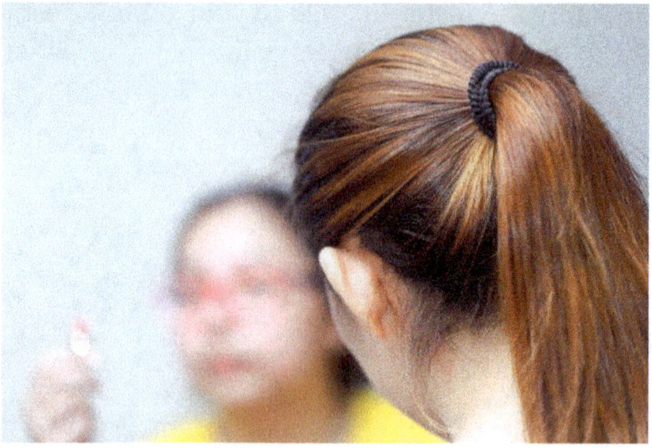

5. Ask for help at the makeup counter. Sometimes it's hard to objectively judge what looks best on ourselves. A professional at the makeup counter can match you with the right color.

Part 5

Matching a Lip Color with the Rest of Your Look

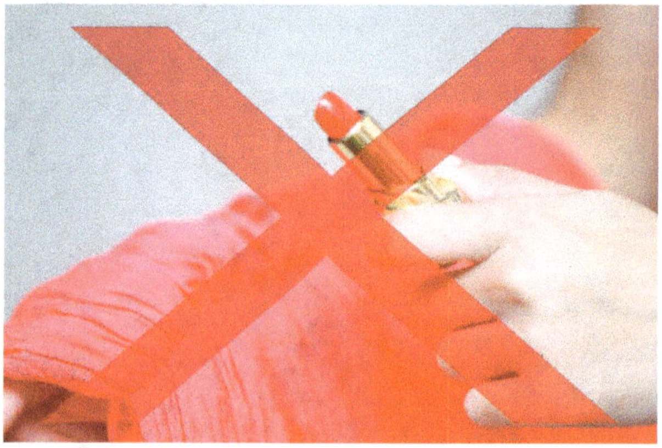

1. Don't match a lip color too closely with your clothing. For example, if you are wearing a fire-engine red dress, wearing the same exact color on your lips will look overwhelming.

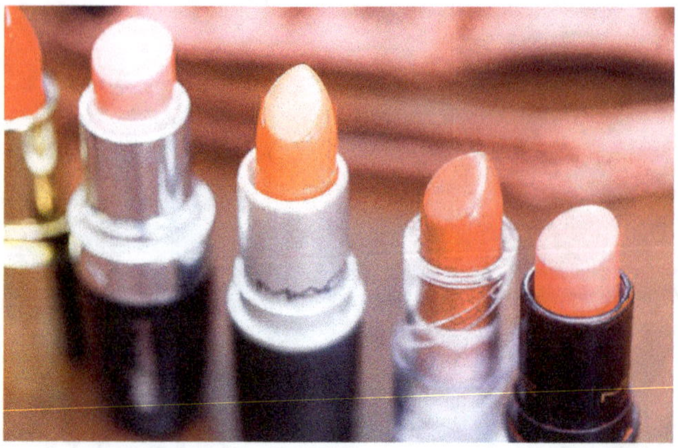

2. Have fun and experiment, but consider these guidelines if you're not sure:

- Nude lips look great with just about anything. It's a great casual look and can help play up dramatic eyes.
- Red can add drama to a fairly plain outfit. Try not to overwhelm by wearing red with very bright clothing or clothes with crazy patterns.
- Pink is versatile because there are so many shades. Pinks that are just a few shades brighter than your natural lip color work for a subtle, everyday look.
- Berries can make a dark ensemble seem sombre and can weigh down an airy, summery look. Try matching berries with mixed neutrals.

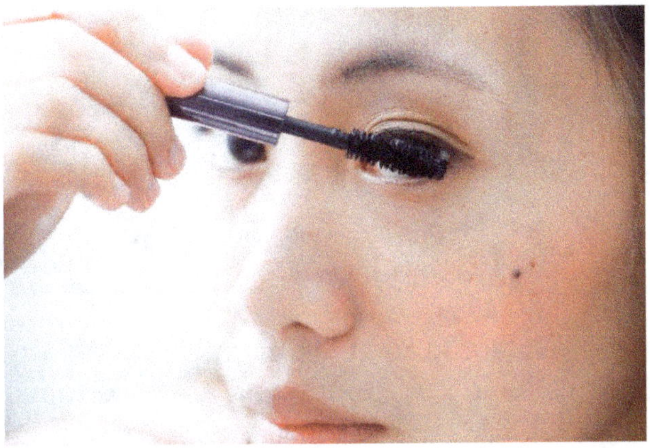

3. Go for dramatic lips or eyes; not both.

- Stick to just mascara on the eyes, or just a bit of dark brown eyeliner in between your lashes.

How to Buy Lipstick

Part 2

Finding the Right Texture

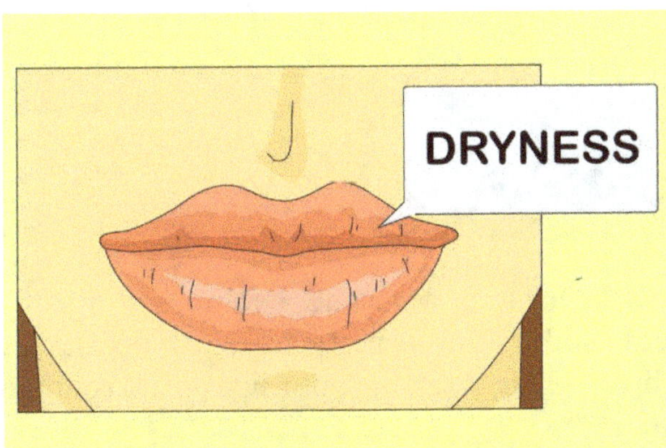

1. Determine your lips' dryness. Different lipsticks suit different hydration needs. If you have very

dry lips, you will need to avoid many shimmery and long-wear lipsticks, as these will dry out your lips even faster.

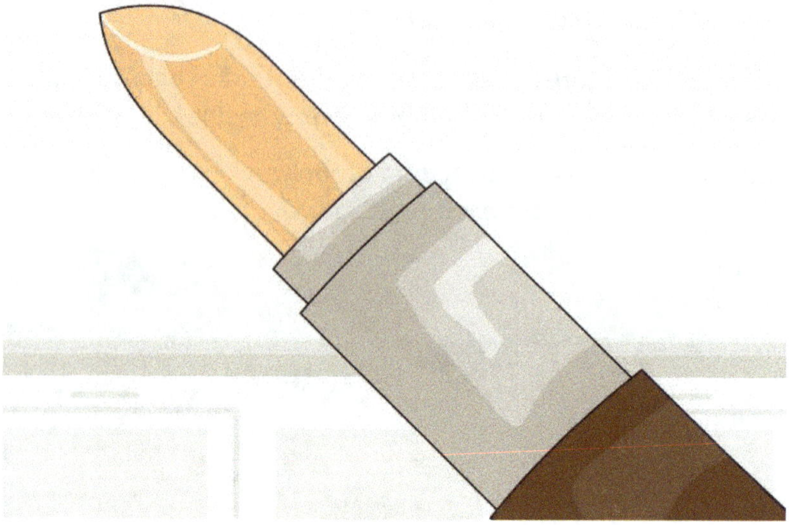

2. Choose cream lipsticks for casual looks and maximum hydration. Cream lipsticks are intended for everyday wear. They often come in nude tones, and are used to make neutral looks look finished.

- If you choose a nude shade, make sure it is a little bit darker than your skin tone.

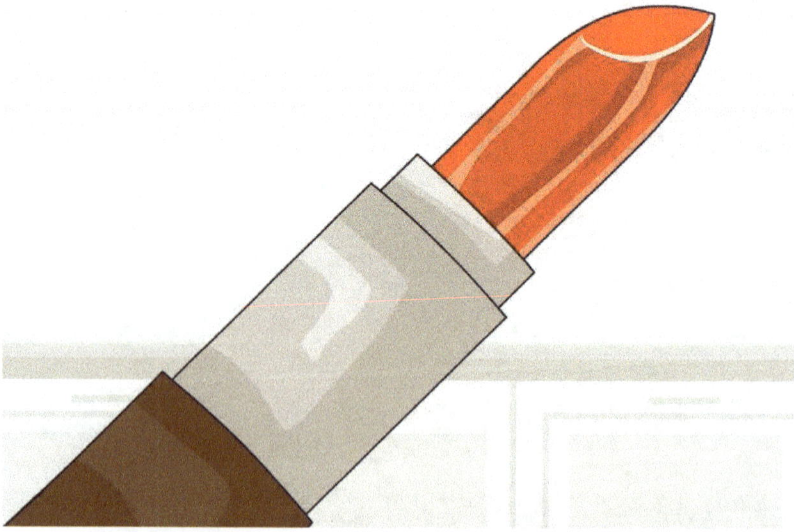

3. Choose satin or gloss lipsticks for long wear and a shimmery finish. Glossy lipsticks add shine to your lips, which gives them volume. Unlike matte or cream lipsticks, glossy lipsticks hide all the lines and wrinkles on your lips with light, giving your lips a full, round feel.

- Glossy lipsticks are not casual. They may also dry out your lips, so do not use them if you have naturally dry lips.

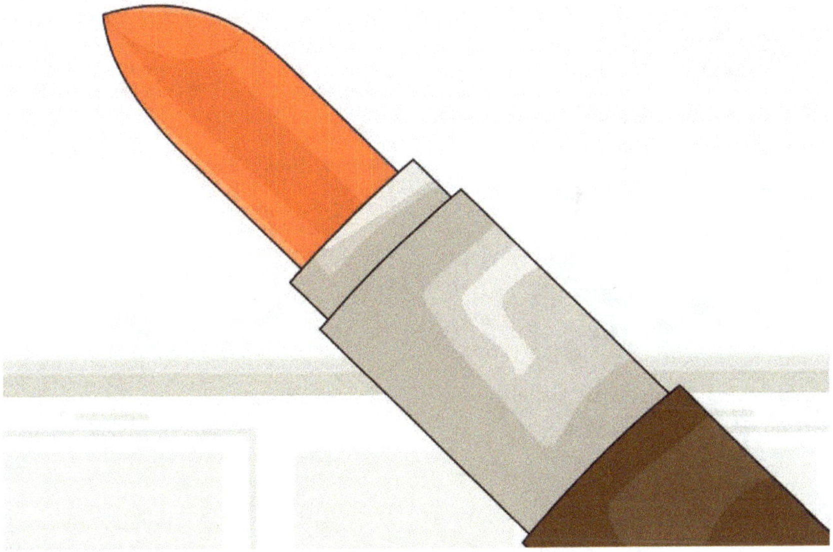

4. Choose matte lipsticks for a velvet finish. These are very popular right now, and they are often long-lasting. Be careful using matte lipsticks if you have dry lips.

- Matte lipsticks accentuate every line and wrinkle on your lips, because they have no shine to gloss over details. If you use matte lipstick, make sure to hydrate your lips beforehand.

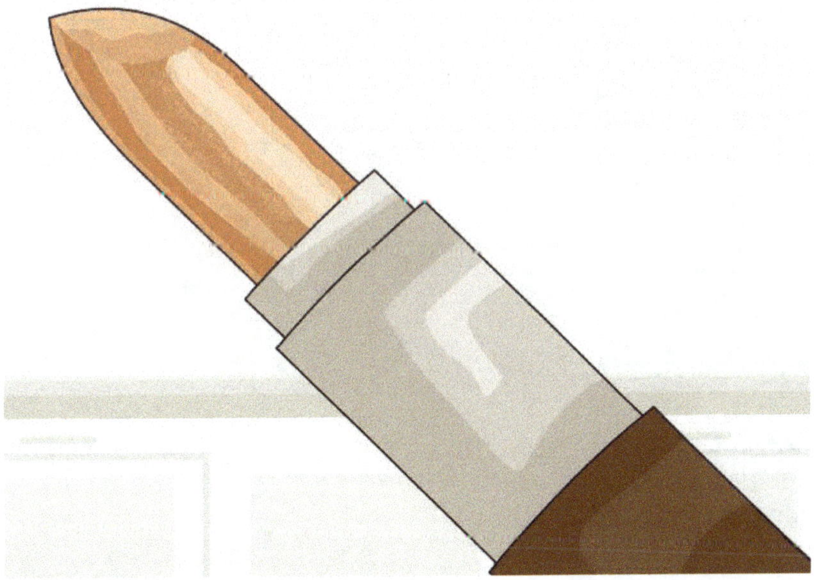

5. Choose frosted lipsticks for a retro look. These are very shimmery lipsticks that were popular in the 1980s and 1990s. They were often chosen a few shades lighter than the wearer's skin tone. Some looks from the '90s like jelly shoes and crop tops have returned, and some celebrities are now wearing frosted lipstick.

- Frosted lipstick is not for casual wear.

Part 3

Choosing the Right Brand

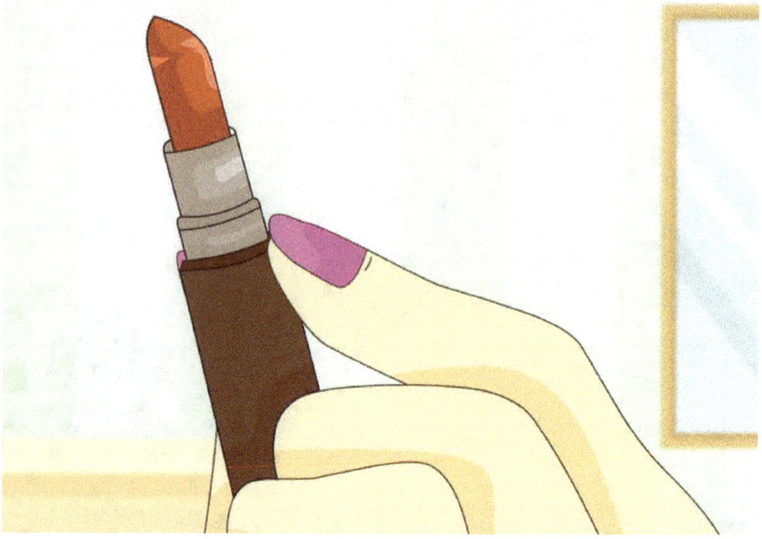

1. Check the pliability of the lipstick. A high quality lipstick should be somewhere between rigid and oily. It should be stiff but not crumbly, slick but not greasy.

- If the feeling of a lipstick makes you uncomfortable don't buy it. It might be a high quality product, but you will not use something that is not enjoyable to apply.

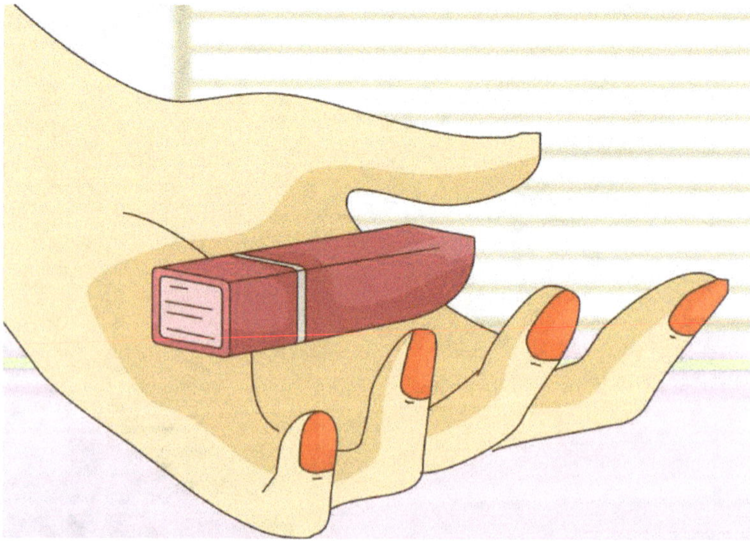

2. Look at the packaging. Packaging isn't just about creating the world of the makeup brand. It also plays a key role in how long you will be able to keep your lipstick after buying it. If the cap is very easy to move, it is likely that the bullet of your lipstick will get broken, or leak into your bag.

- If the packaging is light and cheap with a metallic finish, it will likely begin to flake after a week of bouncing around in your bag. This can be an indication that the brand is not worth buying.

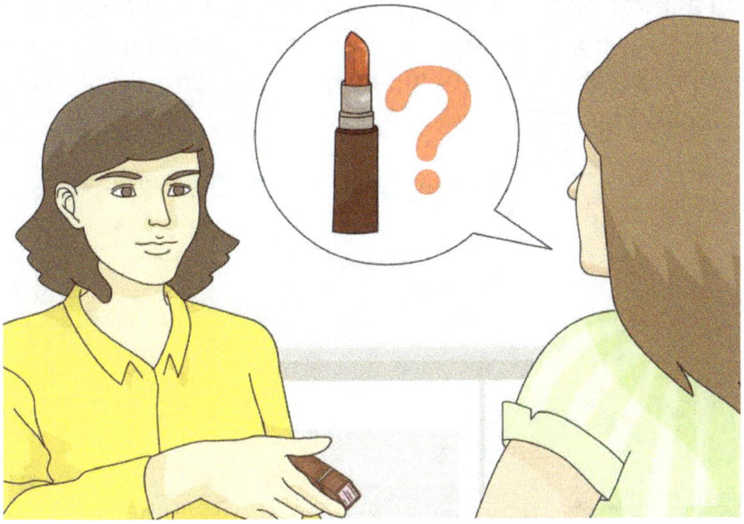

3. Ask for samples or a return policy. If you're still not sure you like the color and texture, big makeup and department stores will have samples for you to take home. If at a drugstore, ask about their return policy. Most will let you return it if you don't like it.

- Never be afraid to ask. If you don't ask, you may miss an opportunity.

How to Apply Lipstick

Exfoliate your lips and some lip balm. Prime your lips with foundation, if desired, then apply lip liner. Apply two coats of lipstick; you can apply it straight from the tube, or use a lipstick brush for more precision. Pull your finger through your lips, then set the lipstick with some powder, if desired.

Part 1

Getting Your Lips Ready

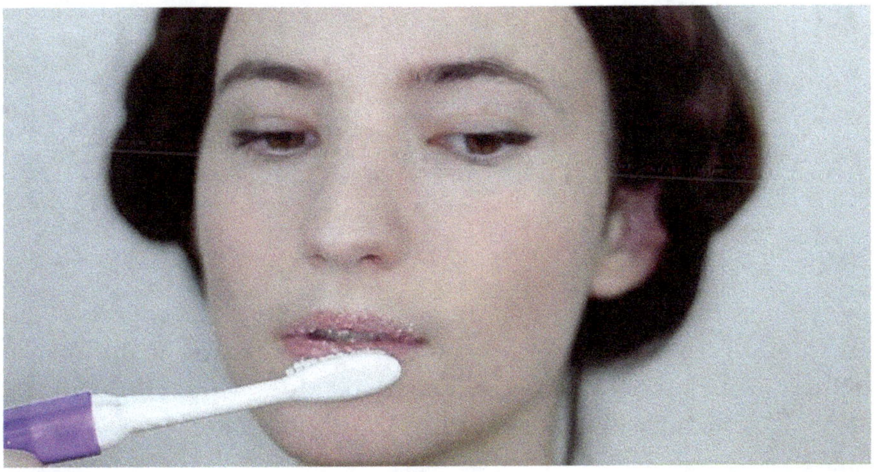

1. Exfoliate your lips. This will help remove any dead skin cells and give you a smooth canvas to work on. It will also help your lips feel softer. You can exfoliate your lips by gently brushing them with a toothbrush for a few seconds, or rubbing them with a damp towel. You can also make a lip scrub using one part oil and one part sugar.

- Good oils to use in lip scrubs include jojoba oil, oil, olive oil, or coconut oil. Even honey works for those who don't want to use an oil.

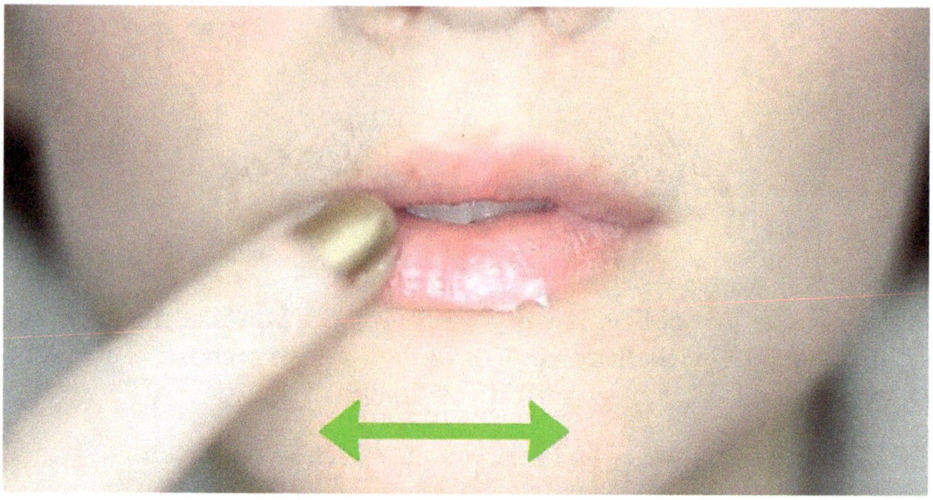

2. Moisturize your lips with some lip balm. Open the lip balm and run the stick across your bottom and upper lip; if it comes in a little jar, use your finger to apply it instead. This will not only help soften your lips and make them smooth, but it will also help the lip liner and lipstick go on more evenly. Leave the lip balm on for a few minutes; you can do the rest of your makeup while you wait.

- Try to choose a waxy, non-oily lip balm. This will be less likely to leave behind oily residue.

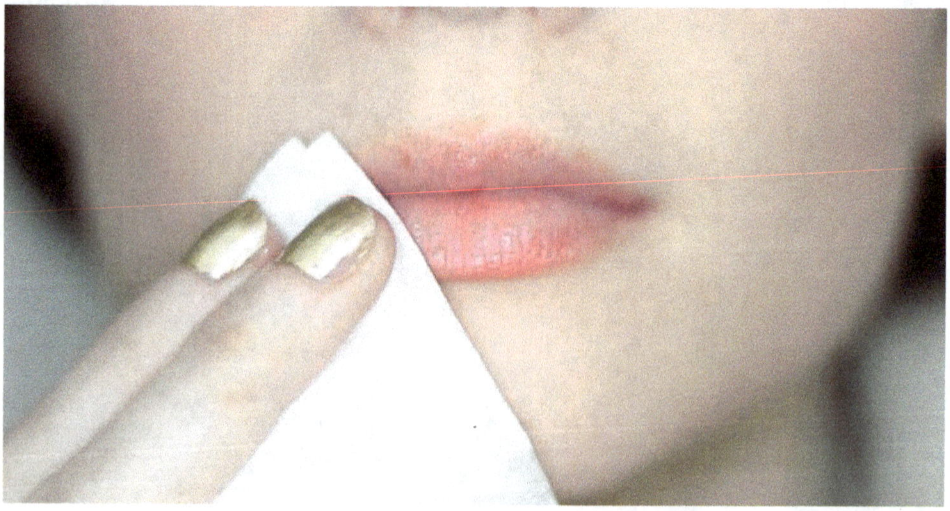

3. Wipe the lip balm off, if necessary. Before you apply any lipstick or lip liner, check and see if there is any lip balm on your lips. If there is still some residue, wipe it off using a tissue or cotton bud. Any lip balm that's leftover will make your lips too slippery and prevent the lip liner and lipstick from sticking.

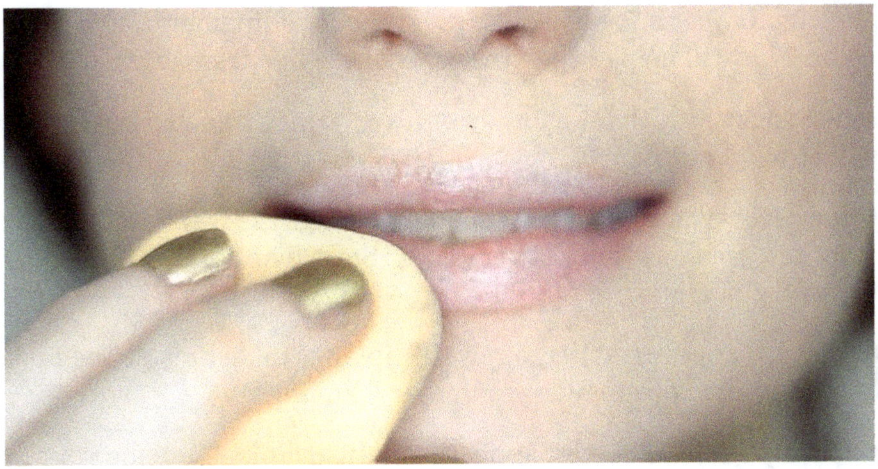

4. Consider priming your lips with foundation. This will help bring out the natural color of the lipstick, but it is not necessary. Use the same color that you use on the rest of your face, and apply it with a makeup sponge. Be sure to smile while doing this; it will help you fill in all the little cracks.

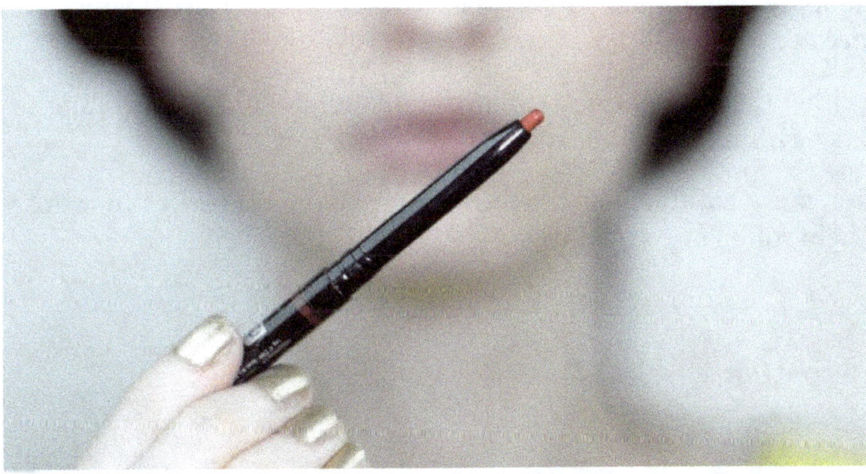

5. Choose your lip liner. Lip liner is very important. It gives the lipstick something to grip on to and makes it last longer. It also helps the lipstick go on more evenly and prevents it from bleeding.

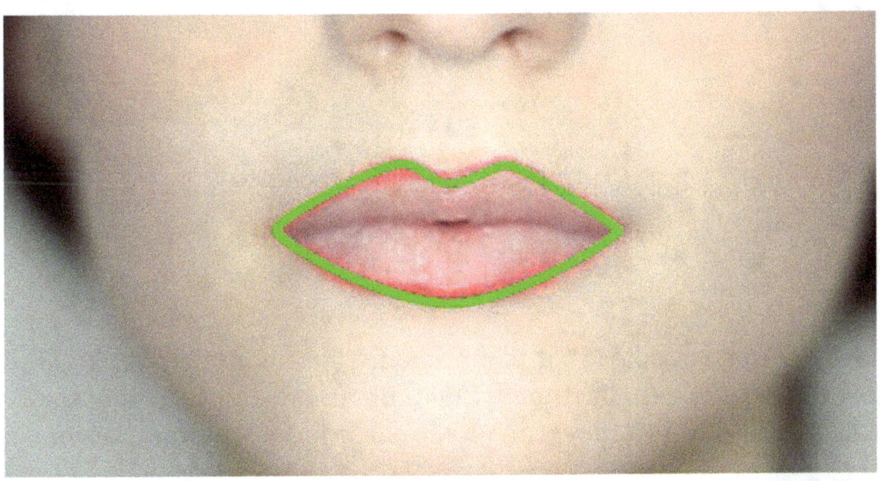

- If you are going to wear a bold color lipstick, choose a lip liner that is a bit darker than the lipstick color. This will help deepen the color of the lipstick and make it more opaque.
- If you primed your lips with foundation, or if you want a more neutral look, match the color of the lip liner to your lips.

6. Apply your lip liner. How you apply the lip liner can change the way your lips look. You can make your lips appear bigger, smaller, rounder, or wider. Start by outlining your lips, then fill them. Here are some tips and guidelines:

- To make your lips appear smaller, apply the lip liner to just inside the lip line. Apply some concealer around your lips to hide your natural lip line.
- To make your lips appear bigger, apply the lip liner to just outside your lip line; it should still be touching your natural lip line.
- To make your lips appear wider, apply the lip liner along your natural lip line, but then extend it just past the corners of your lips. To make them appear narrower, do the same thing, but apply the lip liner to just inside the corners. Conceal your natural lip line with some concealer.
- To make either the upper or bottom lip appear fuller, apply the lip liner to just outside the lip line. Stay within the lip line for the rest of your lips.
- For a softer, more natural look, tap the lip liner on the corners of your lips with your finger. This will help soften any sharp edges.

Part 2

Applying the Lipstick

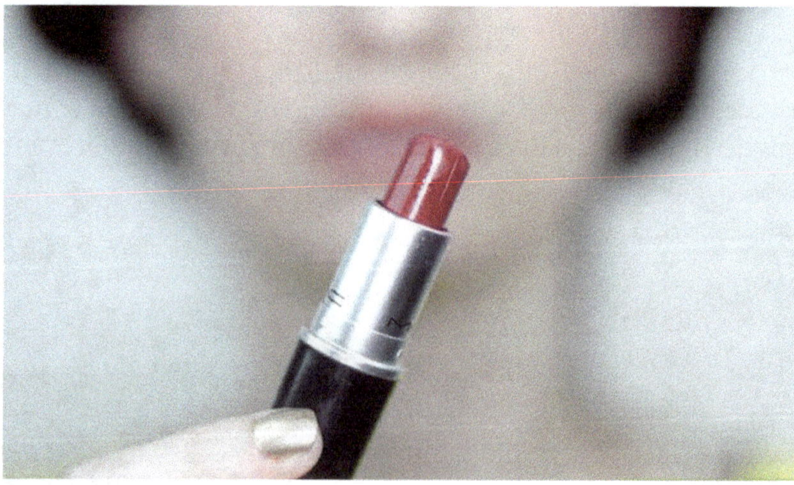

1. Consider choosing a lipstick color that compliments your complexion. You'll be a lot happier with the results of your lipstick application if you understand which lipstick shades and compositions complement your skin tone and texture. Keep these factors in mind when you're picking out lipstick:

- If you're dark-skinned, choose a bold color that provides a pretty contrast. If you're pale-skinned a lighter pink or neutral color may stand out enough for you. For a medium complexion, go for mauve, cinnamon or plum.
- If your lips are on the dry side, you may not want to use matte lipsticks since matte lipsticks can dry lips out. Look for lipsticks that contain emollients and conditioners or use a lip primer to create a barrier between the lipstick and the skin of your lips.
- If you have thin lips and want to make them appear larger, avoid using very dark colors; they tend to make lips appear smaller.

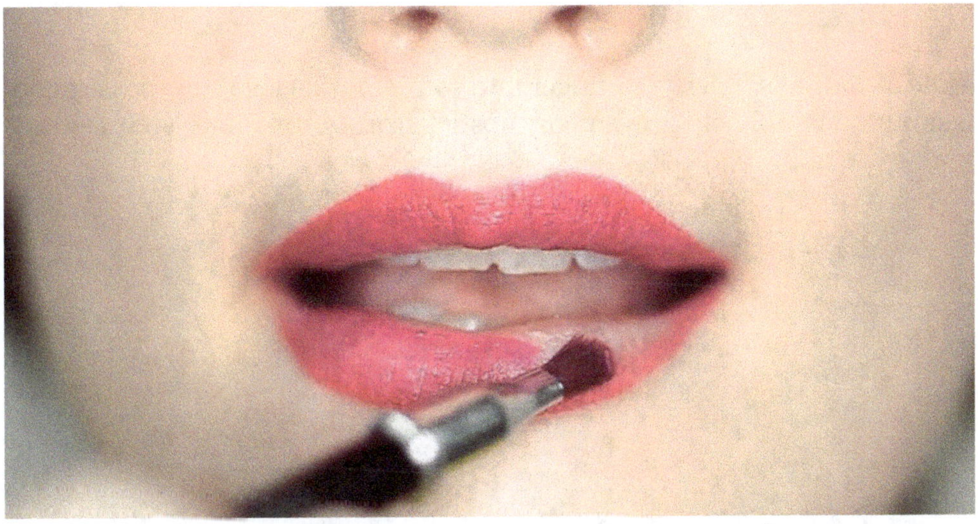

2. Apply the lipstick. Start from the center of your lips and brush the lipstick outward, filling in all the gaps. You can apply the lipstick directly from the tube, or you can use a lipstick brush for more precision.

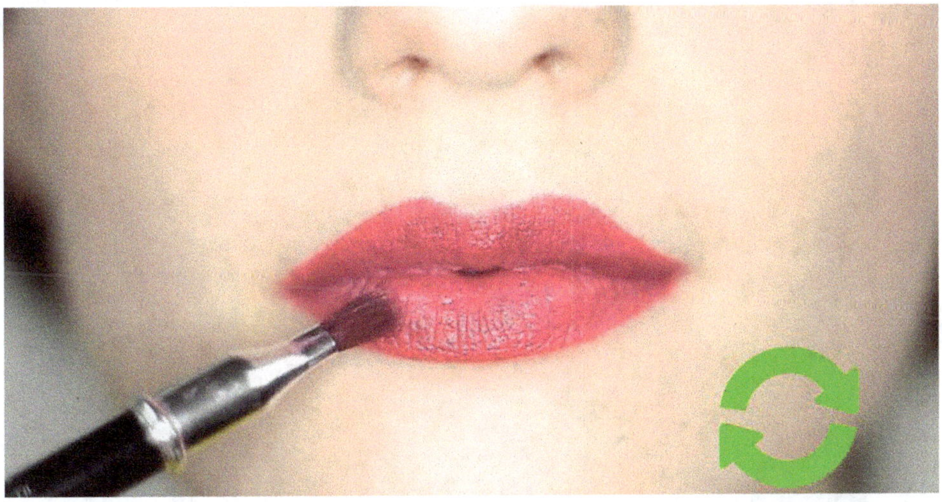

3. Put on a second coat. The first one acted as a sort of base; this second coat will give you a lasting, more intense color.

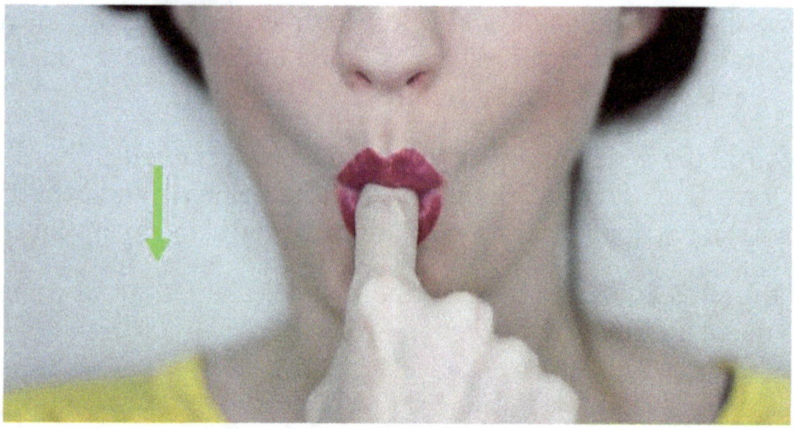

4. Blot the inside of your lips. Stick your finger into your mouth, close your lips around it, and then pull your finger out. This will help prevent any lipstick from getting onto your teeth.

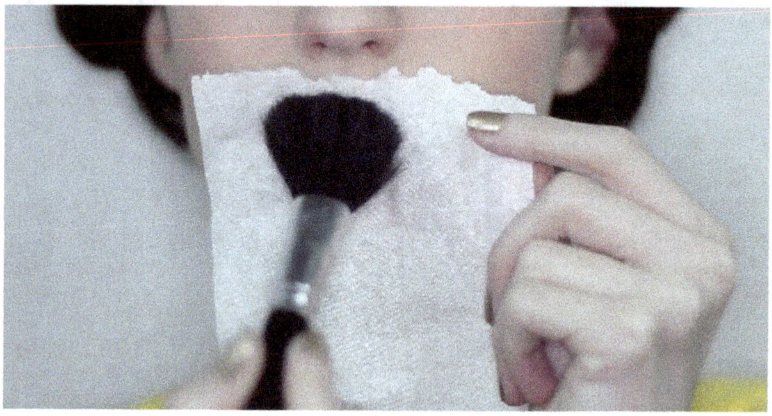

5. Make your lipstick last longer by dusting it with powder. Gently pull a tissue apart so that you end up with two, thin sheets. Press one of the sheets against your lips and lightly dust it with some translucent setting powder. Pull the tissue away and apply a second coat of lipstick.

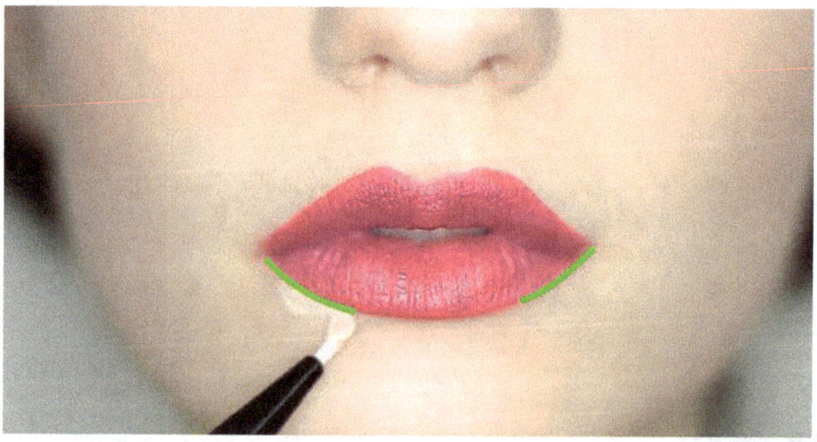

6. Clean the outer edges of your lips with some concealer. Dip a thin brush into a concealer that matches your skin tone, then outline your lips with it. Blend it outward into your foundation. It will not only give your lips a nice, crisp outline, but it will also prevent the lipstick from smearing.

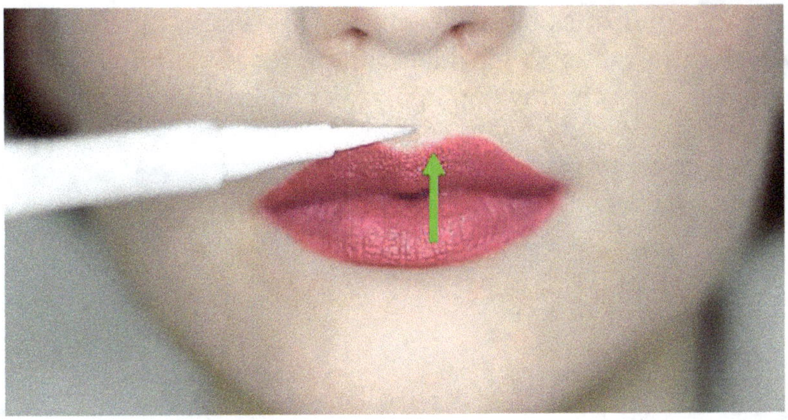

7. Consider using a highlighting pencil on your cupid's bow. This will help accentuate the natural shape of your lip. Simply outline your cupid's bow using a white or ivory pencil. Do not draw over the lipstick; draw above it.

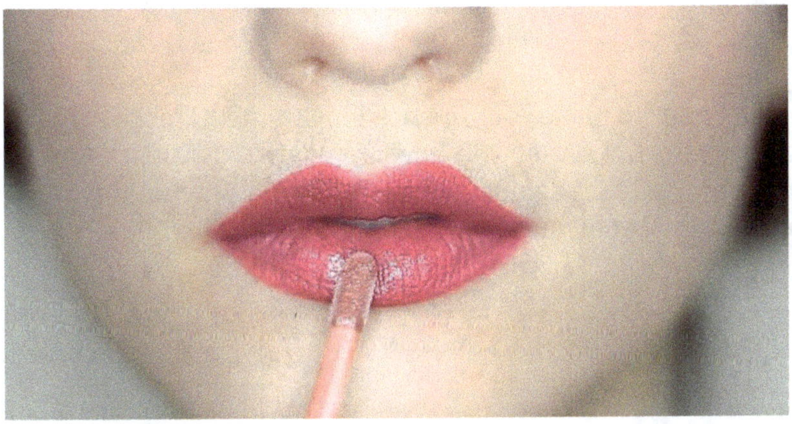

8. Try adding some shimmer with lip gloss. It is not necessary, but it will add some sparkle and shine. It will also help your lips appear plumper. You do not need to apply the lip gloss all over your lips; you can just dab a small amount to the center of your bottom lip.

Part 3

Trying Classic Variations

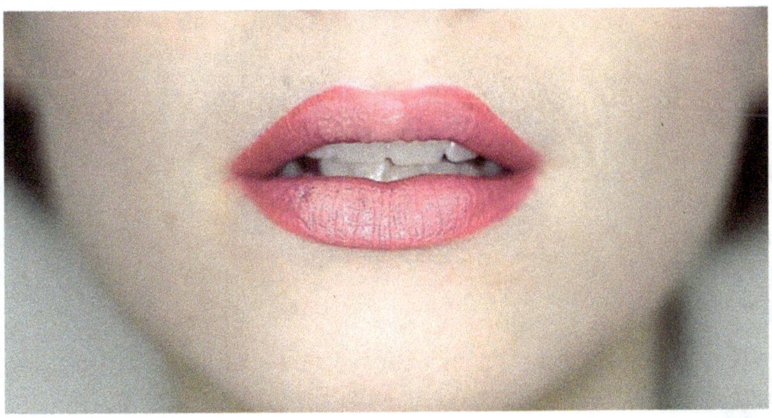

1. Use two different shades of lipstick to make your lips appear plumper. Apply your usual lipstick to your lips, but use a slightly lighter shade down the center of your upper and bottom lip. Be sure to blend well. You can also use a creamy highlighter pencil instead.

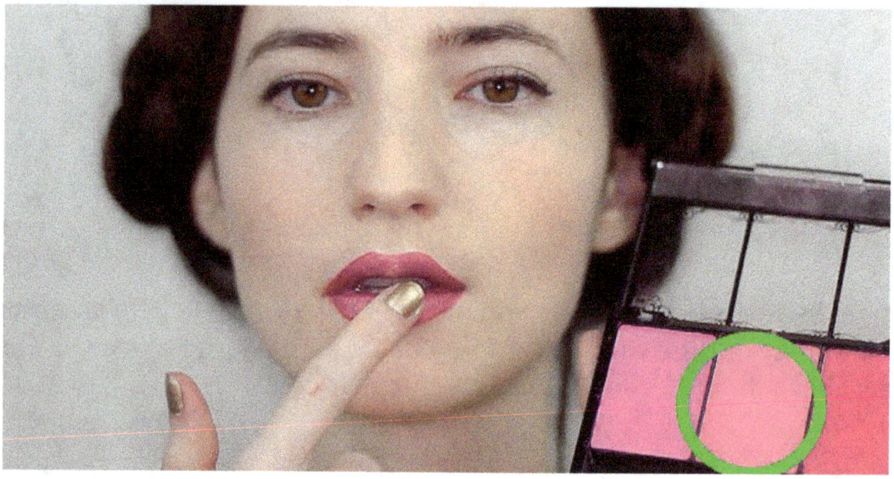

2. Use blush in a similar color to make your lipstick look matte. Choose a matte, powder blush that is the same color as your lipstick. After you have applied your lipstick and lip liner, sweep your finger across the blush and press it against your lips. Keep applying the blush this way until it is completely covering your lips, and your lipstick is matte.

- Do not use shimmery blush.
- This will not work for all lipstick colors; it is only dependant on what colors of blush are available.
- If you cannot find blush in the right color, you can try using matte eye shadow in a matching color instead.

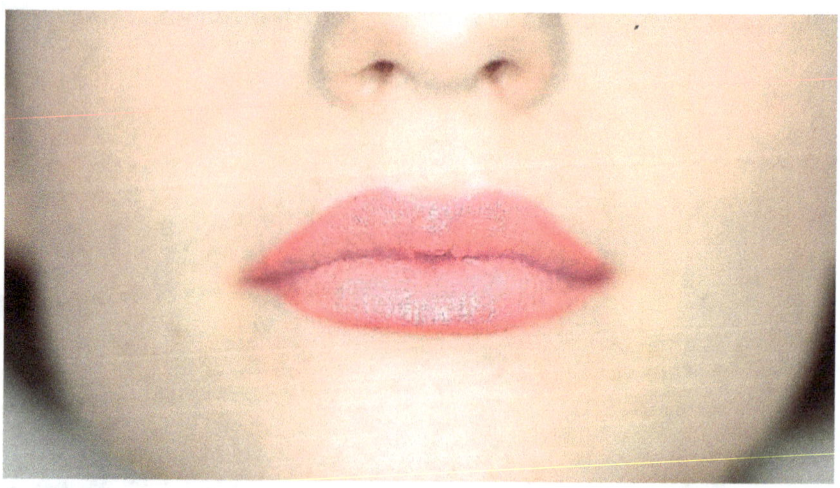

3. Create ombre lips. Choose a lip liner color that is darker than your lipstick color. Outline your lips using this lip liner, then fill your lips in with your lipstick. For an even more exaggerated om-

bre effect, apply an even lighter shade of lipstick to the innermost part of your lips. Blend everything together by applying a clear gloss.

- For a reverse ombre, use a lip liner that is lighter than your lipstick, and outline your lips with it. Fill your lips in with your lipstick; for a more exaggerated look, apply an even darker shade of lipstick to the innermost part of your lips.

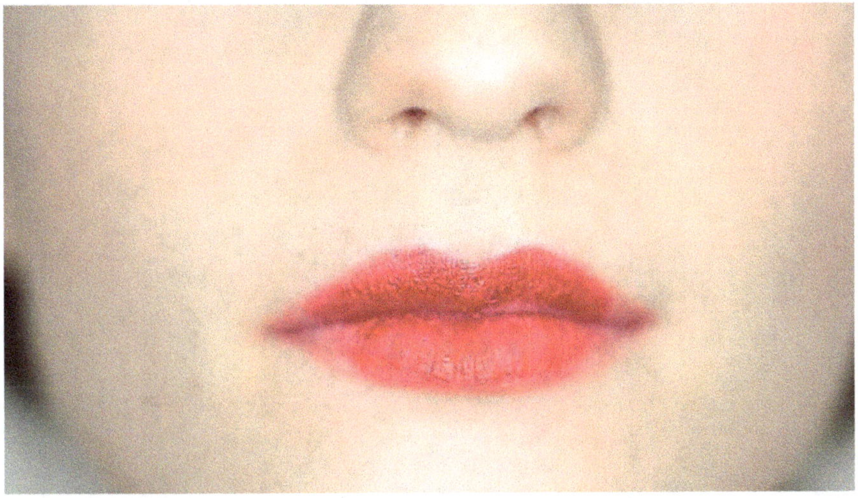

4. Create rosebud lips. This chic, feminine look was popular in the flapper era. It's perfect for a theme party or nights when you want to try something new. Outline the middle of your lips, but stop short of the corners. Fill in the outline with a bright red lipstick. Finish the look with a 1930s finger wave hairstyle.

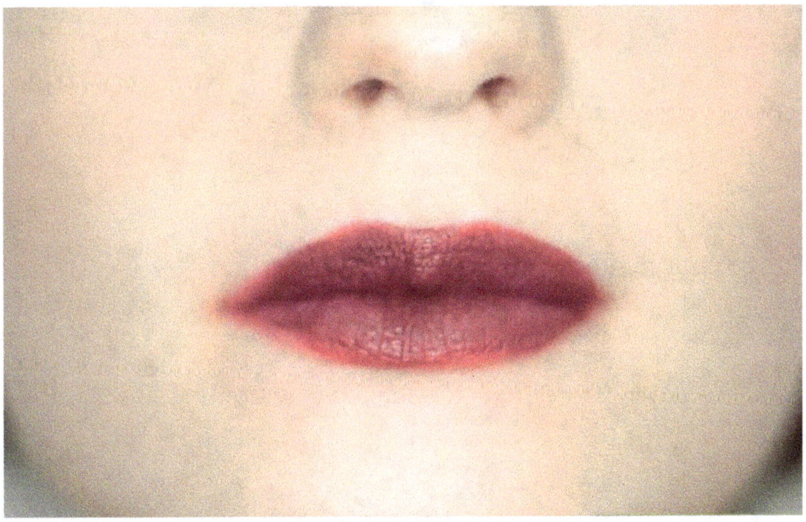

5. Go for goth. Choose a dark lip shade like black, dark red, or maroon. Find a lip liner that matches the lipstick color and outline your lips with it. Fill your lips in using the lip liner, then apply the lipstick. Wear this style with a goth outfit and hairdo.

How to Apply Lipstick with a Makeup Brush

Here is The Method for Applying Lipstick with a Makeup Brush.

Steps

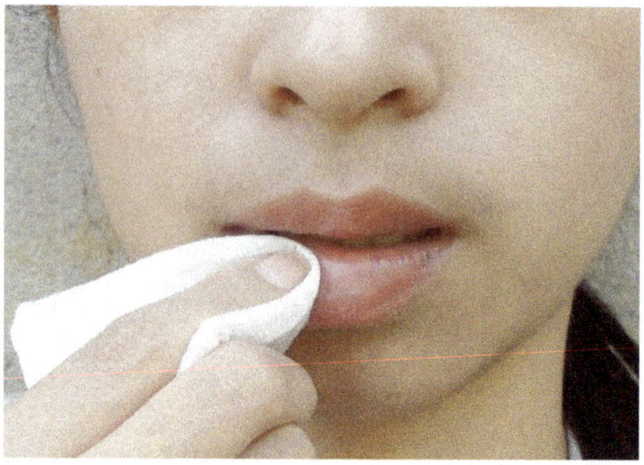

1. Clean your lips.

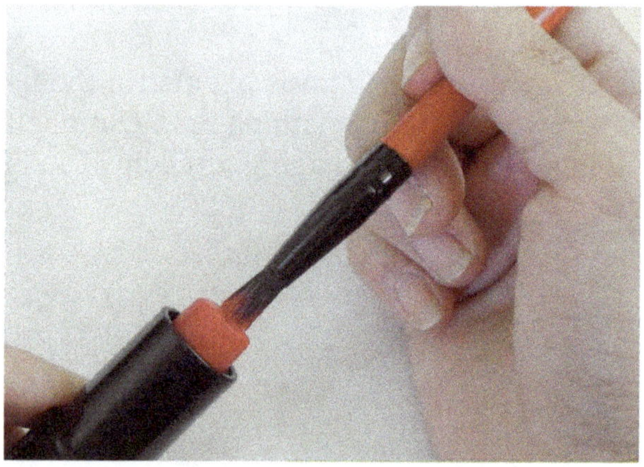

2. Add a little lipstick to your makeup brush.

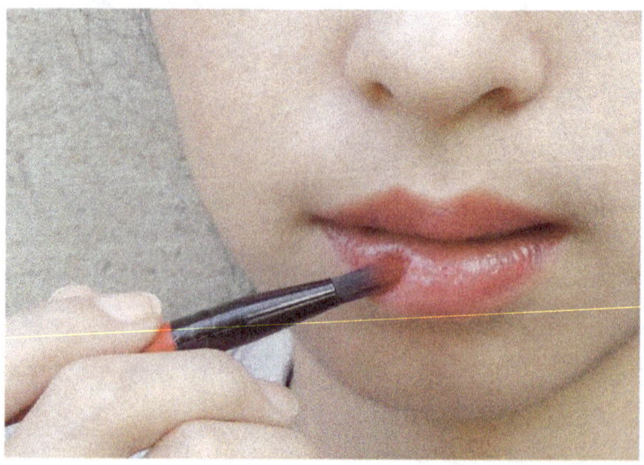

3. Brush the lipstick color onto your lips. Be careful not to press too hard or you might damage your lips. Simply put the brush on your lips and move it gently.

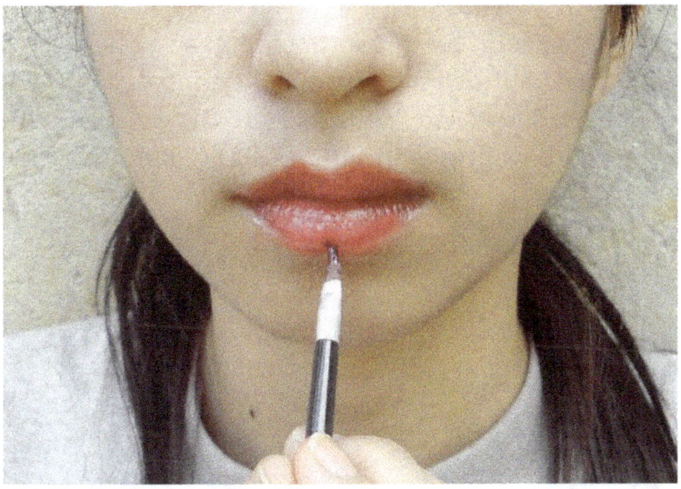

4. Use painting brush. Put lip gloss at the tip of it, then use it like a lip liner. If you want to make your lips look much bigger, put more on your lower lips.

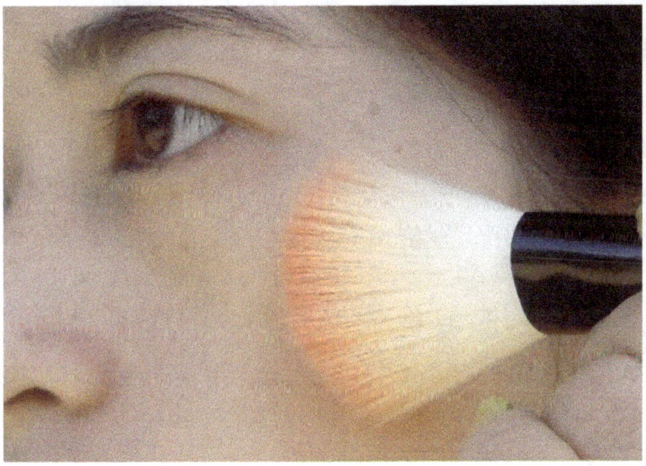

5. Put some purple lip gloss on a bigger brush. Put it on your cheeks and chin to look gorgeous.

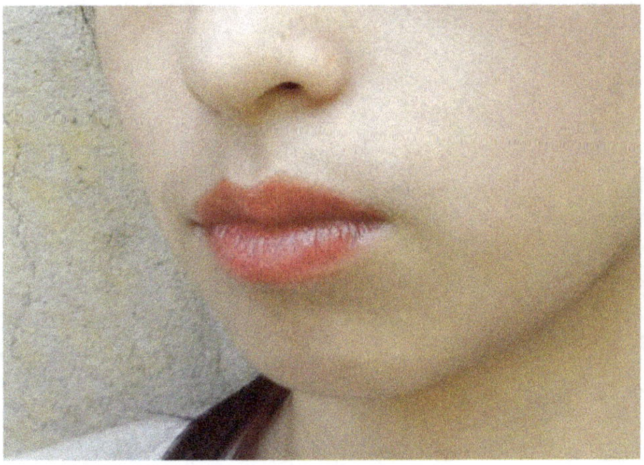

How to Blur your Lipstick

The blurred lipstick trend appeared on the runways several seasons ago and the look is still going strong. The effect is achieved by creating an intentionally soft focus lip, without the definition that lipstick and lip liners typically produce. After muting your natural lip color with concealer, a bright lipstick hue is applied to the center of the bottom lip and blended out so the color does not reach the lip line, creating a soft hazy stain.

Part 1

Creating a Muted Base

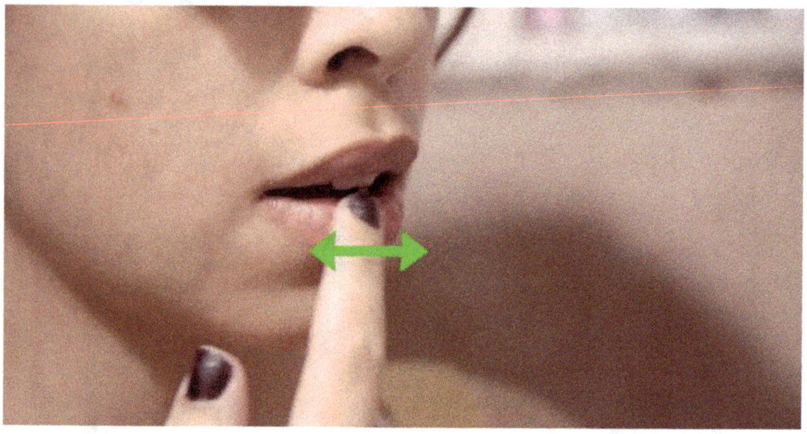

1. Exfoliate your lips with a scrub. The blurred lipstick look can emphasize lip flaws and dryness, especially if you use matte lipstick, so exfoliate them first with a gentle lip scrub. Dry and peeling skin will be removed, leaving your lips smooth and soft – the perfect canvas for applying lipstick.

- If you don't own a lip scrub product, whip one up at home. Mix a small amount of sugar with equal parts olive oil and honey, then gently massage your lips with the mixture for about 60 seconds.
- The lips are very delicate, so use a light touch when applying a scrub.

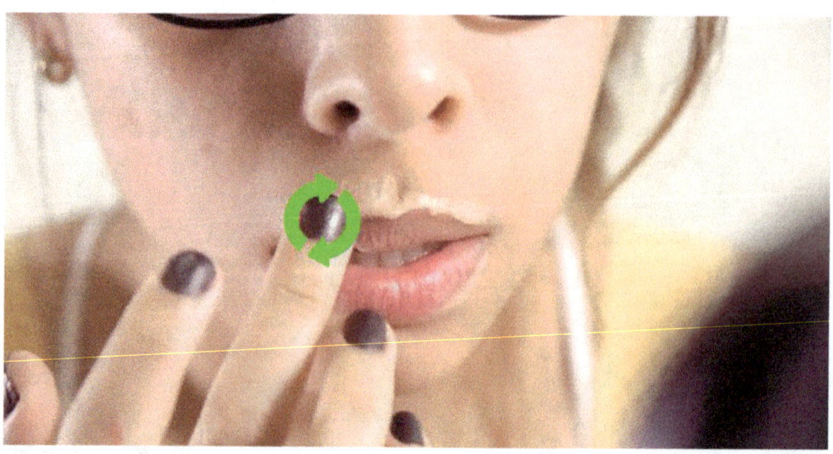

2. Mute your natural lip color with concealer. Dab a small amount of concealer around your lip line. Use a makeup brush or your finger to gently blend the concealer into your skin. Work the makeup slightly above your lip line, and then blend it right below the lip line, so that the majority of your natural lip color is obscured.

- For those with dry lips, it may help to apply lip balm or a tiny dab of coconut oil to your lips for moisture before you add concealer, which can be drying.
- If you don't have concealer on hand, a nude lipstick is a great substitute. This will be a little more moisturizing, as well.

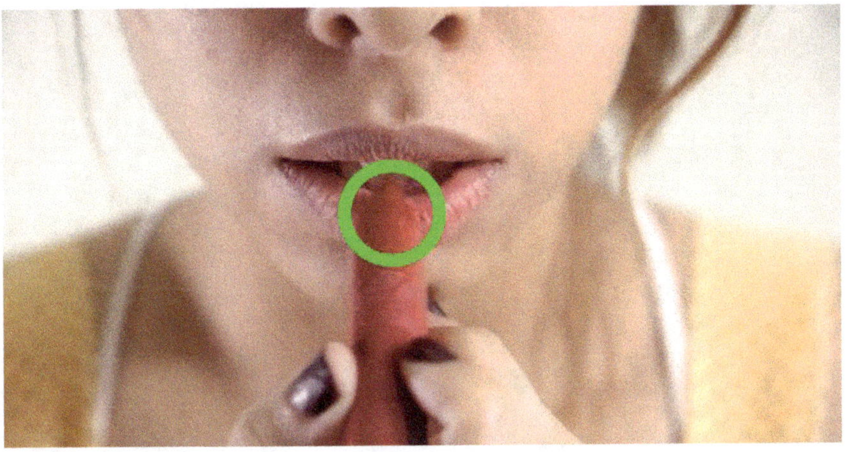

3. Apply a bright lipstick shade to the center of your bottom lip. Popular hues are deep berry or bright red, but you can use any highly pigmented lipstick color you like. Use the fleshy part of your index finger or a lip brush to dab the lipstick right in the center of your bottom lip. Make sure you apply it so that it reaches the very inside edge of your lips.

- Do not apply the lipstick close to your lip line or bring it out to the corners of your mouth.
- To get an intensely blurry result, use a lipstick with a matte finish. However, any finish you like will work for this look.

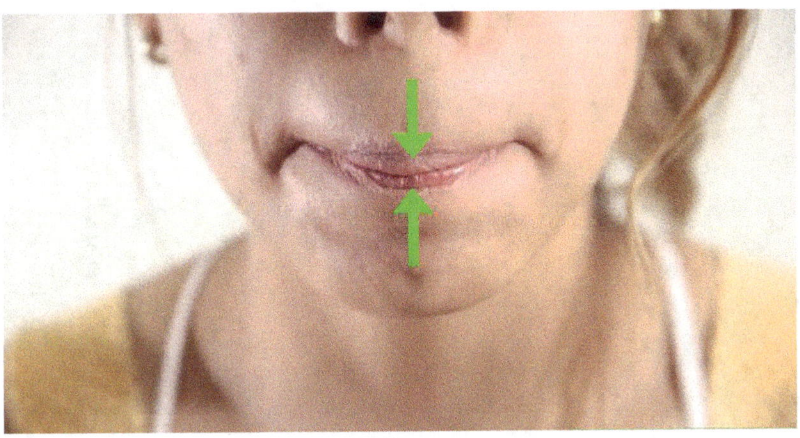

4. Press your lips together. This will transfer some of the bright color to the center of your top lip. Do not rub your lips together or smack them. Press them together once or twice with a small

amount of pressure. Then use your finger or a lip brush to pat a small amount of lipstick in the center of your bottom lip again, to play up the contrast and add depth.

- For a more intense result, tap a loose pigment in a similar or slightly amped up color right in the center of the bottom lip.

Part 2

Blurring the Color

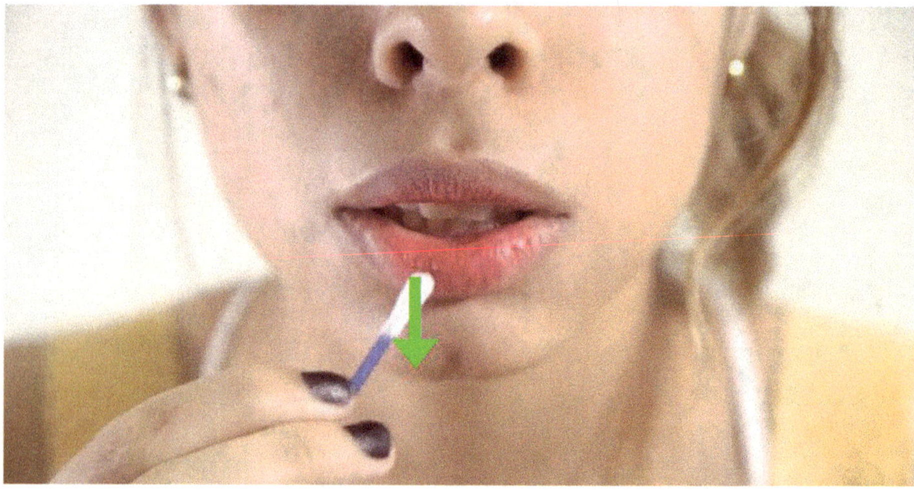

1. Blur the lipstick out toward your lip line. Working with a lip brush or cotton swab will give you the most precision and control, but your finger also works well. Pat the lipstick gently, blending it out toward your lip line on the bottom lip. Do the same for your upper lip. Try to blend so that the hue appears as a gradient, with the brightest color right in the center, and growing increasingly fainter as it gets closer to the lip line.

- Keep blending until the lipstick appears to fade into your skin.

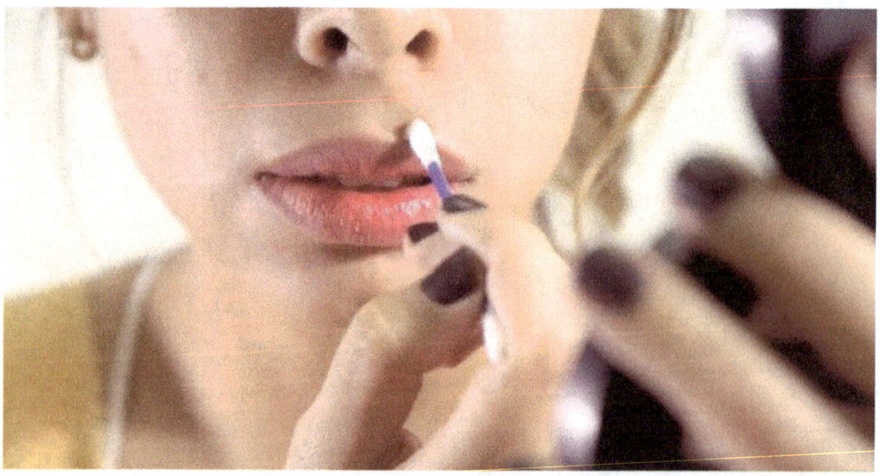

2. Use translucent powder to intensify the effect. Dip a clean cotton swab into translucent face powder, then tap it against the edge of your compact or sink so that the excess falls off. Dab the end

of the cotton swap around the outermost edges of your lips, following your lip line. Flip the swab over to the clean end and gently blur the powder into your mouth.

- Imagine that you're trying to "erase" the appearance of your lip line. Blend it gently, taking care to preserve the gradient effect you created with the lipstick.

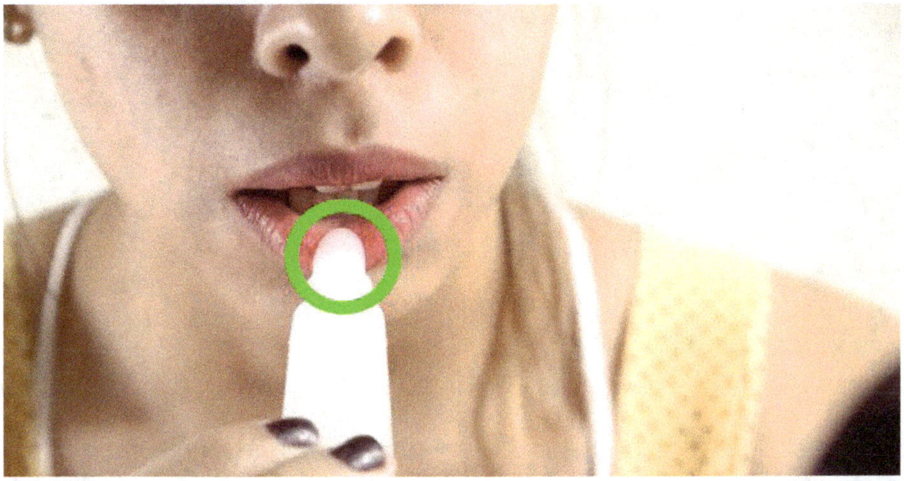

3. Finish with lip gloss, if desired. A matte finish will have a more blurred effect, but adding gloss will intensify the bright color in the center and create more dimension. Dab the lip gloss on lightly, taking care not to smudge or change the work you've done with your lipstick. Use your finger to pat the gloss all over your lips.

Part 3

Experimenting with Other Variations

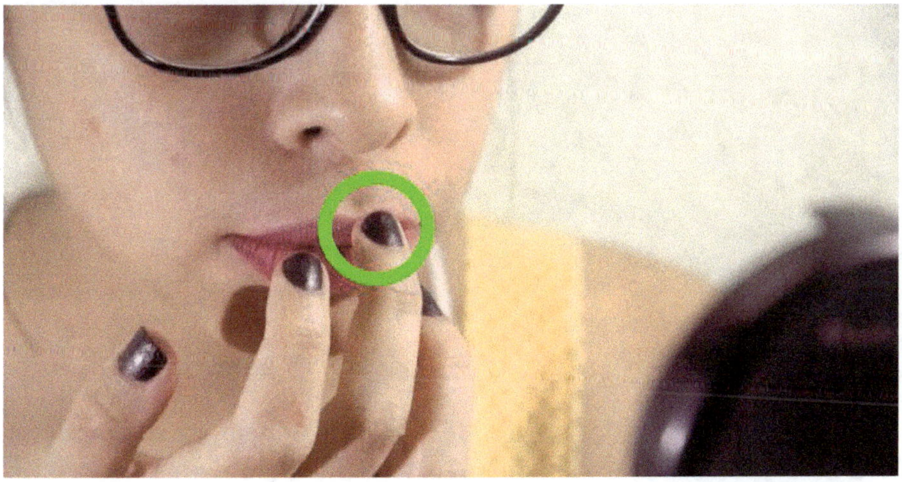

1. Try the faded lipstick trend. This is very similar to the blurred look, but less pigmented. It creates more of a washed out effect and the illusion of thinner lips. Apply a matte lipstick in a bright color all over your lips, as you normally would. Pat a small amount of translucent powder on top and then blot your lips on a tissue to mute the color. Pat concealer around the other edges of your mouth to remove the definition of your lip line.

- Do not apply lip gloss or balm on top of the lipstick, since this will ruin the faded effect.This look is meant to de-emphasize the fullness and color of the lips.

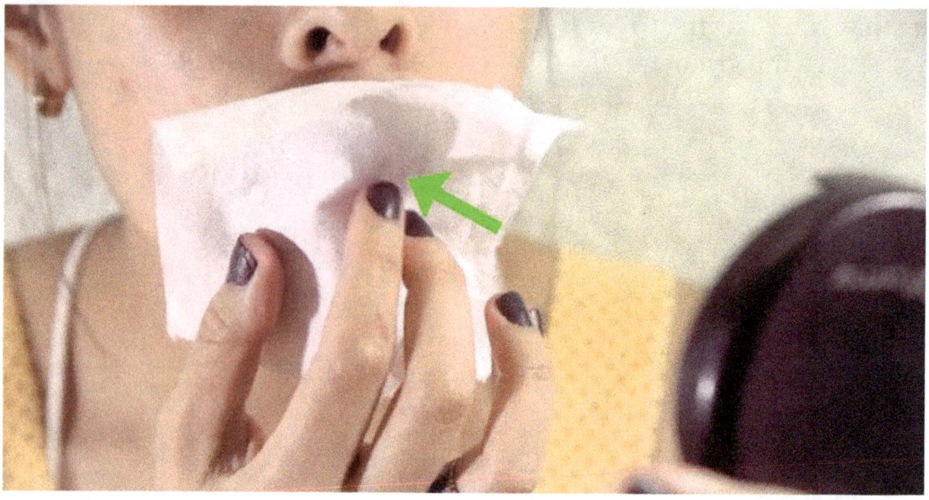

2. Create an undone "stained" look. This is a very subtle look and the technique involves working backwards, applying pigment and then removing most of it. Apply your favorite lipstick to your lips, as usual. Use only a thin layer, or use your finger or lip brush to control the amount of lipstick you use. Hold a tissue over your lips and use your fingers to press down several times, which will blot away pigment.

- Lift the tissue to check your progress. If necessary, keep blotting until your lips have achieved a barely there "stained" appearance.

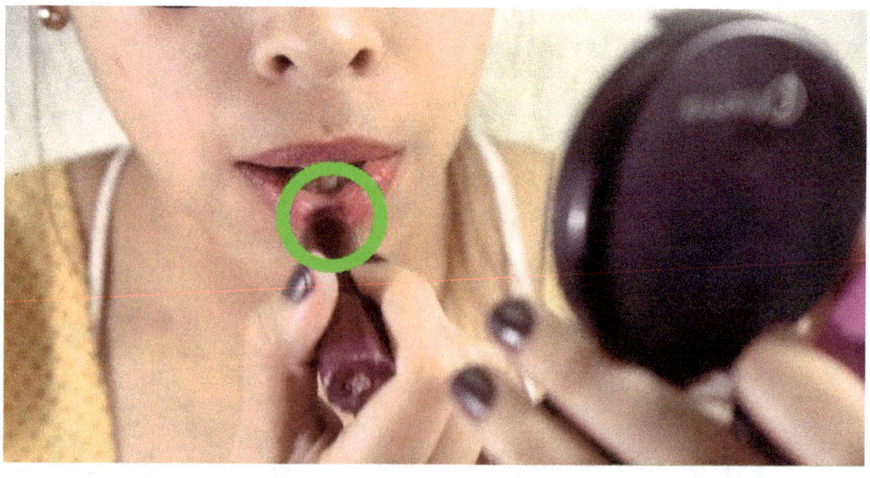

3. Try a dramatized version of the blurred lipstick trend. Apply a lip balm that has a subtle hint of color, such as a berry hue, all over your lips. Then apply a highly pigmented lipstick in a dark wine or berry color to the center of both lips. Dab the lipstick, but do not rub or blend it in. Avoid bringing the color out to the corners of your mouth.

- If the result looks too dramatic for you, blend out the lipstick slightly. However, the effect is intended to be obvious and unnatural.

Lip Liner

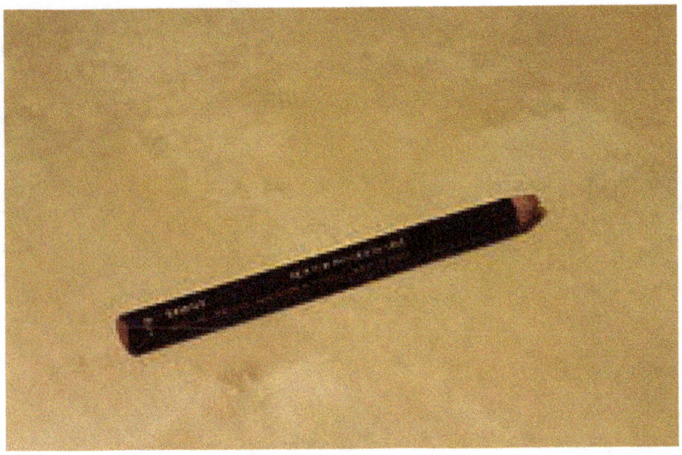

Lip liner

Lip liner, also known as lip pencil, is a cosmetic product. It is intended to fill uneven areas on the outer edges of the lips before applying Prost lipstick, therefore giving a smooth shape. It is also used to outline the lips, keeping lipstick inside the lip area and preventing it from "bleeding", therefore creating a bigger contrast and making the lips stand out more. Alternatively, lip liner can be used to fill in the entire lip before the application of lipstick and in some cases, worn as a lipstick on its own. The product is usually sold in a retractable tube or pencil form which can be sharpened. Lip liner is usually available in the same range of colors as lipsticks: e.g., reds, pinks, browns, plums, etc. Lip liner also comes in invisible, for giving the illusion of smooth lips without adding or affecting color.

Ingredients

Like lipstick, lip liner is composed of waxes, oils, and pigments. Compared to lipstick, lip liners are firmer in consistency and deeply pigmented, making them suitable for drawing on to the lip with precision. For these reasons, lip liners have less oils and more waxes and pigments than a lipsticks. A popular wax is Japan wax.

Brands

Designer brands such as Chanel, Dior, and Marc Jacobs produce their own lip liners. Other brands include but are not limited to Urban Decay, Clinique, and MAC Cosmetics.

How to Apply Lip Liner

Applying lip liner correctly can be a challenge for even the most experienced makeup user. Done correctly it can increase the wear of your lipstick, prevent color feathering, prevent color bleeding, provide more definition to your lips, and enhance or hide lip features.

Part 1

Preparing to Line Your Lips

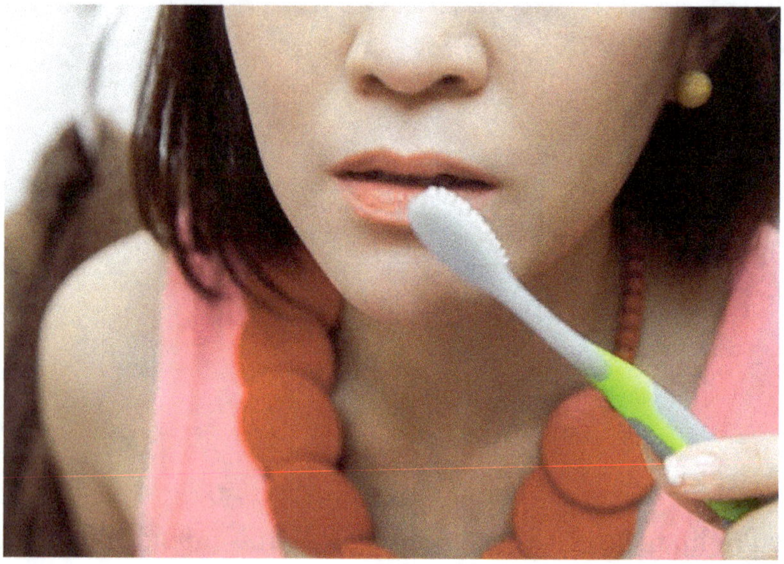

1. Exfoliate your lips (optional). If you don't have an exfoliating balm or scrub (available at most drug stores and shops that sell makeup), you can exfoliate your lips by applying a moisturizing lip balm and then gently scrubbing them with a clean toothbrush.

- Some experts recommend against exfoliating your lips, as this can cause small tears in the skin of your lips, making them dry and chapped in the long term.
- Having healthy, well moisturized lips is better than exfoliating your lips, but if your lips are flakey, exfoliating is a quick way to make them smooth.

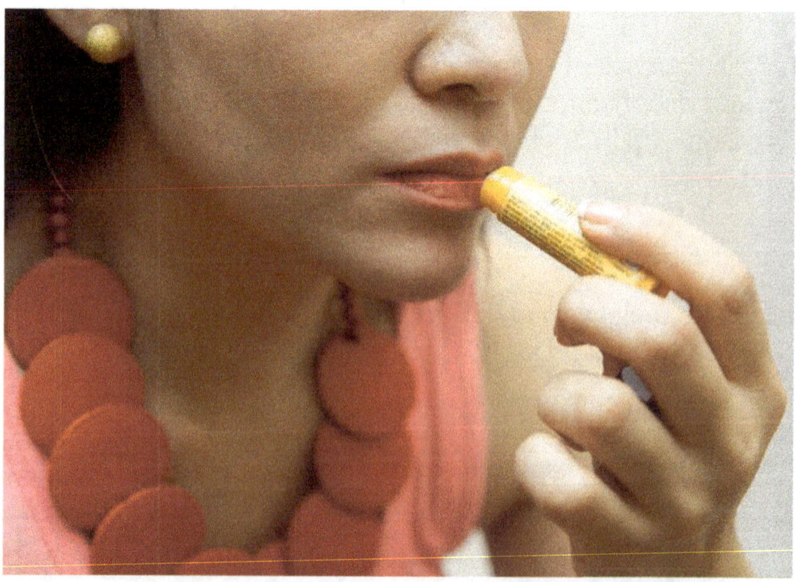

2. Moisturize your lips. Before applying anything else to your lips, apply a light moisturizing balm. Make sure the balm isn't too waxy — you want it to sink into your lips, not sit on top of them.

- If your lips are dry, chapped, or cracked, it will be difficult to apply a smooth line to them, particularly if you intend to fill them in completely with liner.

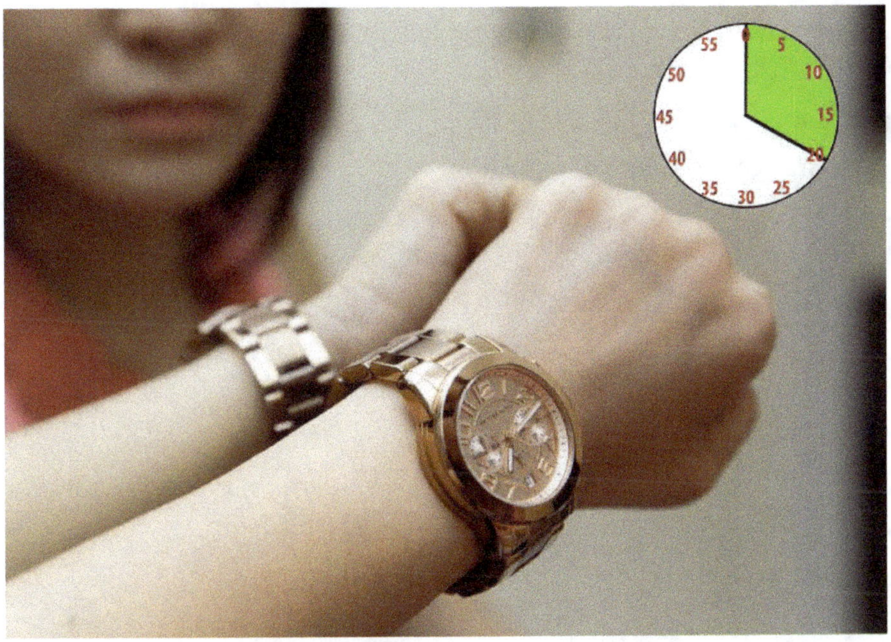

3. Wait for the balm to dry. Some experts recommend waiting 20 minutes to apply anything else to your lips after putting on a moisturizer.

- If you don't have that kind of time, wait at least a couple of minutes, and then dab your lips with tissue to remove any excess moisturizer.
- You want your lips to dry but well moisturized before you apply anything else to them.

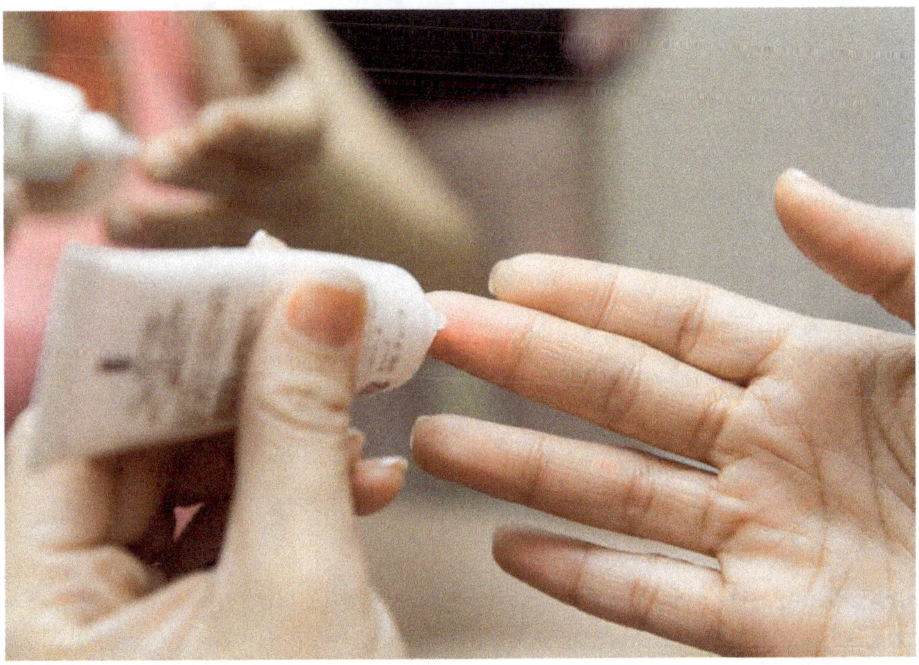

4. Prime your lips (optional). A primer isn't 100% necessary, but some makeup artists do recommend it, as it can help smooth your lips and hold both the liner and lipstick on your lips longer.

- If you intend to wear lipstick, you can apply a lip liner to your entire lips, and this will also help hold the lipstick in place.
- Concealer or foundation can be used in place of primer. These are good options if you're planning to change the shape of your lips.

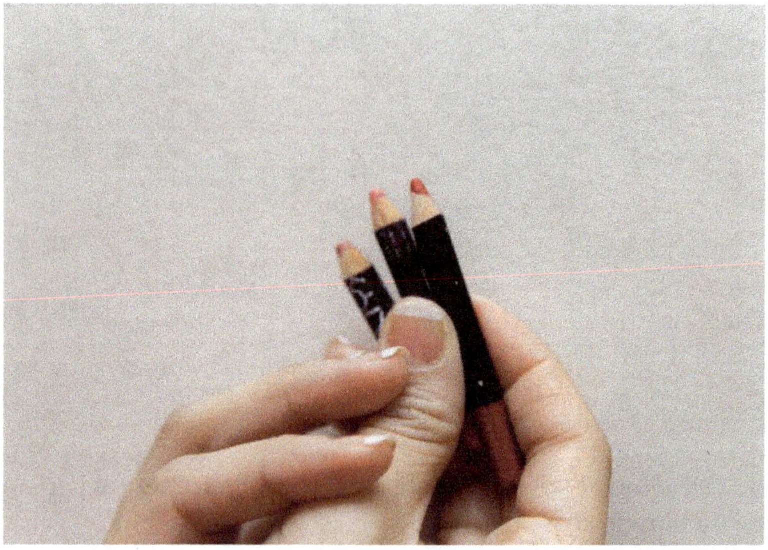

5. Choose your lip liner color. Choose your lip liner color based on what you intend to do with it. If you're planning to wear red lipstick, go for a red liner; if you're planning to keep your lips looking natural, go for a nude or soft pink liner.

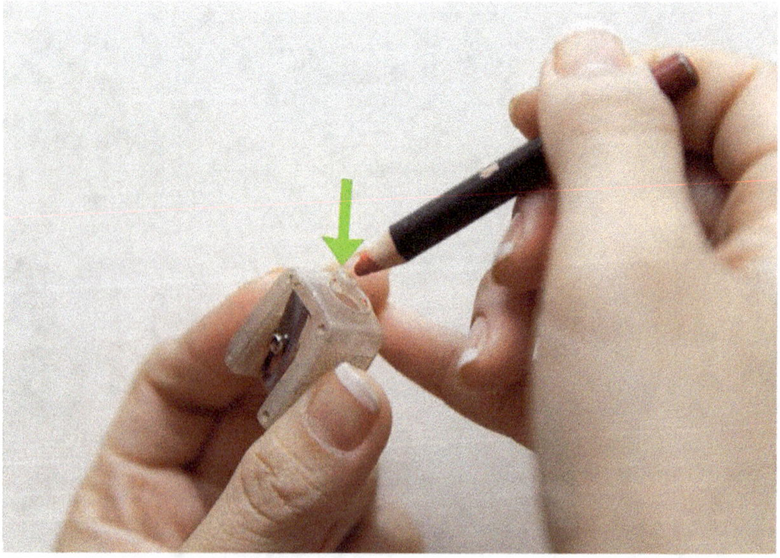

6. Sharpen your lip liner. Always sharpen your liner before using it. A sharp liner will give you a good, precise line. When your liner is dull, it's closer to the wood of the pencil, and if any pieces are sticking up from the wood they might scratch your lips.

- Some people suggest that sharpening your liner before each use removes bacteria from it.
- A trick to make sharpening easier is to place your lip pencil in the freezer 20 minutes before sharpening it. This is supposed to help prevent the tip from breaking off, and should produce a cleaner, sharper point.

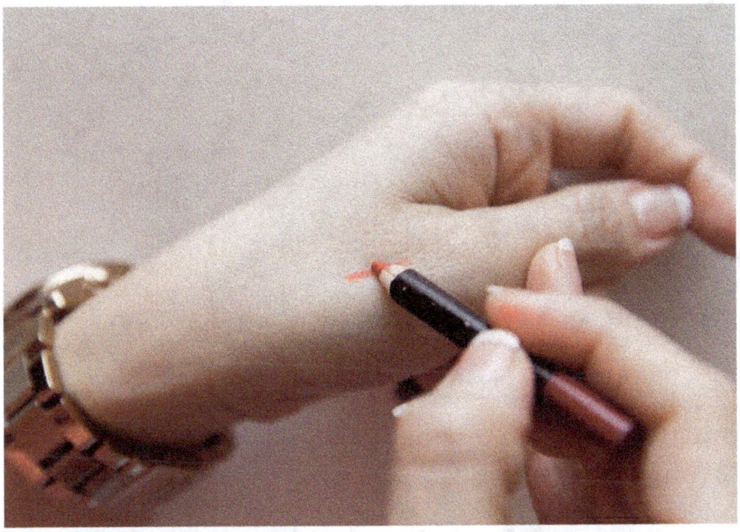

7. Warm up the lip liner. Before using your lip liner, warm up the tip by drawing on the back of your hand. This way it will go on to your lips more smoothly.

- Another way to warm up your lip liner is to rub the tip between your thumb and index finger.

Part 2

Applying Lip Liner to Your Natural Lip Line

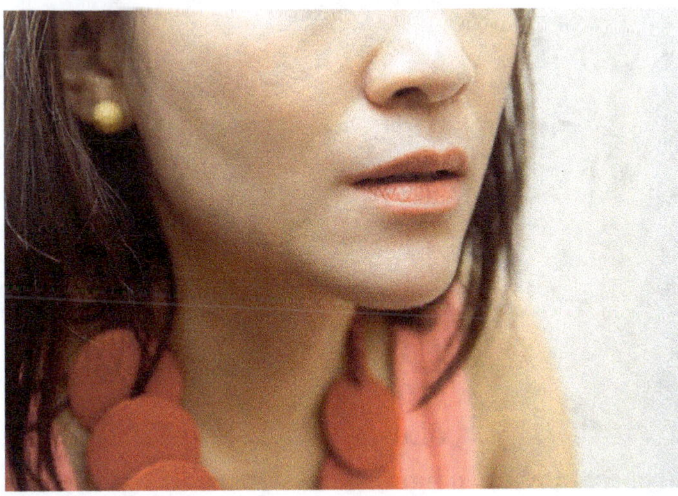

1. Part your lips slightly. Parting your lips slightly will help you stick to their natural shape as you line them.

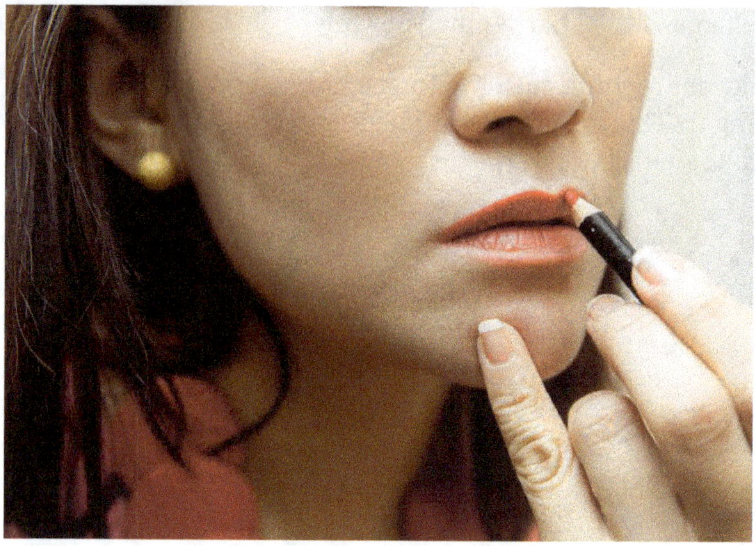

2. Trace your natural lip line. Many artists recommend sticking to your natural lip line, as overdrawn lips can look unnatural. A common thing to do is to start at the center-top and center-bottom of your lips and then work outward.

- Another common lining method is to start at the center, drawing an "x" at your cupid's bow, and then outline the corners and bottom of your mouth before lining the rest of your lips. Unless you're filling your lips in with lipstick, this isn't a good option.
- As you trace your natural lip line, be extra careful to ensure that you've applied liner to any creases or cracks in your lips; this will help prevent your lipstick from bleeding.

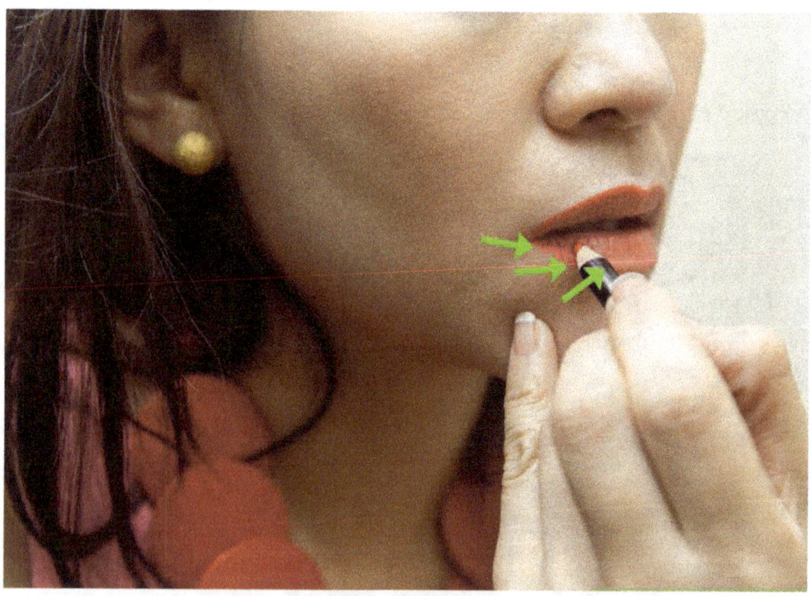

3. Move in light, short strokes. Moving in light, short strokes will give you a more precise line than trying to trace over your line in one smooth movement.

- If the liner tugs at your lips at all, it's too hard. Try warming the tip up by rolling it between your thumb and index finger, or drawing on the back of your hand; you can also see if sharpening it helps.

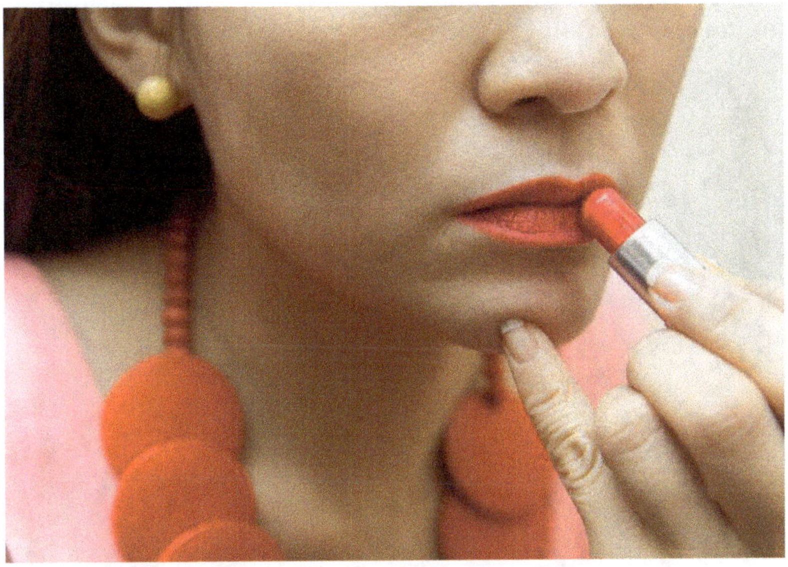

4. Complete your look. What you do after lining your lips depends on whether you plan to keep your lips looking natural, or to wear lipstick.

- If want a natural look, you'll blend the liner into your lips and follow it up with gloss.
- If you want to wear lipstick, you'll fill in your lips with liner before applying the lipstick.

Part 3

Filling in Your Lips

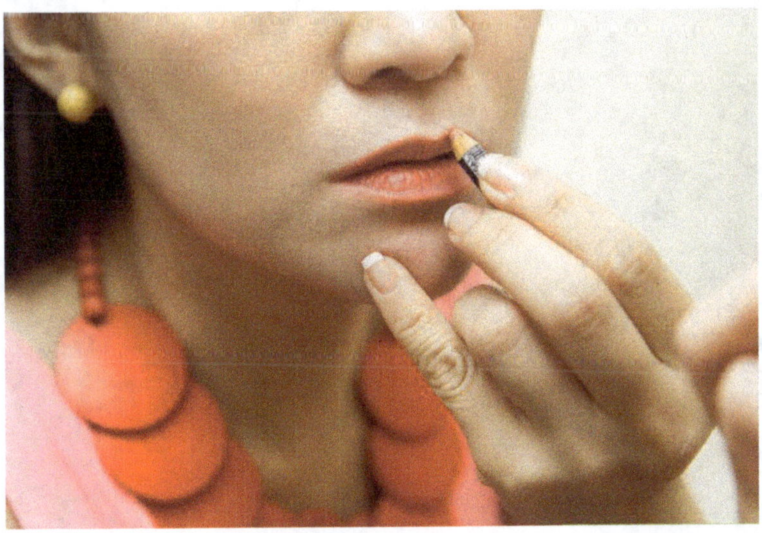

1. Blend a nude liner into your lips for a natural look (optional). If you're not wearing lipstick and simply want to use liner to define your lips, use a nude liner and then a brush to gently buff the line out into the center of your lips. You would then finish the look off with a clear gloss.

- Even if you're not wearing lipstick, a little bit of lip liner lightly applied to your natural lip line can do wonders for helping to define your lips.
- If you're going for a natural lip, your lips should now be done!

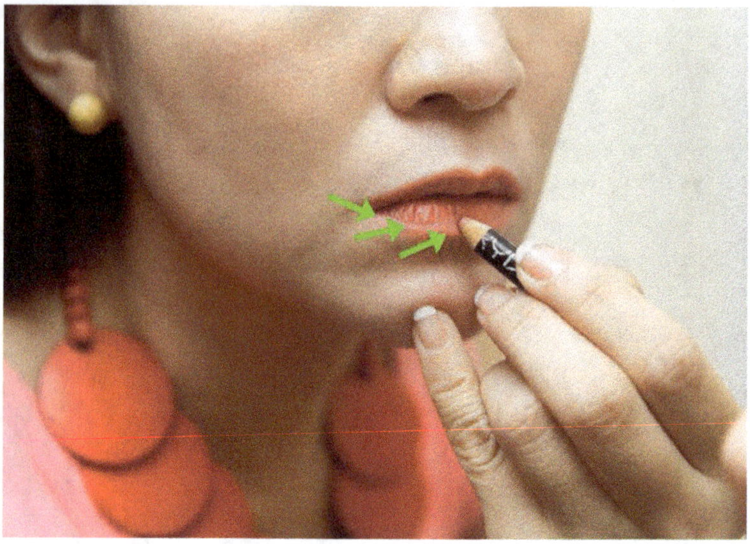

2. Fill in your lips with liner. Using swift, short strokes, fill in your entire lips with liner. This will give you a good base that will help your lipstick stay put longer. It will also help keep the lip color even, meaning the lipstick won't change color where it overlaps with the liner.

- Some people fill their lips in with liner and just wear the liner itself. If you do this, consider using a gloss or similarly colored lip balm over top of the liner to help it look smooth and even.

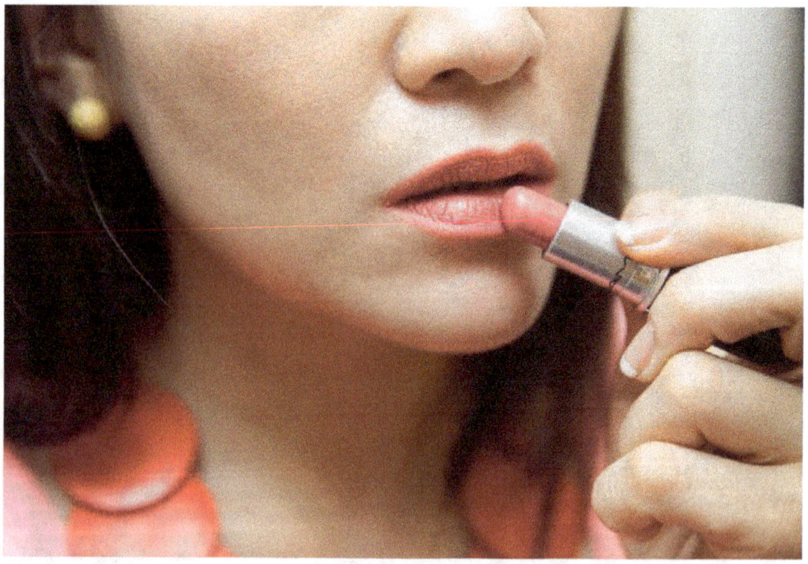

3. Apply your lipstick. Starting at the center of your lips and working outwards, apply your lipstick to your lips. For a lighter and/or more precise application, use a lip brush to apply your lipstick.

- Even if you want your lipstick to go on thick, you can use a brush — it'll just take a couple of layers to get the same thickness as using the lipstick.

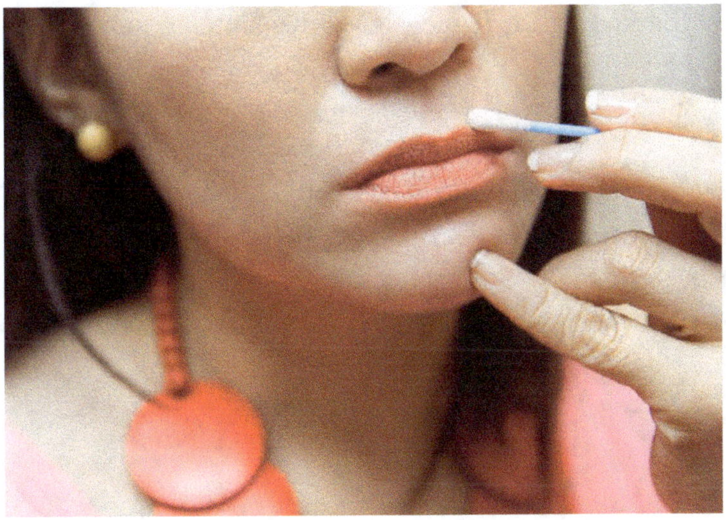

4. Refine your line. Once your lips are lined and filled, the last think you'll want to do is clean up and even out your line.

- You can clean up the line with a bit of moisturizer or makeup remover on the edge of a cotton swab or kleenex.
- If you need to refine the line, simply draw over the necessary areas with your lip liner, then use your lip brush to blend where needed.

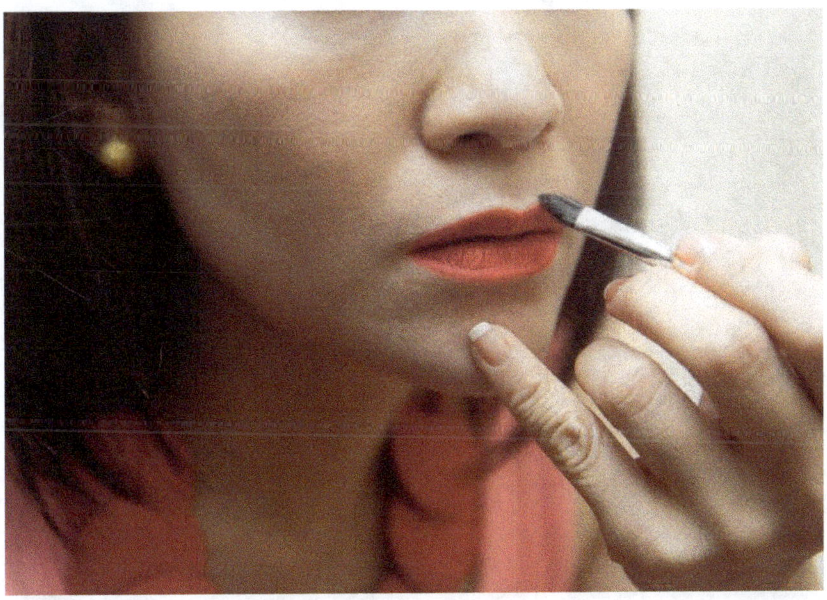

5. Apply concealer or foundation around lips (optional). This is particularly helpful if you're wearing a dramatic color that has left small stains around the edges of your lips; it also helps prevent your lip color from bleeding out to the skin around your lips.

- Use a small brush or a foundation brush to paint a small amount of concealer or foundation around your lips, as needed.
- You can also set the foundation/concealer with a small amount of powder.

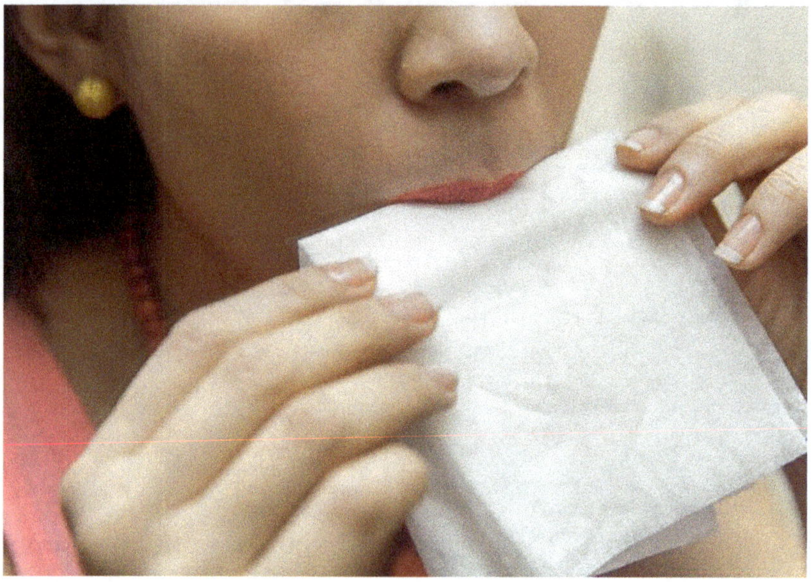

6. Blot between applications (optional). It's really common to apply one layer of lipstick, blot it and then apply another layer. To blot your lips, open them, stick some tissue or blotting paper between them, and then close them gently in an "mmm" position.

- If you're going to use tissue paper, make sure it's a thick, good-quality tissue that won't leave any bits of fluff on your lips.

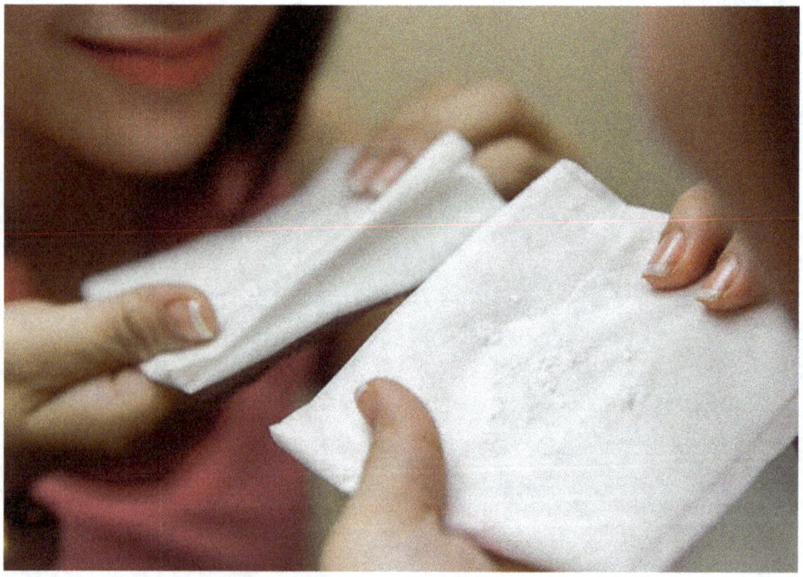

7. Set your lips (optional). Makeup artists often set lipstick by laying a thin layer of tissue over the lips and then dabbing a translucent powder over the tissue so that a small amount of powder gets on to the lips and helps hold the lipstick in place.

Part 4

Making Your Lips Look Larger

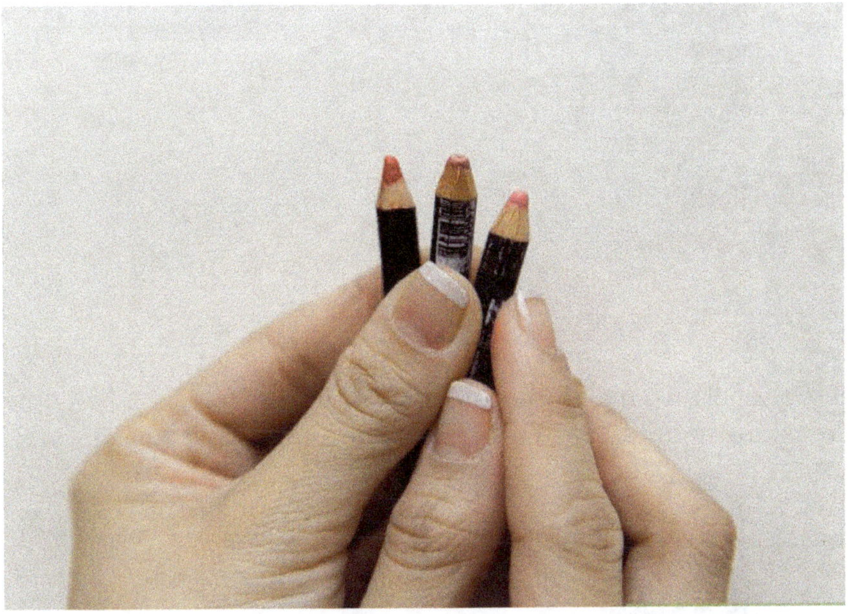

1. Choose your colors. Choose a nude liner and nude lipstick for a natural look, or a more dramatic liner and matching lipstick if you're feeling more adventurous.

- Note that darker colors and mattes can make lips look smaller.

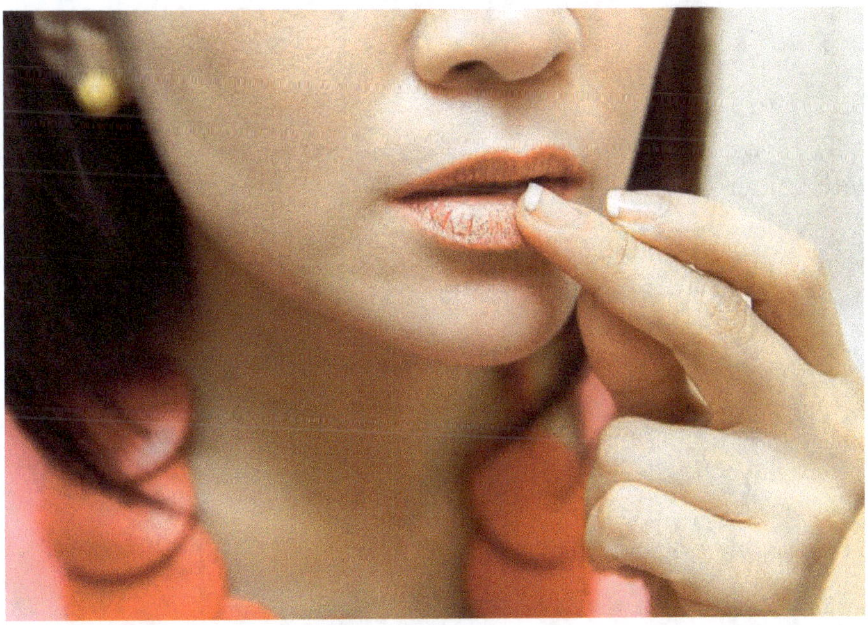

2. Apply a concealer to your lips and the surrounding area. This will help blur your natural lip line. It will also help your liner and lipstick stay put.

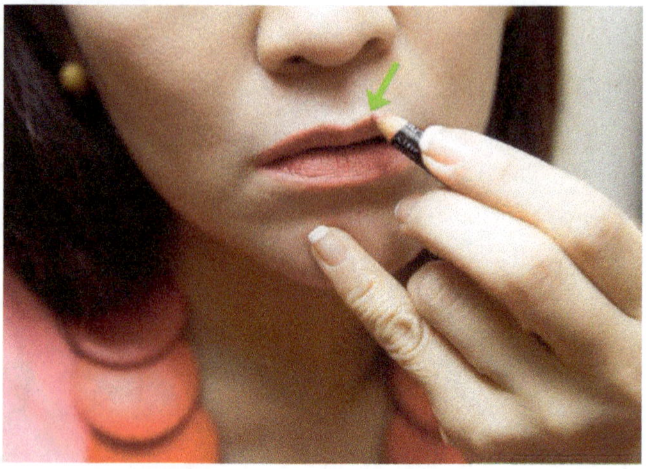

3. Keep it natural (optional). To make your lips look slightly larger, line just outside your natural lip line. To keep it looking natural, only go a very small step beyond your natural lip line.

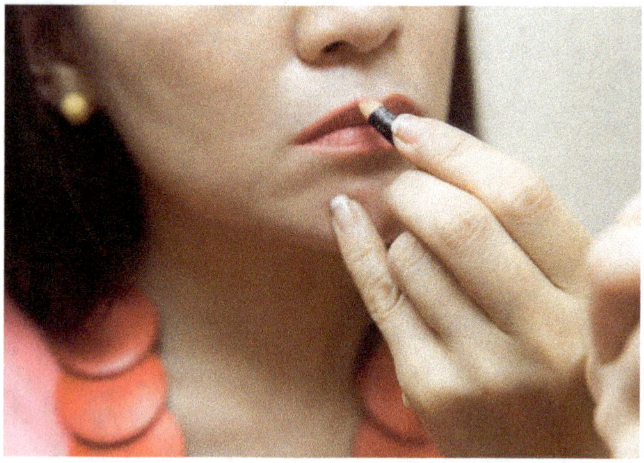

4. Go big (optional). If you want your lips to look significantly larger, you're better off using a two-toned method, with a liner that's slightly darker than your lipstick.

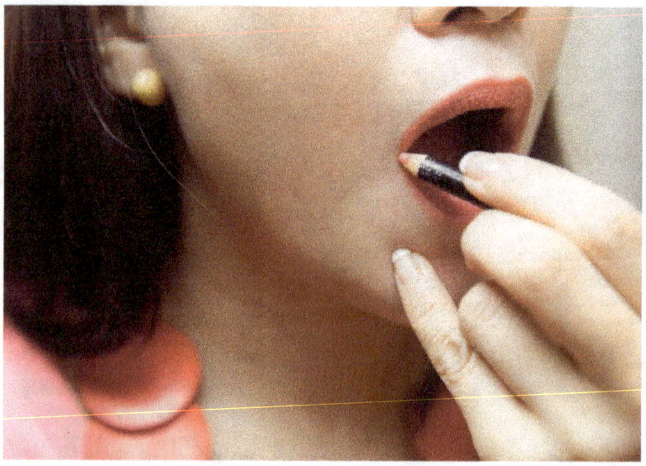

- In 2014 Kylie Jenner sported newly plumped lips with a '90s-inspired lining style of having a darker liner and a lighter lipstick. Experts say it's important to use a darker liner and then lipstick that's only slightly lighter (e.g., a burgundy liner and a cranberry lipstick) for this look.

5. Return to your natural lip line at the corners of your mouth. Regardless of what size you go, make sure that you return to your natural lip line as you near the corners of your mouth. If you don't, you'll end up with clown lips.

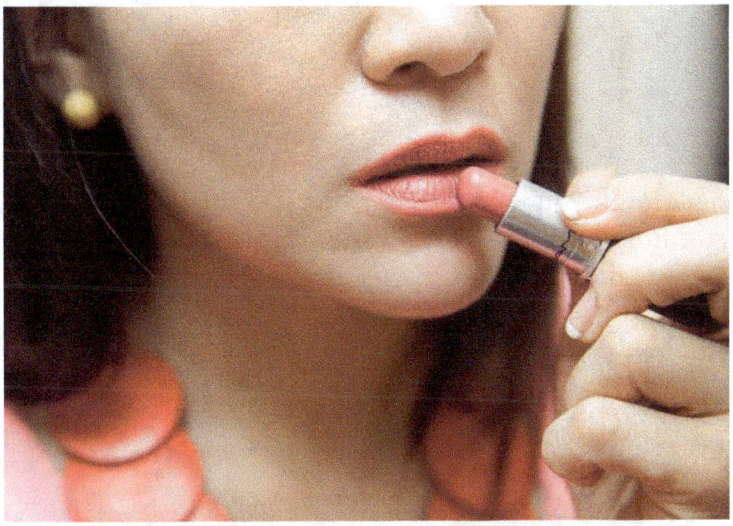

6. Heavily apply lipstick to the center of your lips. As you do this, be sure to leave space between the lipstick and the lip liner, as you'll be pulling the lipstick up into the liner and blending the two in the next step.

- Go thick with this application, as you'll need to be able to drag it up and blend it into your lip line.

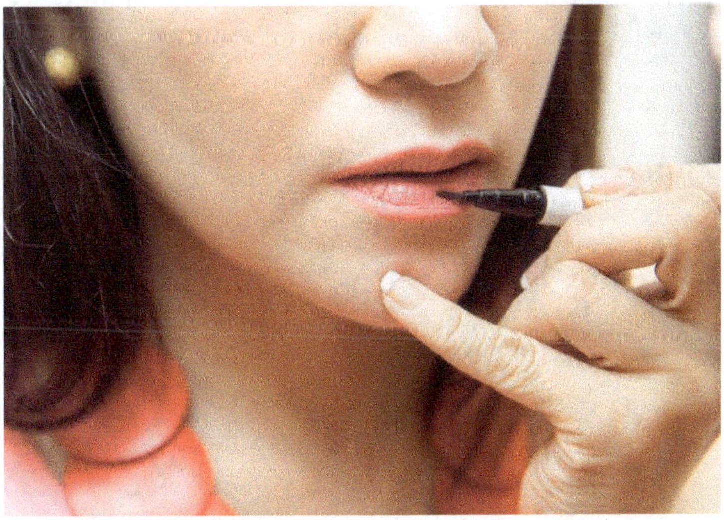

7. Blend the liner and lipstick together. Use a lip brush to pull the lipstick up to your lip liner, and blend the two.

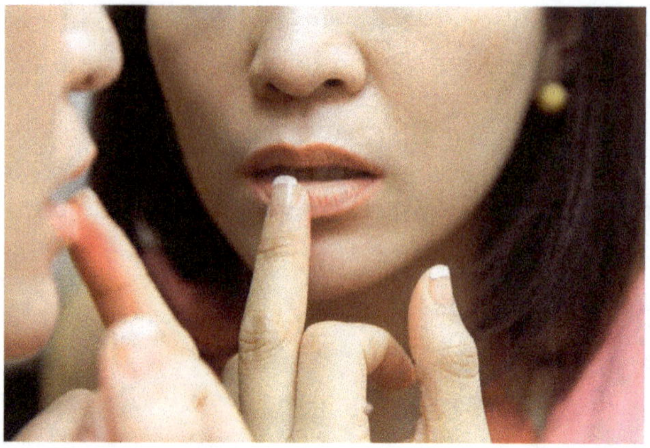

8. Run your ring finger or pinky finger over your lips. Do this gently back and forth until you've smoothed out any remaining hard lines. You want your lips to look smoothly graded, with just slightly darker edges leading into a lighter, plump center.

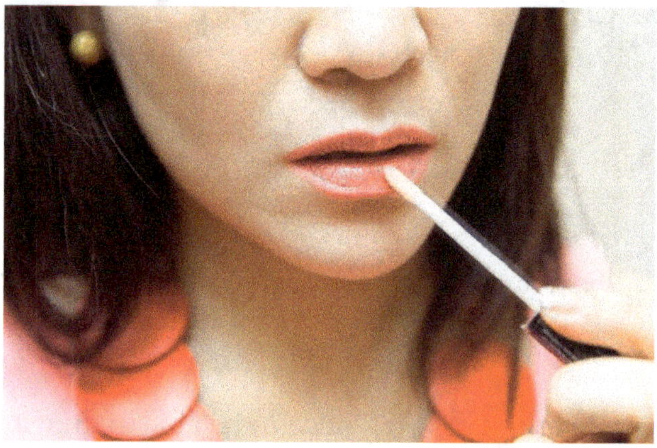

9. You're done! If you'd like you can dab a tiny amount of gloss or shimmery powder in the center of your bottom lip, which will help make it look a bit more plump.

Part 5

Making Your Lips Look Smaller

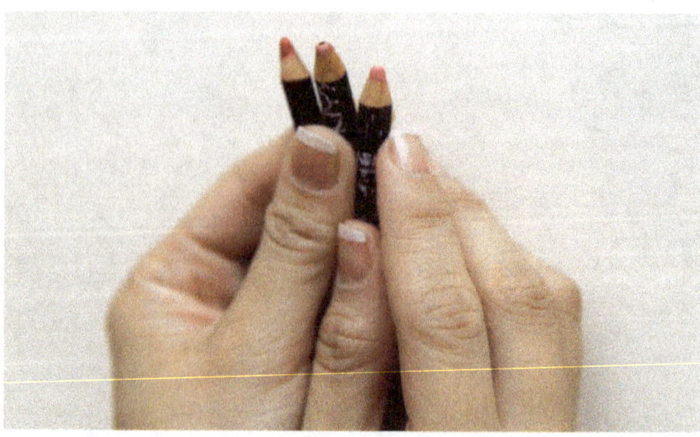

1. Choose your colors. Choose a nude liner and nude lipstick for a natural look, or a more dramatic

liner and matching lipstick if you're feeling more adventurous.

- Note that darker colors and mattes can help make lips look smaller.

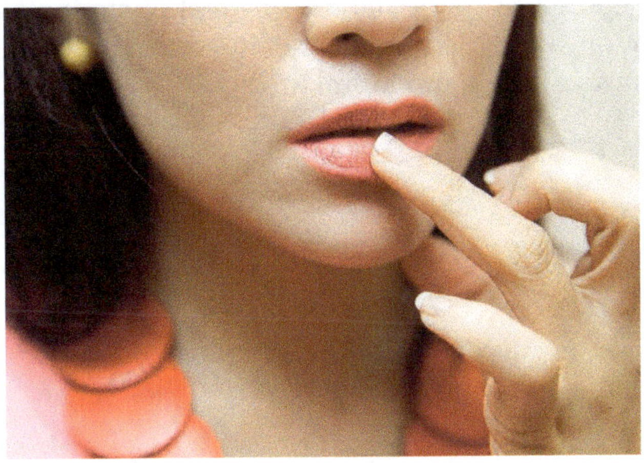

2. Apply a concealer to your lips and the surrounding area. This will help blur your natural lip line. It will also help your liner and lipstick stay put.

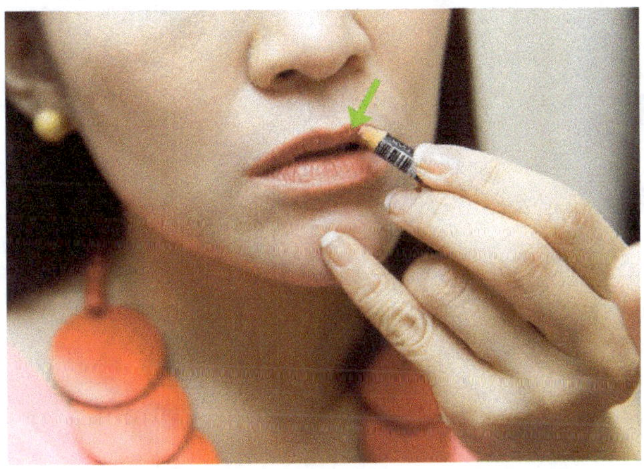

3. Draw slightly inside of your natural lip line. Using short and swift strokes, line just inside of your natural lip line.

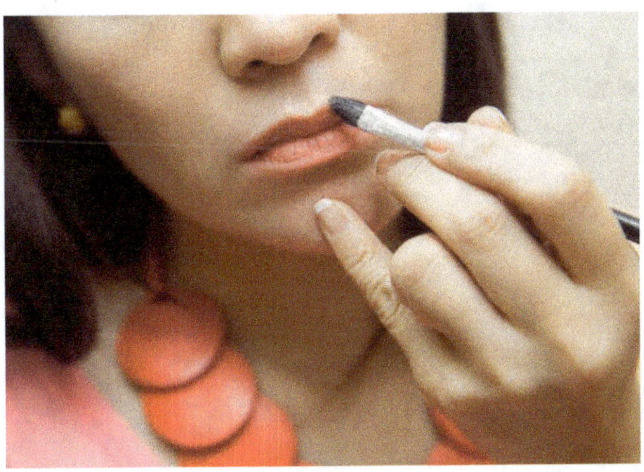

- Use a nude lip liner for nude-looking lips, or a darker shade for a more dramatic effect. Darker colors can help make lips look smaller.

4. Clean up around your lips. Once you're done lining and filling in your lips, remove any stray lines with a kleenex or cotton swab, then use a concealer brush and some foundation to clean up around the lip liner and further hide your natural lip line.

Part 6

Choosing the Right Tools

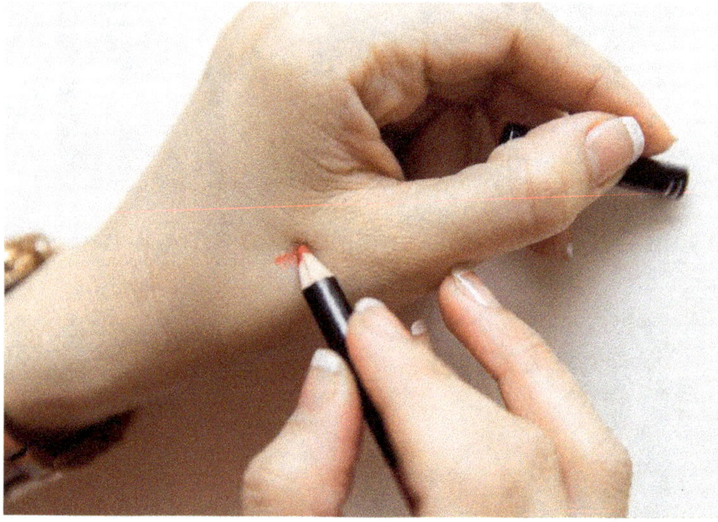

1. Buy a good-quality lip liner. Good-quality lip liners are available at drug stores and makeup shops: you just need to know what to look for. Always try before you buy. A good liner should easily draw a smooth, richly colored line on your hand.

- Avoid liners that go on translucent, chalky, and/or crumbly.
- If it's at all difficult to draw a line on the back of your hand with a liner, avoid it.

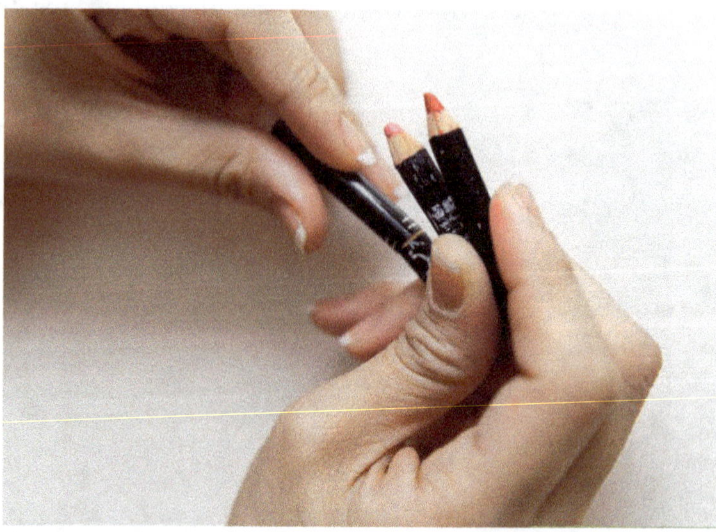

2. Know what colors to buy. Some makeup aficionados have a matching lip liner for every color of lipstick they own. If you only buy one color of lip liner, however, make it a nude or natural one.

- A solid beginner's set of lip liners would include one nude, one red, and one pink.

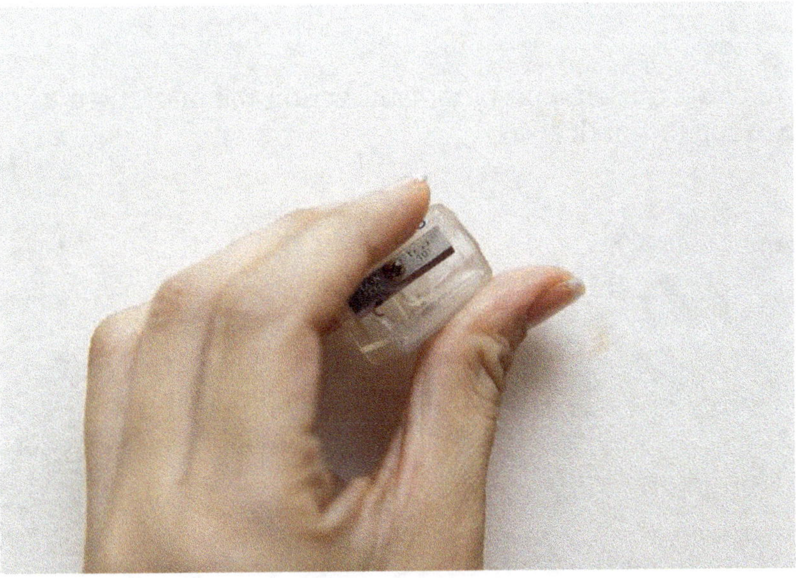

3. Get a good sharpener. Unless you're using a liner stick that twists up (these usually come in plastic casings), you'll be using something similar to a pencil crayon. You'll need a pencil sharpener to keep your liner in good shape.

- There isn't a lot of advice available as to how to purchase a good-quality sharpener; it's best to ask friends or do an online search for highly reviewed sharpeners within your price range.
- Sharpeners can cost anywhere from $2 to over $40, but it's certainly possible to get a good-quality one for under $10.

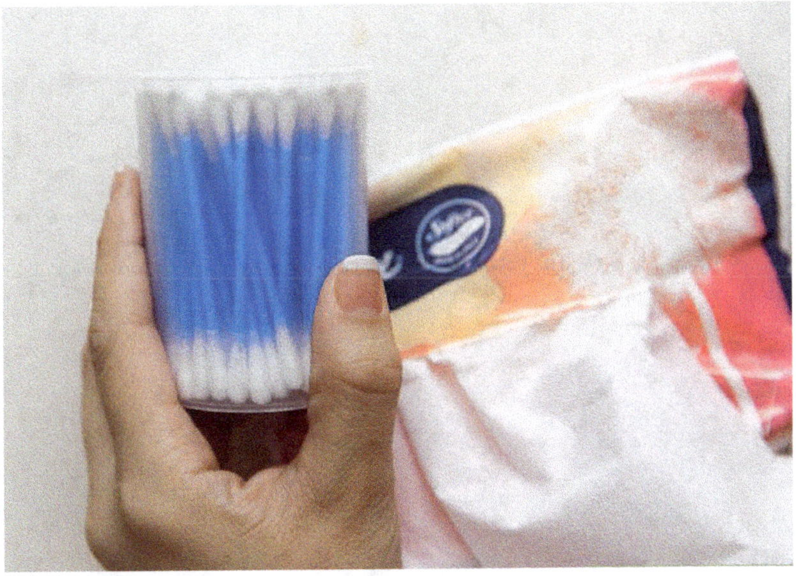

4. Have some tissue paper or cotton swabs available. Especially when you're new to lining your lips, you may need to clean up the lines. It's a lot easier to do if you have a cotton swab or tissue paper handy.

- For particularly stubborn marks, put a little bit of moisturizer or makeup remover on some tissue paper or the tip of a cotton swap, and gently rub at the mark until it disappears.
- It can help to dab a tiny amount of moisturizer on the mark then use the dry side of the cotton swab to rub the mark away.

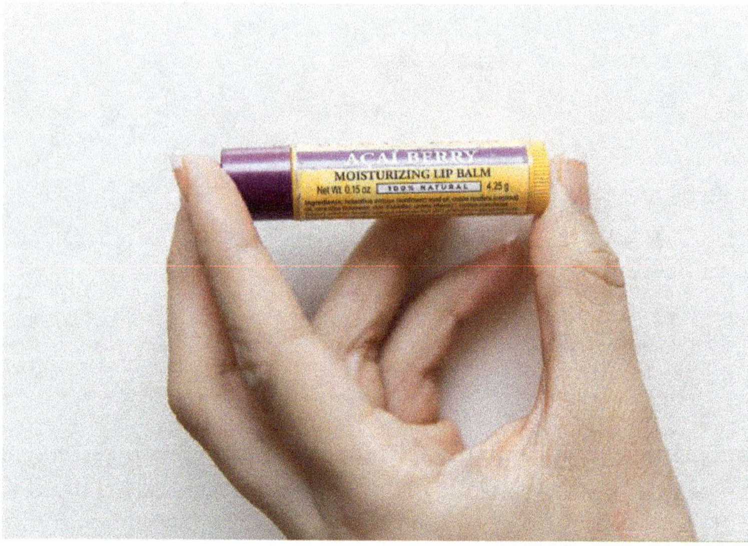

5. Get a good lip balm. Moisturizing your lips before applying a liner can help prevent them from drying out, which can make your liner look dry and crumbly when it sinks into the cracks that form in your lips when they're dry.

- A good lip balm will sink into your lips and make them feel moisturized. Avoid anything too goopy, which will make it difficult to apply anything else to your lips.

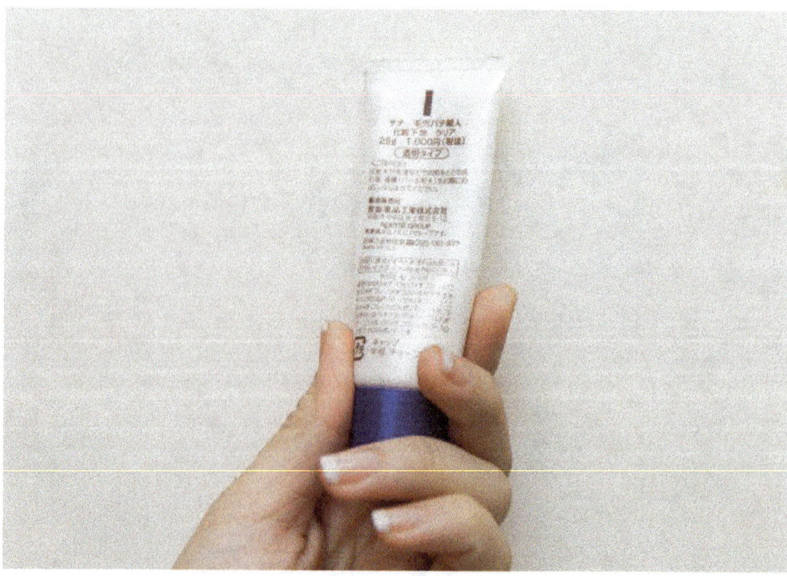

6. Get a lip primer (optional). Some makeup artists suggest applying a lip primer to your lips before doing anything else, as this can help lengthen the life of your liner and lipstick once they're on your lips.

- If you don't have a primer, you can also use concealer or foundation to prime your lips.

Lip Gloss

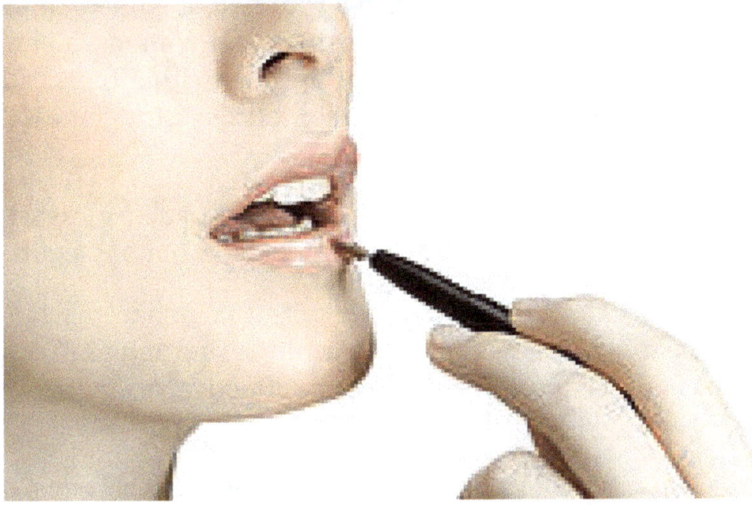

Lip gloss being applied with a retractable lip brush.

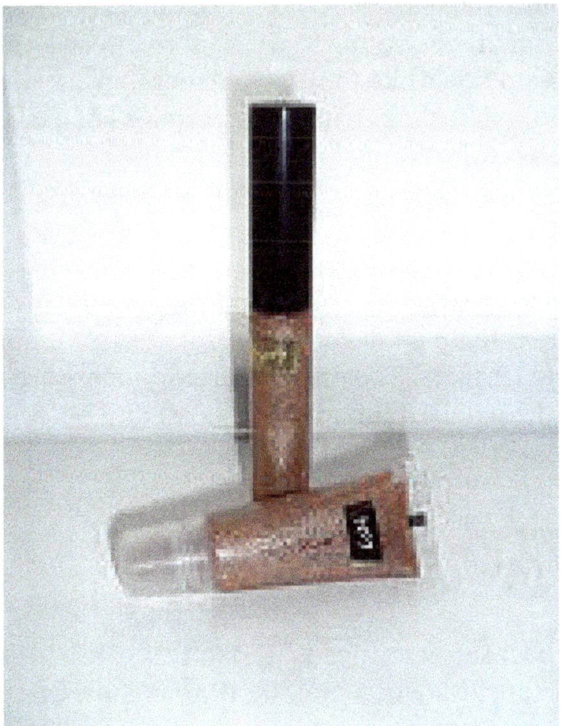

Lip gloss in squeezable tube and wand applicator formats

Lip gloss is a product used primarily to give lips a glossy lustre, and sometimes to add a subtle color. It is distributed as a liquid or a soft solid (not to be confused with lip balm, which generally has medical or soothing purposes)or lipstick, which generally is a solid, cream like substance that gives off a more pigmented color. The product is available in ranges of opacity from translucent to solid, and can have various frosted, glittery, glossy, and metallic finishes.

Types

Like lipstick, lip gloss comes in a variety of forms and may be applied in different ways. It can be contained in a small cylinder and applied with a rounded or sloped applicator wand (known as a doefoot applicator) or with a built in lip brush. It can come in a small, soft, squeezable plastic tube designed to be passed over the lips or applied with a fingertip or lip brush. Solid or semisolid glosses come in boxes or tubes and sometimes blur the distinction between lip gloss and lip balm.

Basic lip gloss: adds basic shine to your lips without color. Colored lip gloss: adds a combination of color and shine. Glittery lip gloss: can be with or without color, but has a glitter base.

New types of "plumping" lip gloss contain ingredients that make the lips appear softer and plumper. These are a cheap, easy, and usually harmless alternative if compared to collagen, Restylane, Juvederm, or fat injections. They are not as effective, however because the effects are temporary.

Lip gloss is often used when a person wants to have some color on their lips, but does not want an intense, solid lip color effect (i.e., a more "made-up" look), as lipstick would create. Lip gloss is also often used as an introduction to makeup. It is often used by preteen and young teenage girls who want to wear some makeup, but are too young to wear more intense lipstick colors. Lip gloss is also common for young women who don't like to wear makeup but have to attend a formal occasion. Lip gloss can be applied on top of lipstick to increase the gloss of a color, or to add depth as in the case of glitter gloss.

Ingredients

Like lipstick, lip gloss is a mixture of waxes, oils, and pigments. However, lip gloss contains less pigments, and those used are often pale in color or diluted (<3%). Furthermore, the free-flowing nature of the product requires less wax. The principal components are lanolin, which feels good on the lips due to its moisturizing qualities and imparts gloss, and polybutene.

How to Choose a Lip Gloss

Unsure which lip gloss will best suit your needs? It isn't too difficult a choice but there are some things that you will need to consider when making it, to ensure that the lip gloss does what you expect it to.

Part 1

The Basics of Lip Gloss

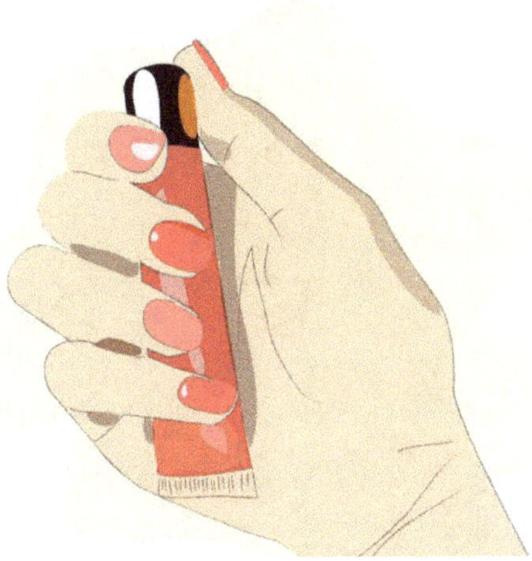

1. Understand what lip gloss is used for. Lip gloss has three main functions, namely: To add luster (shine) to lips, to add moisture to lips and, in some cases, to add just a touch of color. Lip gloss can be used instead of lipstick or over lipstick.

- Some lip gloss contains flavor as well. For some people, this is the reason for wearing it.

2. Know where you can purchase lip gloss from. Pharmacies, drugstores, department stores, beauty stores, local marts, etc. all carry lip gloss lines. You can also buy lip gloss online, but it's best to know what you like first, and just buy top ups of that brand when you're sure it's the right one for you.

Part 2

Choosing Lip Gloss

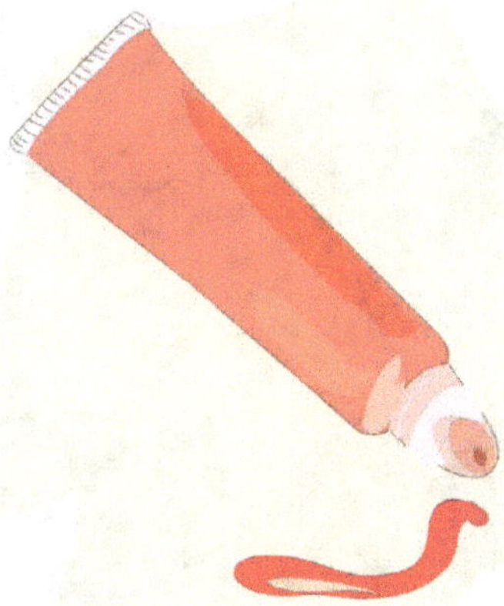

1. Consider what you want from the lip gloss first of all. Do you want it to just add shine? Or, would you like one with color? Perhaps flavor is your preferred reason for using the lip gloss. In some cases, you may wish to combine the reasons. By knowing what you expect the lip gloss to achieve for you, you're all set to start choosing.

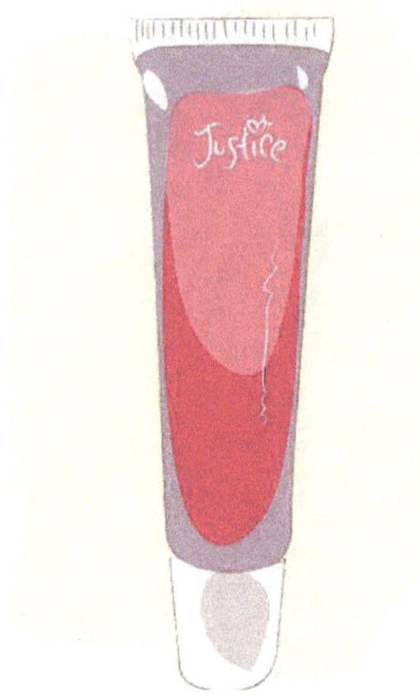

2. Choose colored lip gloss if you don't wear lipstick. This can add a touch of color to your lips, as well as adding shine. Colored lip gloss comes in either full color or sheer; the sheer gives a "hint" of color, while full color will recolor the lips temporarily. Colored lip gloss is best if the color is slightly darker than the natural color of your lips, as well as accounting for your skin complexion.

- If you use a lot of bright colored eyeshadow, it is recommended that you do not wear a colored lip gloss, as this can provide too much color. Pick which feature you want to dominate, and stick with that.
- Decide whether you want glitter in the lip gloss. If you lick your lips often though, the glitter can get stuck in your teeth.

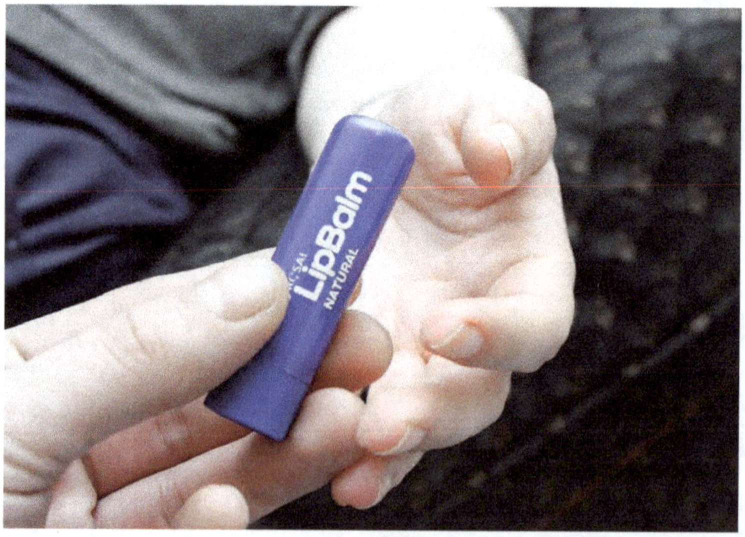

3. Ask the retail assistant for tips and colors that match with your face color, if you are buying colored lip gloss. This will help to ensure that you don't buy a color that isn't well matched to your complexion.

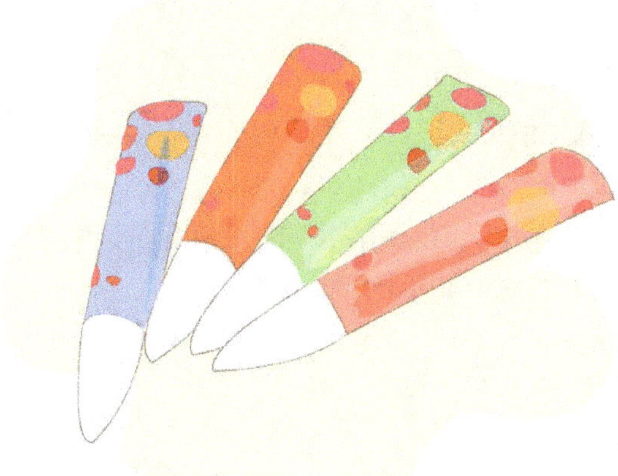

4. If choosing a flavored lip gloss, aim for one that you like. Some of the more commonly used flavors for lip gloss include: Grape, cherry, strawberry, peppermint, and spearmint. In some cases, the suggested flavor may not be what you expected, so don't spend too much on flavored lip glosses.

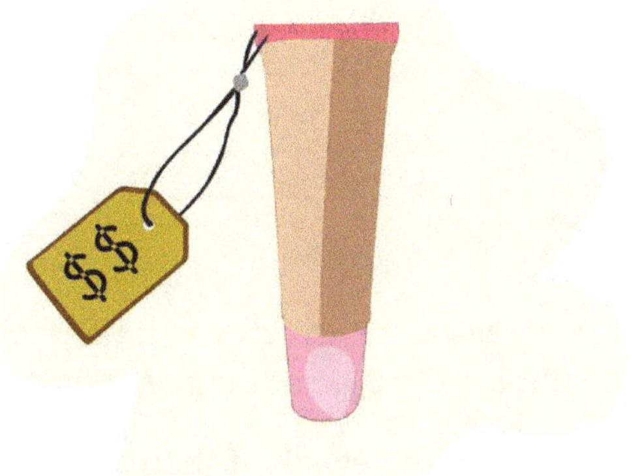

5. Keep your budget in mind. Prices will vary depending on the brand and the type of lip gloss on offer. Don't be afraid to try cheaper versions though; there isn't much to a lip gloss, so a lot of the cheaper lip glosses are just as good as the more expensive ones.

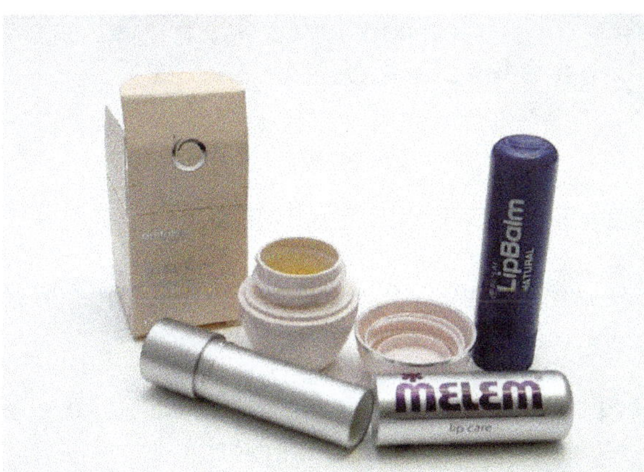

6. Work out which container will fit best with your lifestyle. Lip gloss comes in various forms, including a tube with a brush, a glass container with a roll on feature, a rub-on hard stick, a small pot, or a squeeze tube. It's personal preference as to which way you prefer to apply the lip gloss,

although since you're new to it, it might pay to experiment with each type before deciding on which one works best for you.

- The brush version may feel lighter and in need of less rubbing pressure than the roll-on version.
- Finger applied gloss requires absolutely clean fingers. This might not be as useful if you're not near a bathroom during reapplication time.

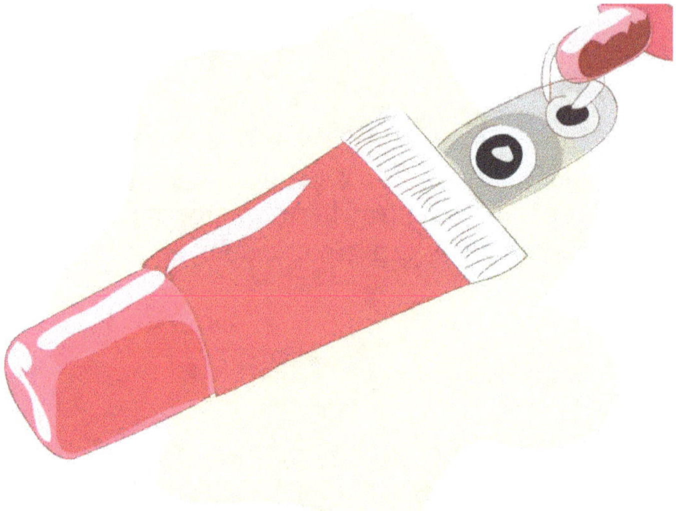

7. Choose a lip gloss suited to the occasion for which you'll be wearing it. Think about where are you will be wearing it, as this can impact the type of lip gloss you need. For example:

- For school: Choose clear lip gloss, especially if there are rules about not wearing makeup. This might also apply in certain workplaces, if makeup is not permitted.
- For dates or events: Choose colored lip gloss (especially for evenings), or a fun lip gloss with glitter in it.
- If you're going to be outdoors a lot, consider using a lip gloss that contains SPF 15 or above in it. Also choose one that is long lasting.

Part 3

Things to be Mindful of

1. Be aware that some lip gloss or its ingredients may not be suitable for you. Take note of the ingredients before purchasing. Some things to consider include:

- There is a risk of allergies: Some ingredients may cause allergies if you're susceptible, such as beeswax, colors (dyes), flavorings or preservatives.
- The ingredients are unacceptable: If you don't like certain ingredients, such as parabens (suspected carcinogens), or non-vegetarian/vegan ingredients, then you'll need to avoid lip gloss containing such ingredients.

- The gloss is uncomfortable: Heavy gloss doesn't work for everyone. If you choose a heavier gloss and find it is unpleasant, try a lighter one instead. Equally, if the glitter lip gloss feels like sandpaper, choose a different one.
- The gloss doesn't last: If you are using lip gloss to add color, it won't last as long as lipstick. Either reapply frequently, or change to a lipstick and only use lip gloss for added shine.

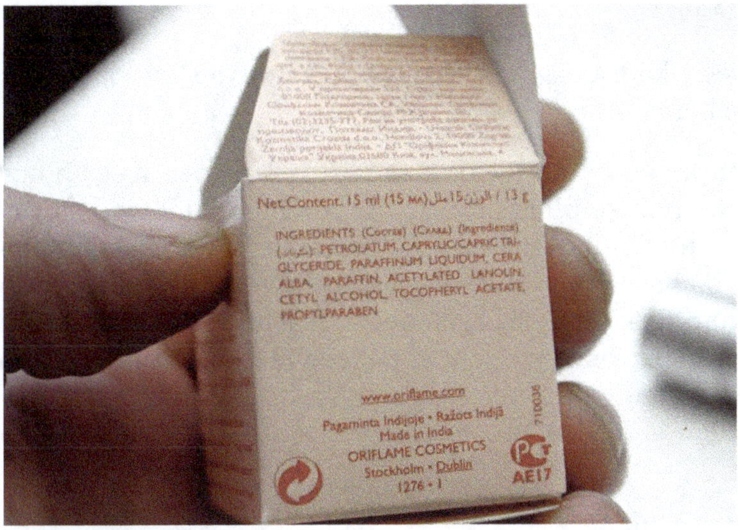

Lip Balm

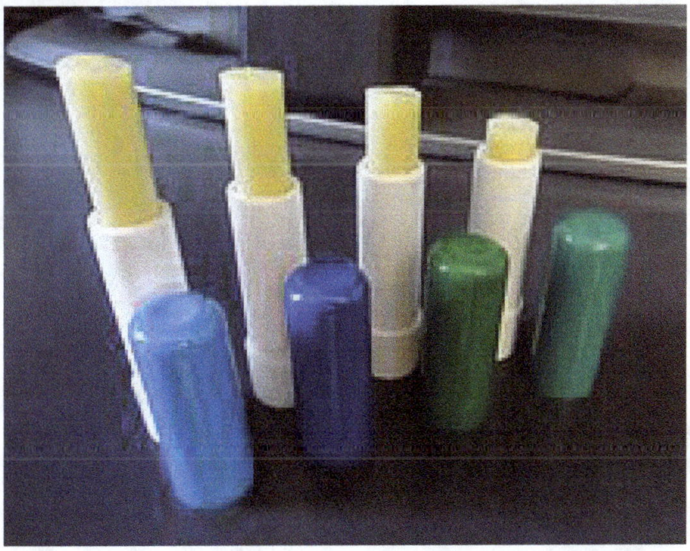

Homemade lip balms

Lip balm or lip salve is a wax-like substance applied topically to the lips of the mouth to moisturize and relieve chapped or dry lips, angular cheilitis, stomatitis, or cold sores. Lip balm often contains beeswax or carnauba wax, camphor, cetyl alcohol, lanolin, paraffin, and petrolatum, among other ingredients. Some varieties contain dyes, flavor, fragrance, phenol, salicylic acid, and sunscreens.

The primary purpose of lip balm is to provide an occlusive layer on the lip surface to seal moisture in lips and protect them from external exposure. Dry air, cold temperatures, and wind all have a drying effect on skin by drawing moisture away from the body. Lips are particularly vulnerable because the skin is so thin, and thus they are often the first to present signs of dryness. Occlusive materials like waxes and petroleum jelly prevent moisture loss and maintain lip comfort while flavorants, colorants, sunscreens, and various medicaments can provide additional, specific benefits.

Lip balm can be applied where a finger is used to apply it to the lips, or in a lipstick-style tube from which it can be applied directly.

Lip balm was first marketed in the 1880s by Charles Browne Fleet, though its origins may be traced to earwax. More than 40 years prior to the commercial introduction of lip balm by Fleet, Lydia Maria Child recommended earwax as a treatment for cracked lips in her highly-popular book, *The American Frugal Housewife*. Child observed that, "Those who are troubled with cracked lips have found this [earwax] remedy successful when others have failed. It is one of those sorts of cures, which are very likely to be laughed at; but I know of its having produced very beneficial results."

Notable brands

- Baby Lips by Maybelline
- Burt's Bees
- Blistex
- Carmex
- ChapStick
- Labello
- Lip Smacker
- Lypsyl
- Tholene
- Vaseline
- Lip balm by Weleda
- Lip care by Nivea
- Revo by Walgreens

Dependency

Some physicians have suggested that certain types of lip balm can be addictive or contain ingredients that actually cause drying. Lip balm manufacturers sometimes state in their FAQs that there is nothing addictive in their products or that all ingredients are listed and approved by the FDA. Snopes found the claim that there are substances in Carmex that are irritants necessitating reapplication, such as ground glass, to be false.

How to Apply Lip Balm

Everyone loves lip balm during the cold, dry months, but using lip balm responsibly is an important part of keeping your mouth and lips healthy. Follow these tips on picking the right lip balm and using it appropriately.

Part 1

Applying Lip Balm from an Applicator

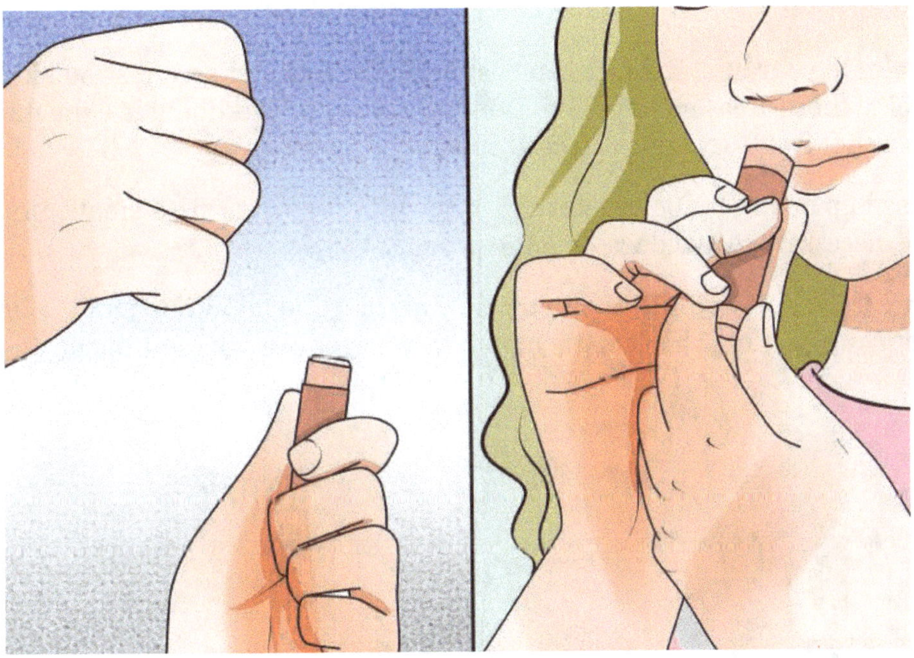

1. Uncap the container and prepare a small amount of balm. Depending on the type of lip balm you selected, you will retrieve the balm in different ways. The most common type of lip balm is the tube.

- For tubed lip balm, use the dial located on the bottom of the tube to raise the lip balm above the brim of the tube. You need only raise the balm by a half centimeter or so.
- Gel-based lip balms are squeezed through a tiny hole in a lipstick-shaped applicator tip. An amount slightly smaller than pea-sized should provide enough coverage.
- Liquid lip balms often come with what is known as a doe foot applicator. These are attached to the cap of the balm and store the balm on a spongy applicator tip.

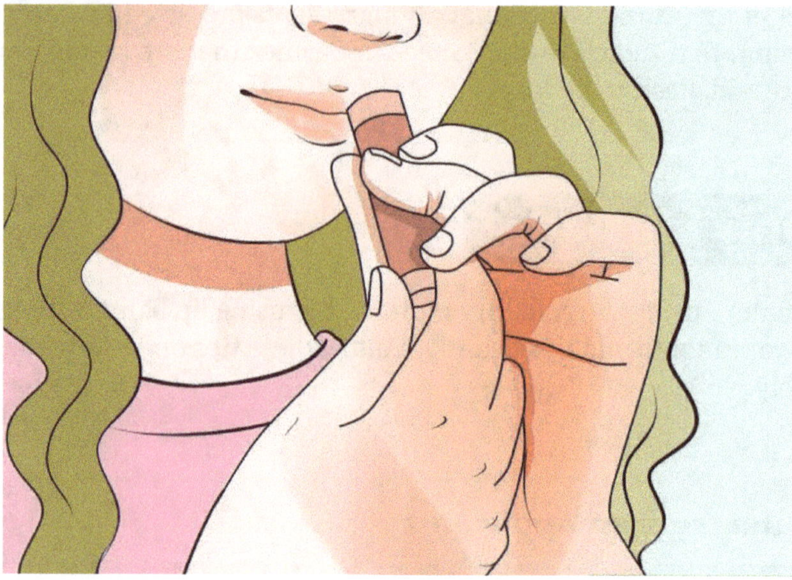

2. Apply the balm to your lips. A thin, even coating to the lips and area just outside of the mouth is best for keeping those areas moisturized. Don't worry about overdoing it – the most you have to worry about is a slightly glossy appearance around your mouth.

- Gel-based lip balm cannot be returned to the tube, so start with a smaller amount and add more as necessary to avoid wasting the product.
- If you wear lipstick, apply the balm to your lips first and allow it to sit for a few minutes before applying lipstick. This lets the moisturizing agents work their magic on your lips first.

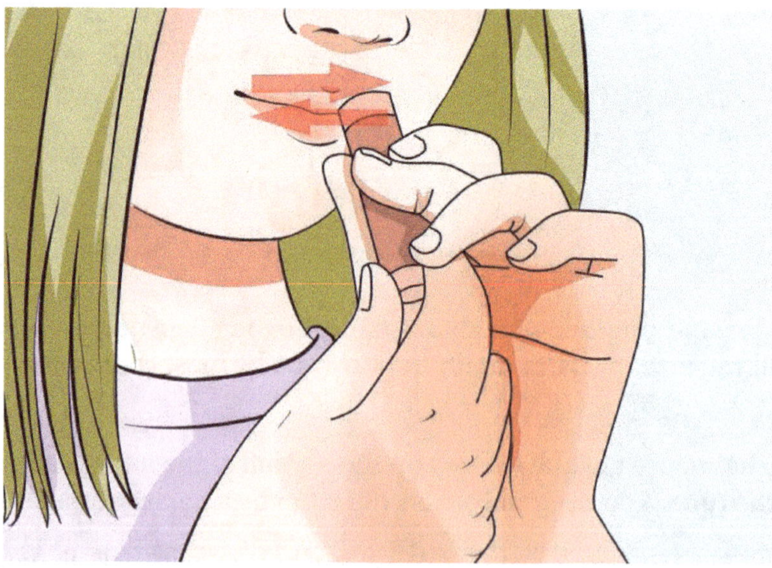

3. Draw in your lips to spread excess balm. You want to "hide" your lips in your mouth. This helps spread the product over areas near the mouth that also become dry or cracked.

- If your lip balm has a tint or coloring, be careful when applying and spreading the balm. Being too imprecise can cause a streaky, smeared mess on your face!

Part 2

Applying Lip Balm with Your Fingers

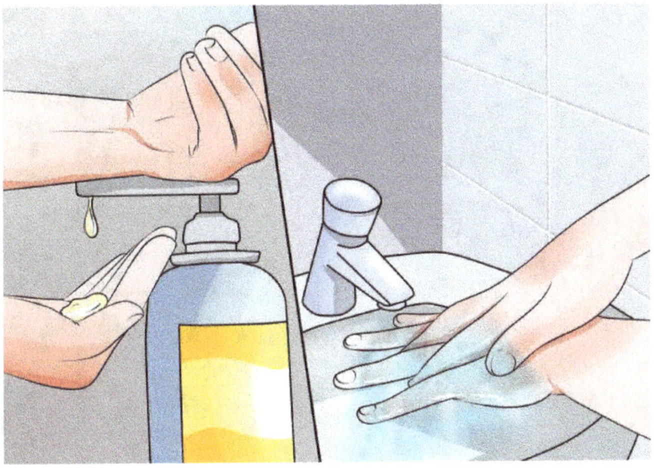

1. Wash your hands. Use soap and water, or an anti-bacterial gel if you're out and about. It's a good idea to wash up properly before you touch your lips (or any other sensitive part of your body).

- Touching your fingers to your lips (in this case, to apply lip balm) increases the chance of spreading germs and infections to your mouth.
- The proper way to wash your hands involves scrubbing the palms, back of hands, each thumb, between the fingers, and under the fingernails for 15 seconds total.

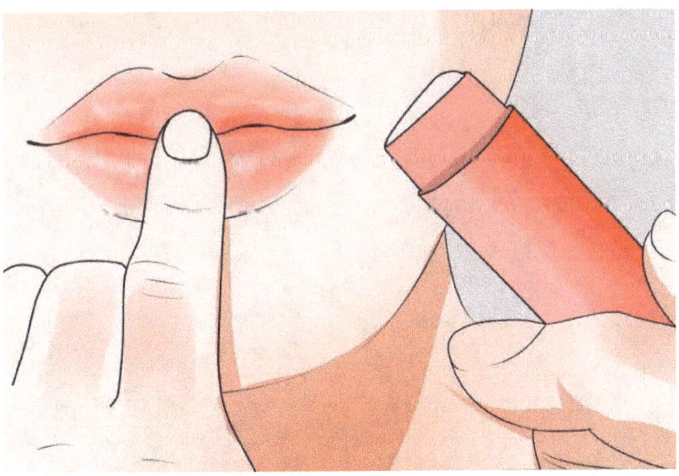

2. Use your fingers to apply the balm to your lips. Use your index finger, applying to the center of the bottom lip first, working your way toward the corners. Use a small amount and apply evenly to the lips, adding more balm as necessary. Balms meant for the fingers are waxy or gel-like in consistency.

- Small balm applicators are available for purchase. These can be carried and dipped into the balm to apply this style of balm without using your fingers. They can be easily cleaned, and will generally stay cleaner than your fingers. Quite helpful if you can't wash your hands!

- Don't use your fingers to apply lip balm when you are sick - you don't want to risk contaminating the balm. Instead, purchase a separate balm, and only use that one while you are sick. Using an contaminated lip balm, even when using an applicator, risks spreading germs.

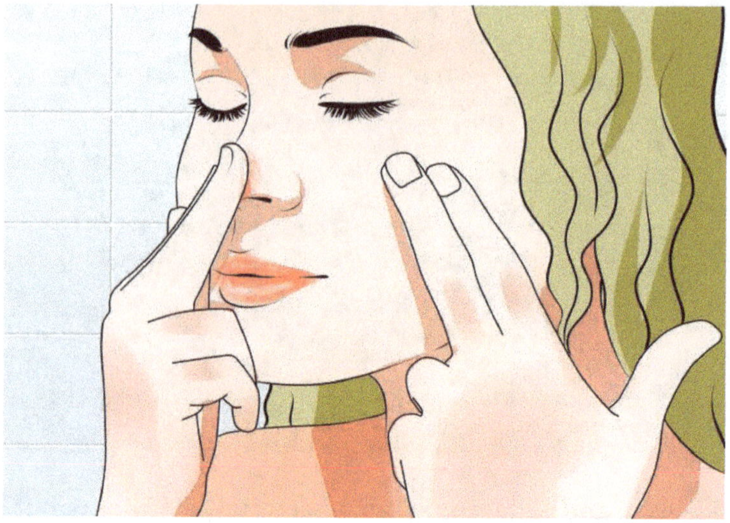

3. Apply to other dry areas (optional). Lip balm can also be applied to other dry areas on the face. Use your fingers to apply a small amount of balm to your nose, cheeks, and other areas that could use moisture.

- Common areas that dry out include just under the nose and the cheeks. This is particularly prevalent during times of cold weather, wind, or if you are prone to rubbing your nose.

Part 3

Using Lip Balm Responsibly

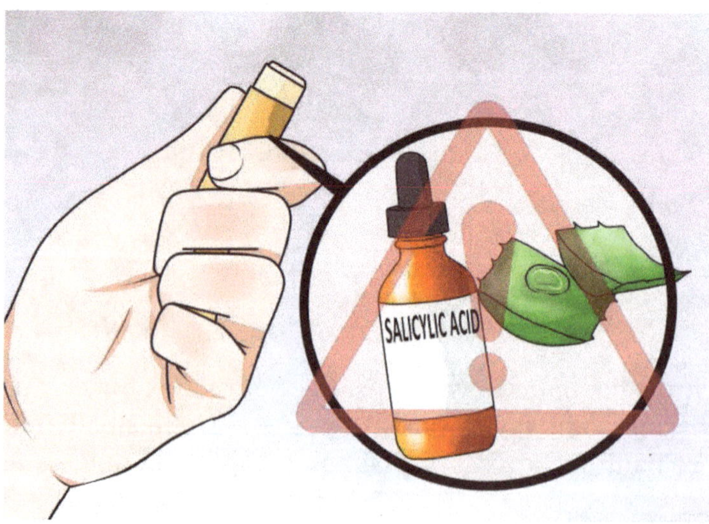

1. Avoid harmful ingredients. Ingredients used for artificial colors and fragrances can cause lip irritation and actually contribute to dryness. Avoid these ingredients to keep from damaging your lips further, which can lead to unnecessary reliance on the balm.

- Menthol, camphor, and phenol cool the lips, but contribute to dryness.
- Artificial colors and fragrances often cause lip irritation.
- Certain ingredients help moisturize, but can irritate lips, depending on your individual reaction. These include salicylic acid, aloe butter, and vitamin E.

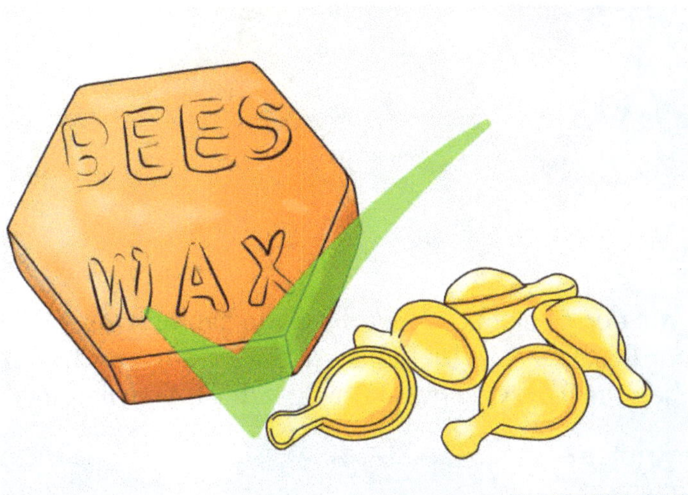

2. Look for ingredients that help moisturize and protect. Ingredients such as beeswax and ceramides help retain water for your lips. Other ingredients to look for include dimethicone, which helps prevent drying and improves longevity of the product, and sunscreen.

- Choose a lip balm that features an SPF rating. This helps protect your lips from getting sunburned, dried out, and cracked. Find a balm with SPF 15 or higher for best results.

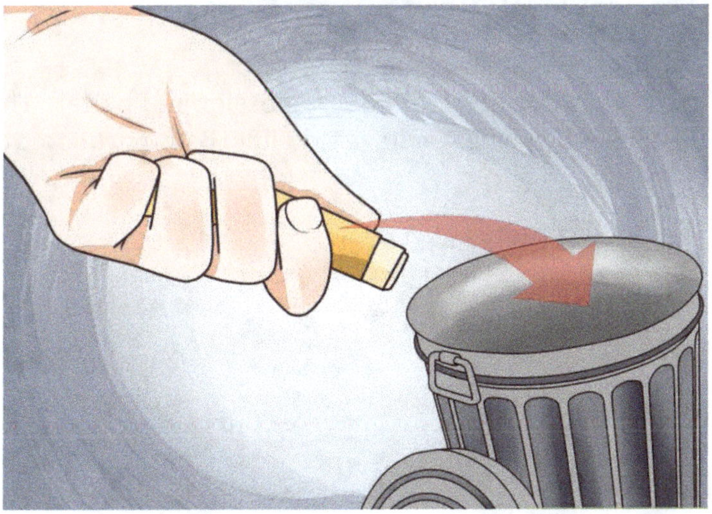

3. Throw away old lip balm. Old lip balm can dry out, losing its moisturizing properties. It can also harbor bacteria and mold if stored in a dark, damp area, so check the expiration date before use.

- Some lip balm comes in packs featuring multiple containers. Consider buying in bulk if you are concerned about "wasting" old lip balm.

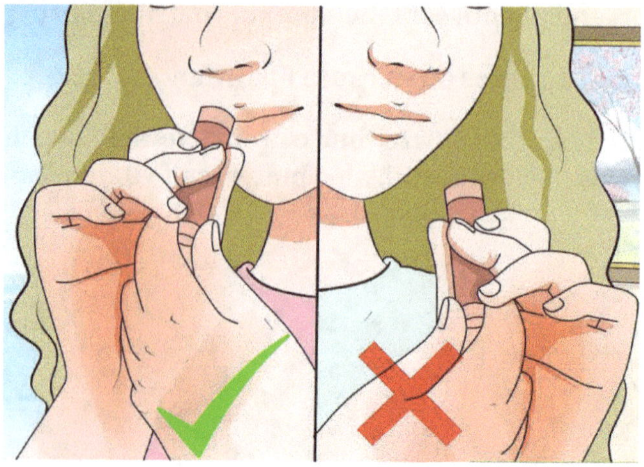

4. Don't use lip balm if you don't need it. Lip balm can be habit forming. Overuse can actually lead to further drying out your lips. Only use lip balm when necessary, such as the cold winter months, or dry season. Ask yourself the following questions to determine whether you might be addicted:

- Do you use it very often?
- Do you spend a lot of money on lip balm?
- Does a lack of lip balm distract you from other activities?
- Do others comment on your use of lip balm?

How to Apply Lip Color

Lip gloss and lipstick can make your lips look fuller, glossier and better! They can add volume to your lips and make them appear bigger if you have thin lips. Below are some steps to apply lip gloss or lipstick.

Steps

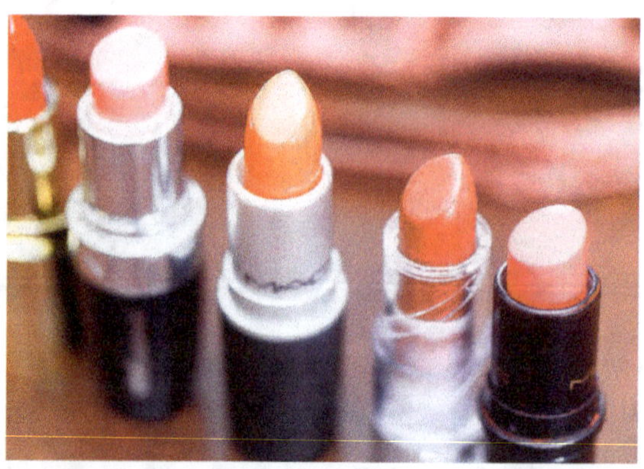

1. Choose the perfect lip cosmetic for you. Do you want it to be shimmer, clear, coloured, flavoured

or sheer? There are many different kinds out there, so go shopping and take a look at what's available!

- Lipstick is usually has a more opaque colour, and a thicker consistency than lip gloss.
- Lip gloss is usually transparent, or with a subtle hint of color. They can be used as an additional layer over the lipstick for an additional shine.
- Lip balms are usually transparent, and are designed to protect the lips from sun and wind, and often to soothe chapped lips and cold sores.
- Lip stains are like a pen. They can sometimes have a strong colour, but they help change the color of your lips without looking like you are wearing lip color.
- Some categories may overlap. You can find lipsticks with SPF protection, lip gloss that is very thick, etc.

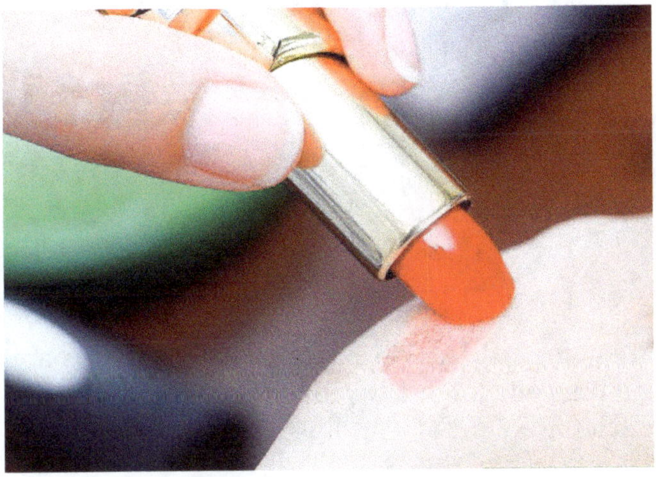

2. Sample lip cosmetics at the store. Sometimes samples are available to comparison shop. You put these on your hand or a testing strip provided by the store, *never directly on your own lips*.

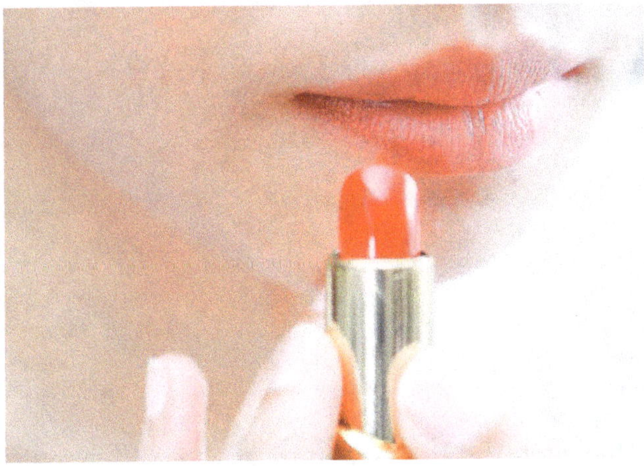

3. Choose a great colour that compliments your skin tone. Find the perfect shade by experimenting with different colours.

- Start with a subtle color, something a few shades darker than your lip color.
- Avoid bright fire-engine-red *at first; a beginner's mistake is going straight for the loudest red you can find to announce, "I'm wearing lipstick!" Even if you* do *look great in that color, any mistake, imperfection, or slightest smudge will stand out.*
- If you have a sister who is experienced with lipstick color, find out her favorite shades. Sisters tend to look good in similar colors, because of their similar skin tones. (But don't share her makeup!)

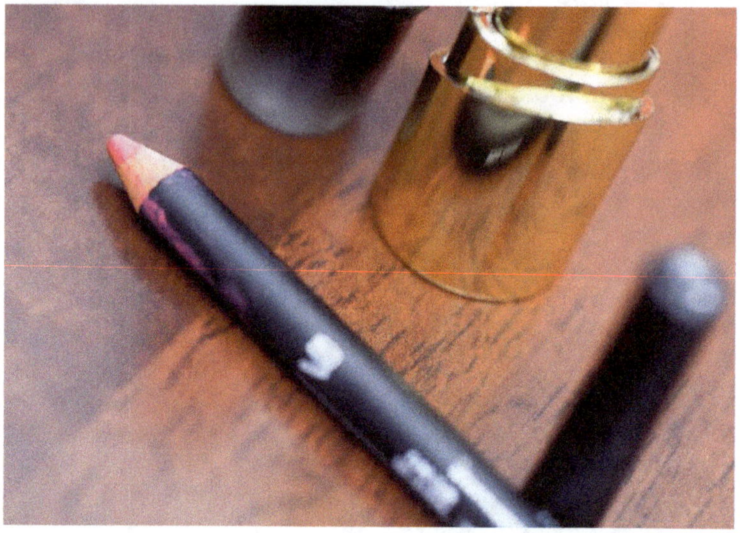

4. Decide whether you are going to wear lip liner. Today's lipsticks are better formulated than those of the past, making it unneeded. For a beginner, it is usually an unnecessary step. If you do, it should be neutral or match the colour of your lipstick.

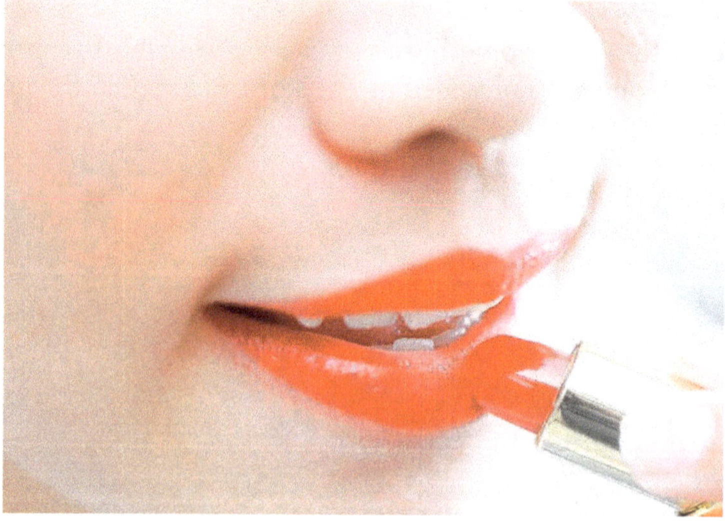

5. Apply your lipstick first. Stretch the lips and start at the center, putting on the lipstick to the corners. Blot the lipstick with a tissue. Make sure the lipstick has not smudged over the line of your lips.

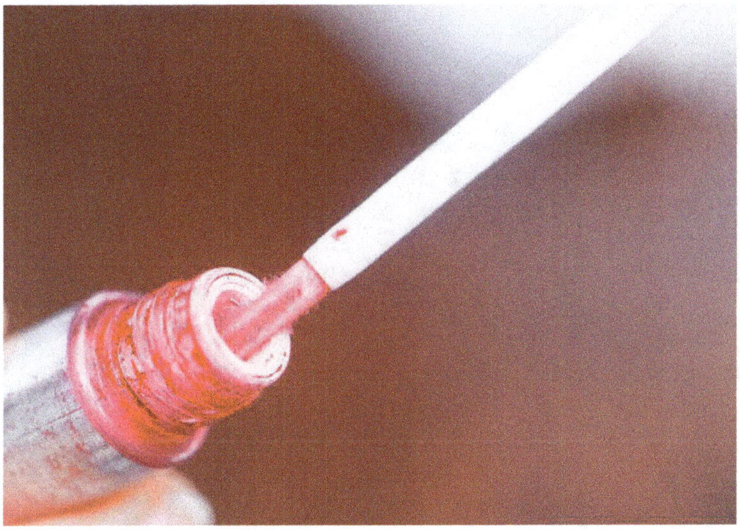

6. You can also apply your lip stain first if you so choose. Stretch your lips and draw the stain in a line in the center of each lip, upper and lower. Rub your lips together and blot.

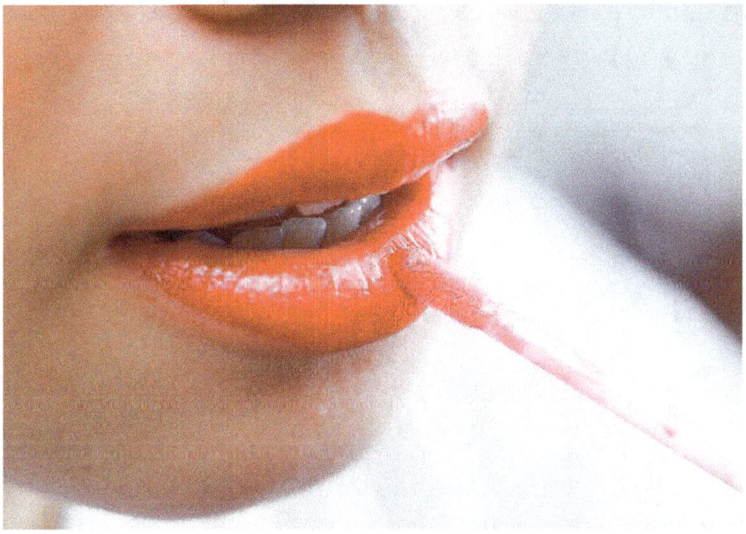

7. Apply your lipgloss. Either apply it all over your lips, or just apply it in the centre of each lip and rub your lips together to apply an even, thin coat. Another option is to apply it in the centre of your lower lip, as this makes your lips look fuller.

How to Apply Lip Stain

Tired of having to reapply lipstick all the time? Use lip stain instead. It lasts much longer, and is also smudge-proof and waterproof. Applied correctly, it can also make your lips appear both full and smooth. This article will show you how to apply lip stain effectively. It will also give you a few tips and pointers on how to get that full, plump look as well.

Part 1

Prepping Your Lips

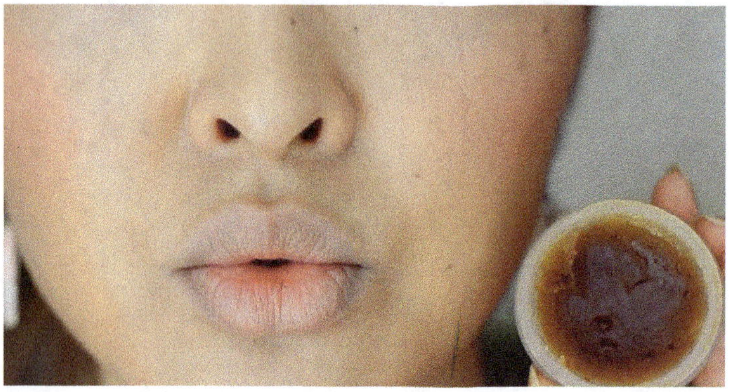

1. Find a lip scrub. A lip scrub will help buff away dead skin cells and make your lips appear smoother and plumper. It will make applying the lip stain a lot easier. If you don't have a lip scrub at home, or don't have time to run out and buy one, you can make your own by combining 1 part honey, 1 part sugar (white or brown), and 1 part oil (almond, coconut, jojoba, or olive) in a small dish.

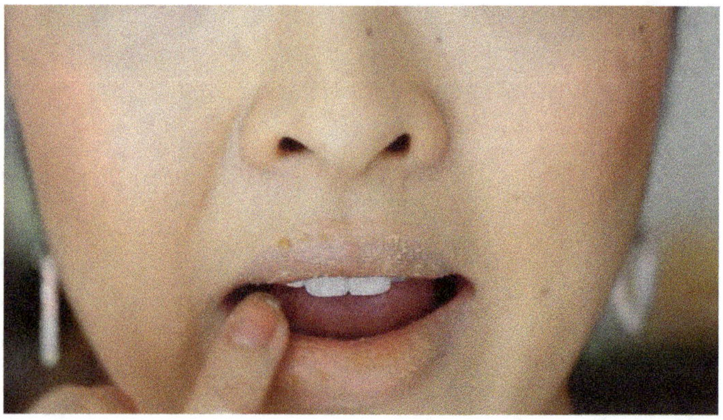

2. Exfoliate your lips with the lip scrub. Apply the scrub to your lips using your fingers. Gently massage your lips using soft, circular motions. A few seconds is all you need. If you have very chapped lips, however, you might need to exfoliate them for up to two minutes.

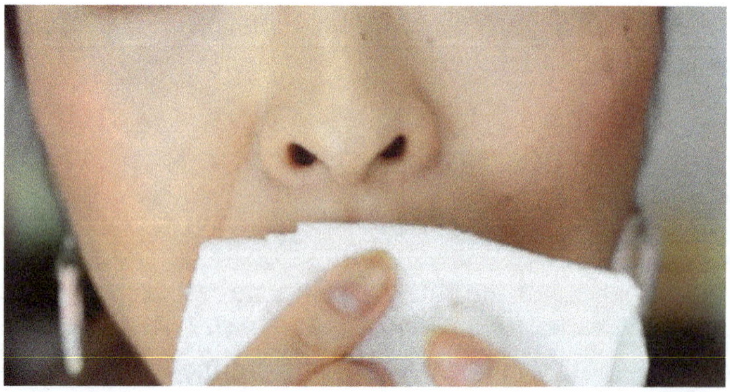

3. Wipe the lip scrub off with a damp towel. Soak the corner of a clean, soft towel with warm water.

Squeeze out the excess moisture from the towel, then gently wipe the excess lip scrub off your lips.

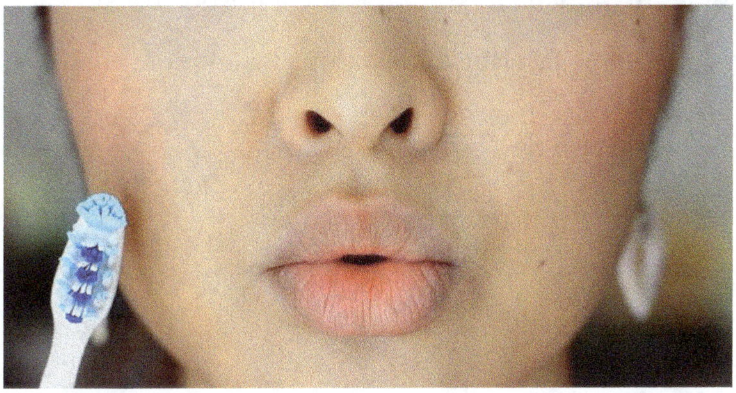

4. Buff your lips with a soft toothbrush. Use a clean toothbrush. This is great for circulation and can help make your lips appear more plump and full.

- Consider getting a separate toothbrush for lip buffing purposes.

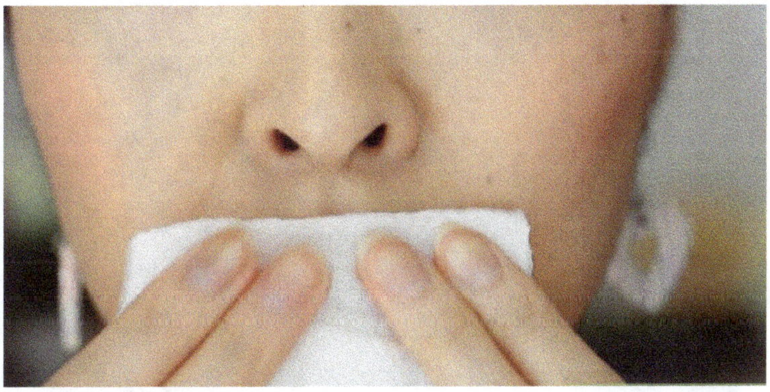

5. Pat your lips dry. Take a soft towel, and gently pat your lips dry with it. You are now ready to start applying your lip stain.

Part 2

Doing the Basics

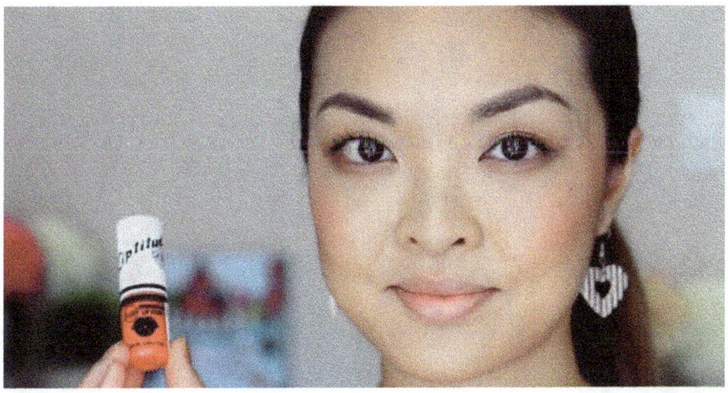

1. Get out your desired color of lip stain. Depending on how your lip stain is packaged, you may

also need a lip brush. Lip stain can come in a bottle with an applicator, in a small jar, and in a small tube. If the lip stain comes in a small jar, you will need a lipstick brush.

- If you plan on doing some layering and contouring later on, choose a lighter shade.

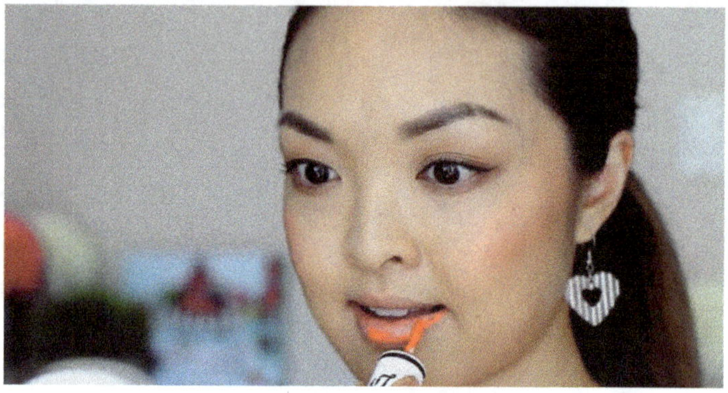

2. Start applying the lip stain to your bottom lip. Simply start from one corner of your lip, and drag the applicator or brush to the other. Follow the curve of your bottom lip. Once you have your lip outline, fill the center part in with more lip stain.

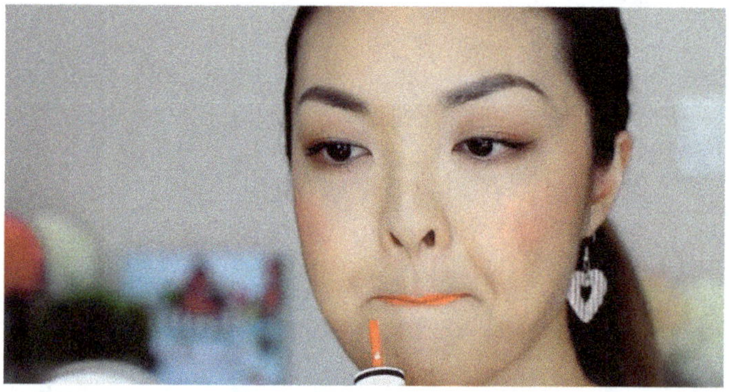

3. Smack your lips. Pull your lips inward, so that you can't see them, and then pop them. This will help transfer some of the excess lip stain from the bottom lip to the upper lip.

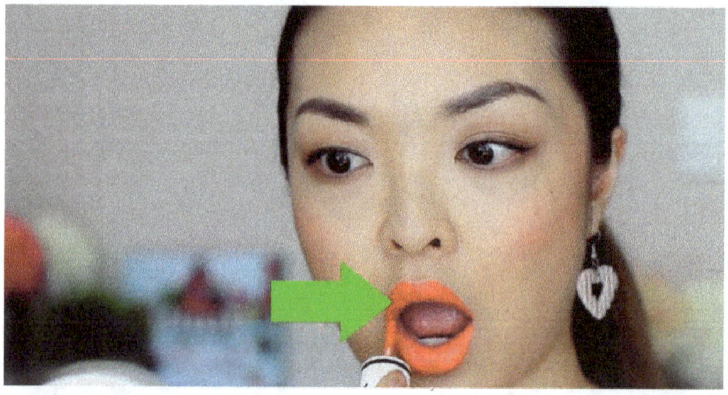

4. Finish applying the lip stain to your upper lip. Start applying the lip stain at the top of your lip. Drag the applicator or brush downward towards the corner. Be sure to fill in the center part of your lip as well.

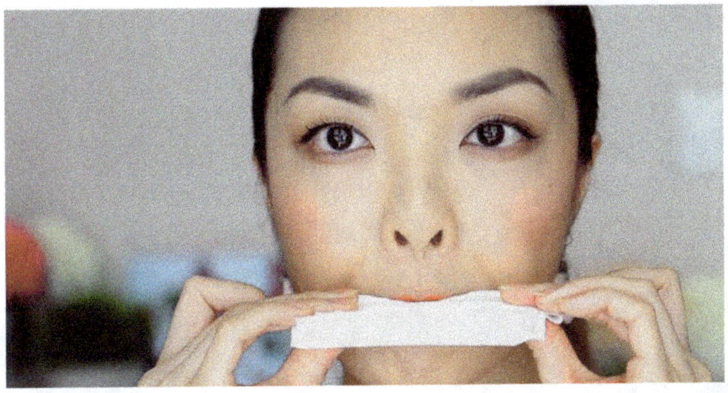

5. Blot your lips with a tissue or paper towel. Take a tissue or paper towel, and fold it in half. Place it between your lips. Close your lips and pull them inward. Open your lips and discard the paper towel. This helps get rid of any excess lip stain. It also helps make your lip stain look more natural.

Part 3

Adding Depth and Shimmer

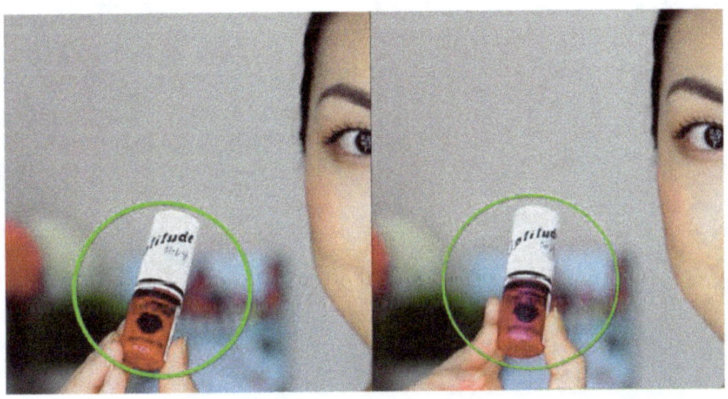

1. Choose a brighter and darker shade of lip stain. You will be applying brighter shade to the outline of your lips, to make them "pop." You will be applying the darker shade to the inner part of your lips to add depth. Combined, this will make your lips appear fuller and plumper.

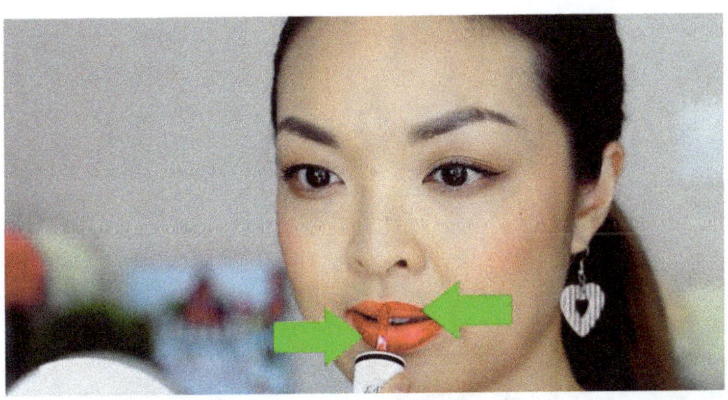

2. Start outlining the inside of your upper and bottom lips with the brighter lip stain shade. Keep the lip stain inside your lip line, not outside. The innermost part of your lips should still have the lighter lip stain color.

- For a sharper, crisper look, use a lipstick brush to apply the lip stain—even if it comes with an applicator.

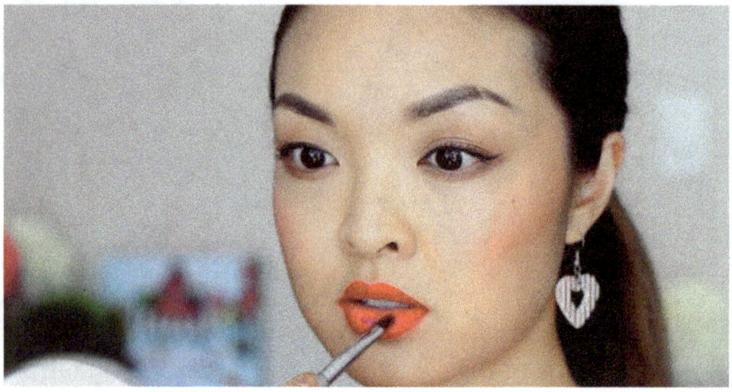

3. Blend the lip stain shade in with a lipstick brush. Once you have outlined your lips using the brighter shade, go over your lips with a lipstick brush. Focus on the transition line, right where the two shades meet. This will create a smoother transition, and make your lip stain look more natural.

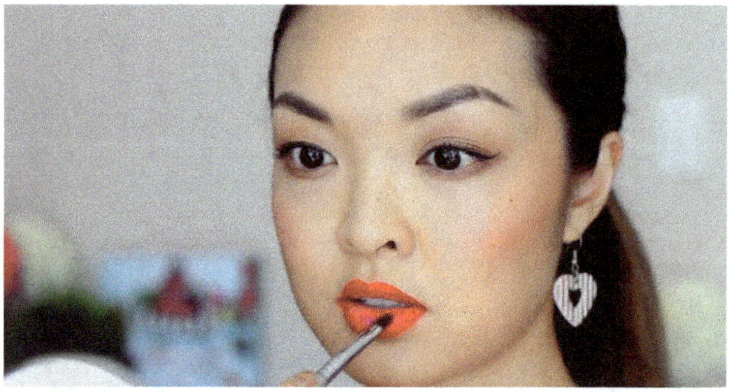

4. Apply the darker shade to center part of your lips using a lipstick brush. Gently dab the lip stain on using a soft, tapping motion. Focus the color on the inner part of your mouth, and work your way to the center of your lips.

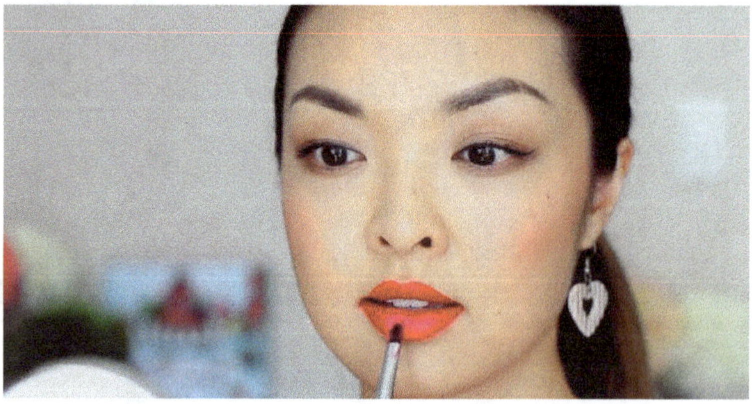

5. Consider adding a dab shimmer on the center of your bottom lip. This will help make your lips appear plumper. Choose a light pink, shimmery shade, and tap it onto the middle of your bottom

lip. This will help give your lips that finally touch of luscious fullness.

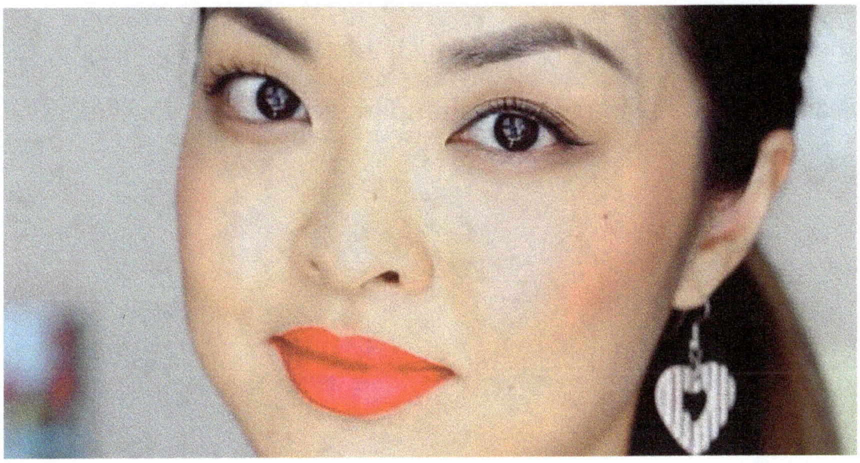

How to Get Pouty Lips

Pouty lips are oh-so-pretty, and if yours are naturally thin, you might be wondering what you can do to plump them up. You can use makeup to make them appear to be fuller, use a lip plumping product, or even dab on a little cinnamon to make them temporarily swell a little. Prepping your lips by exfoliating them well will also help you create a more kissable look.

Method 1

Using Plumping Techniques

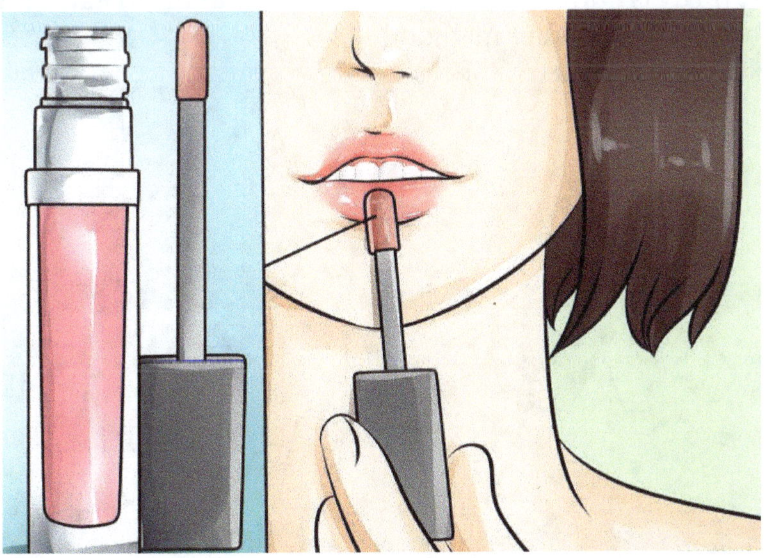

1. Use a lip-plumping product. In the cosmetic section of the drugstore you'll find shelves of products designed to have a lip-plumping effect. These glosses and chapsticks usually contain ingredi-

ents like cinnamon oil or capsaicin, the substance that makes hot peppers hot. These ingredients slightly irritate the skin, causing it to plump up temporarily.

- Lip-plumpers are usually quite glossy, which creates an even poutier appearance.
- Caffeine is also commonly found in lip plumpers, so check the ingredients if you're sensitive to it.

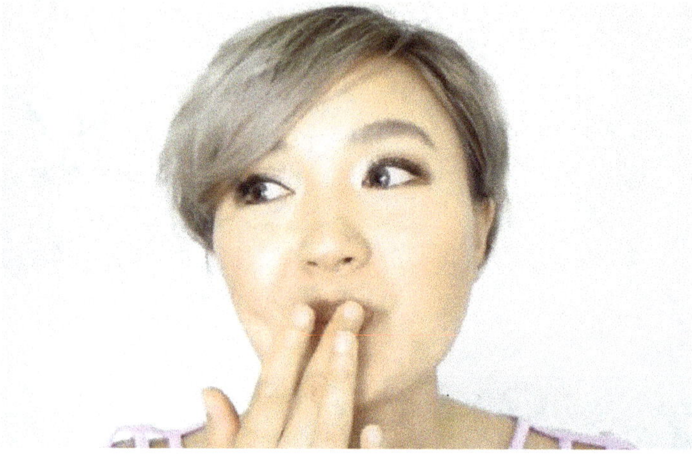

2. Try brushing with a little cinnamon. Cinnamon is a mild irritant that can safely plump up your lips a little. Try sprinkling a little cinnamon powder on your old toothbrush (the one you are not using) then using it to brush your lips. Gently scrub your lips until they become full and flushed.

- Try making your own cinnamon plumping gloss by mixing a little cinnamon into a teaspoon of coconut oil. Place it in an old chapstick jar and use it whenever your lips need a boost.
- Feeling a little tingly is normal, but if your lips feel painfully irritated after using cinnamon, discontinue use and try another method.

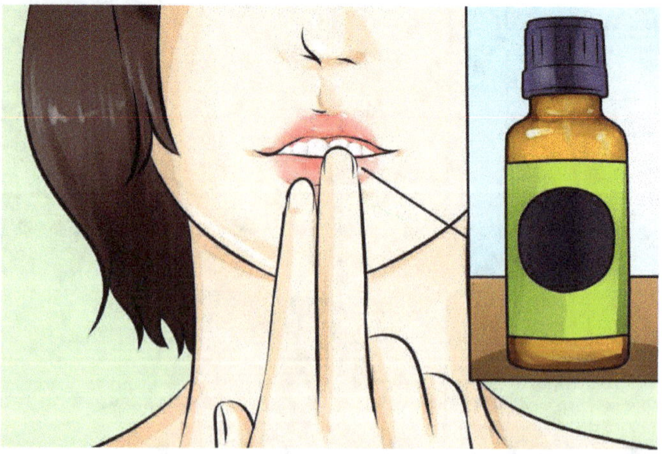

3. Rub on some peppermint oil. Mint, similarly to cinnamon, has a mildly irritating effect that can cause the lips to swell a little. A great natural way to plump your lips is by rubbing on a few drops of peppermint oil.

- Make your own plumping gloss by mixing 5 drops of peppermint oil with a teaspoon of coconut oil. Store it in an old chapstick jar.
- If your lips feel irritated by the peppermint, use another method.

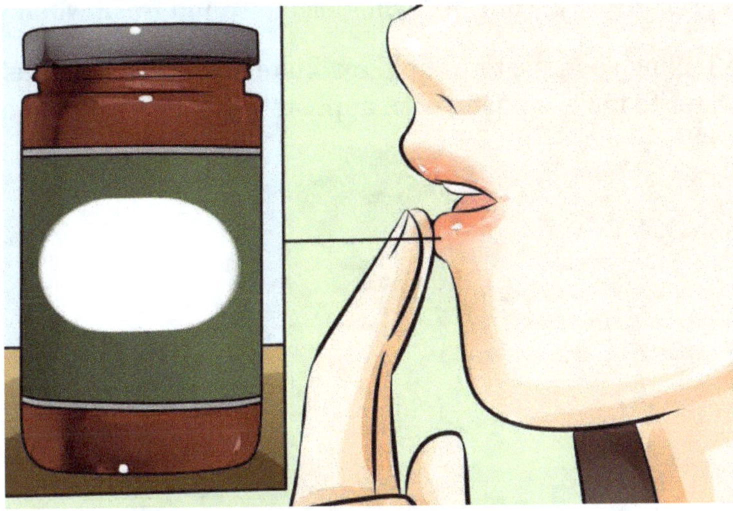

4. Rub a hot pepper on your lips. This method isn't for the faint of heart, but it works! Take a small piece of jalapeno or another moderately spicy pepper and rub it over your lips. In a moment or two, your lips will start to swell, much like they do when you eat hot salsa or hot sauce.

- Don't try this with habaneros or other very hot peppers, since the experience might get uncomfortable.
- You could also dab a little dried pepper powder, such as cayenne, into your lips for a plumping effect.

Method 2

Using Makeup

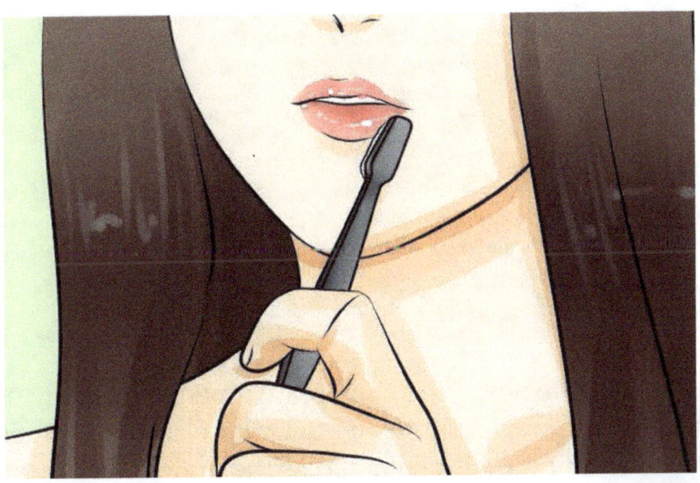

1. Start by exfoliating. Exfoliating your lips increases circulation, helping blood rush to your lips

to make them look fuller. Use a toothbrush to scrub away dry, flaky skin, leaving the fresh skin underneath.

- You can moisturize your lips at the same time by using coconut oil. Put a little on your toothbrush and scrub away. Your lips will look shiny and fresh when you're finished.
- Or try using a baking soda paste to help exfoliate deeper. Mix a teaspoon of baking soda with enough water to make a paste, then apply it to your toothbrush and scrub.

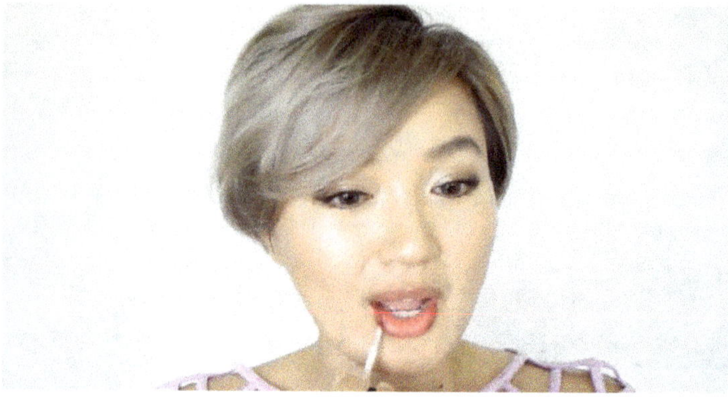

2. Use lip pencil to broaden your lip outline. Choose a lip pencil that's the same color as your lips, a few shades darker than your facial skin tone. Carefully outline your lips just a centimeter or so above and below your natural lip line. Fill in the gap using the lip pencil. This will create the illusion that your lips are larger than they really are.

- Don't be tempted to make them look too big, or it will be obvious that you're using makeup to create fuller lips.
- To make your lips pop, use a colorful lipstick or gloss over the pencil, covering both your lips and the area you drew in.

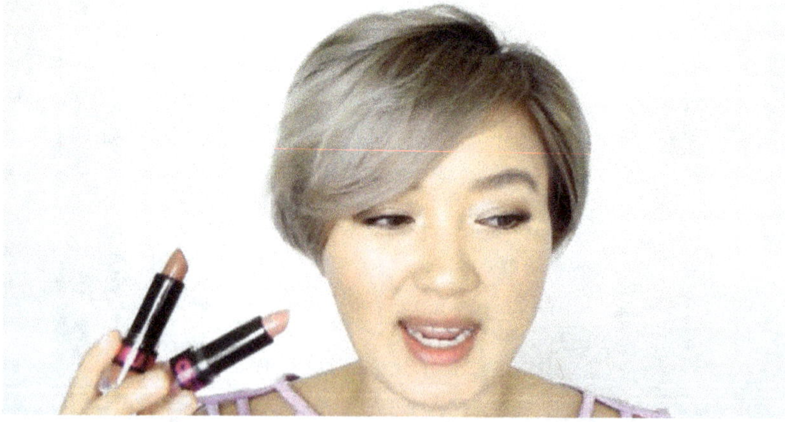

3. Contour your lips with deeper colors. You can create a pouty effect by using a darker color on the underside of your bottom lip, and a slightly lighter color elsewhere. Choose a deep red and dab it on the outer part of your bottom lip. Sweep it across the underside of your top lip as well. Use a slightly lighter red to fill in the rest of your lips, both the bottom and the top. Use your fingers to blend the colors where they meet.

- To create a more defined line, use dark lipliner on the bottom edge of your bottom lip, and a lighter liner on your top lip.
- For a stand-out finish, apply a coat of clear gloss.

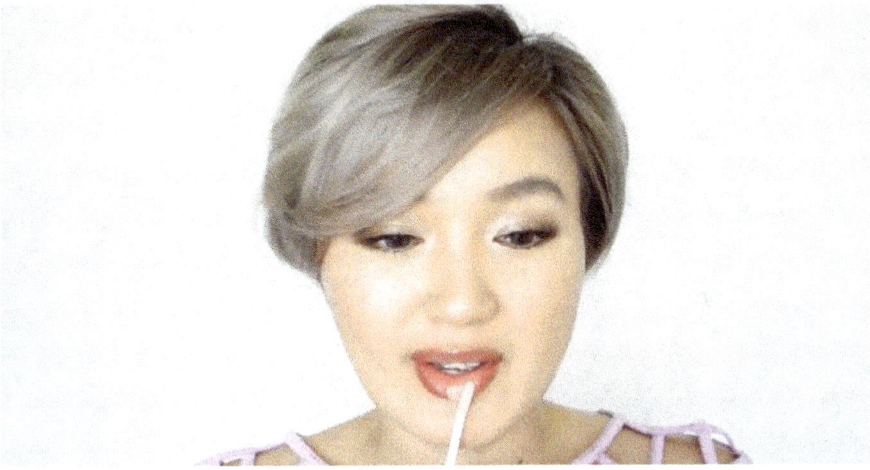

4. Wear shiny lipstick. If you don't have time for lining or contouring, wearing glossy lipstick is a quick way to make your lips look more pouty. Choose a shiny pink, red or even clear gloss that will make your lips stand out from the rest of your face. The contrast in texture will make your lips look fuller than normal.

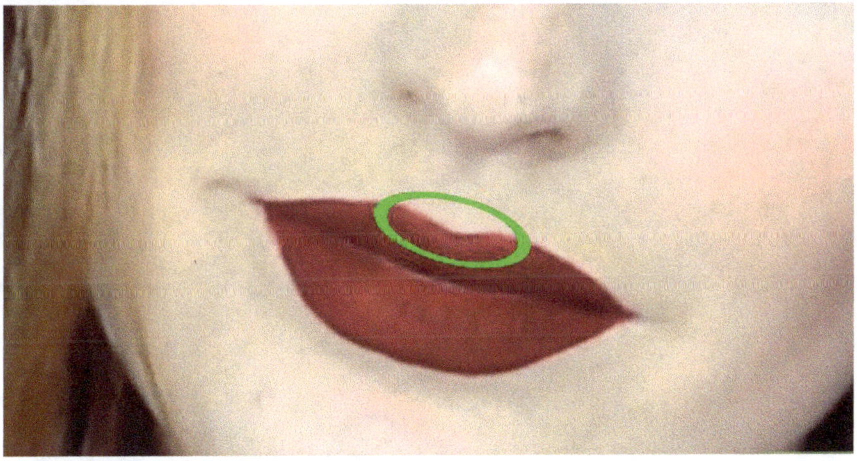

5. Highlight your cupid's bow. This is the ridged area between the bottom of your nose and the top of your upper lip. Highlighting it draws attention to your lips and makes them look fuller and more pouty. Rub highlighter into your cupid's bow, or simply use clear lip gloss there to make it stand out.

Method 3

Trying Long-Term Methods

1. Look into lip fillers. If temporary methods aren't cutting it for you, you might want to research lip fillers. Due to the popularity of the pouty look, there are dozens of options available. The most

famous lip fillers are Botox, but there are other options that use different chemicals to keep the lips full.

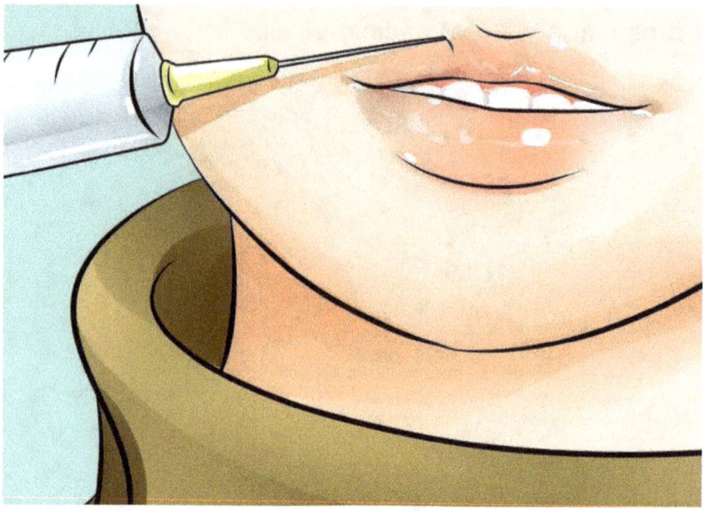

- During treatments, filler is injected into the lips, causing them to plump. The effect usually lasts for several months.
- Be sure to conduct plenty of research and choose a technician who is well reviewed and very experienced.

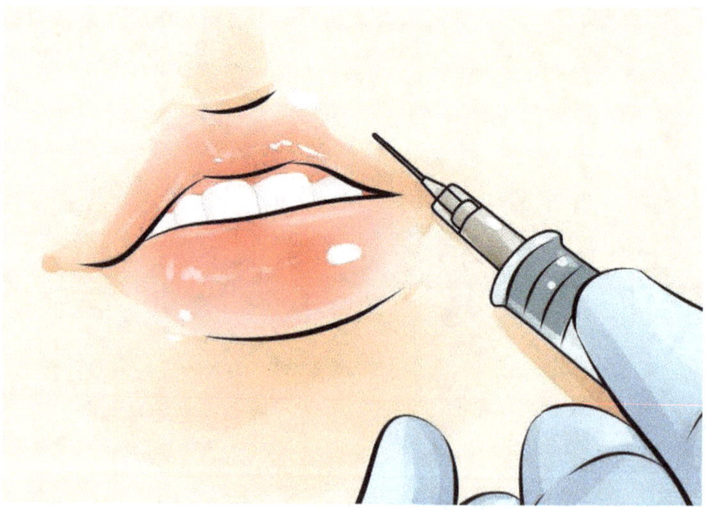

2. Look into permanent makeup. If you're tired of lining your lips all the time, maybe permanent makeup is the right choice for you. It involves essentially tattooing the area around your lips to make them appear fuller or more colorful.

- If you've given it a lot of thought and permanently pouty lips are what you want, do plenty of research to find a technician who will help you achieve the right look.
- It's very difficult to remove permanent makeup, so don't go this route unless you're absolutely sure it's what you want.

How to do Galaxy Lip Makeup

Intricate lip art has been all the rage lately. From ombre to tie dye lips, makeup artists are finding all new ways to turn their pout into a masterpiece. If you're looking for an extremely unique and attention-grabbing look, search no further than these galaxy lips. With a handful of different lip products and some creativity, you can make your lips look out of this world (pun fully intended).

Part 1

Prepping the Base

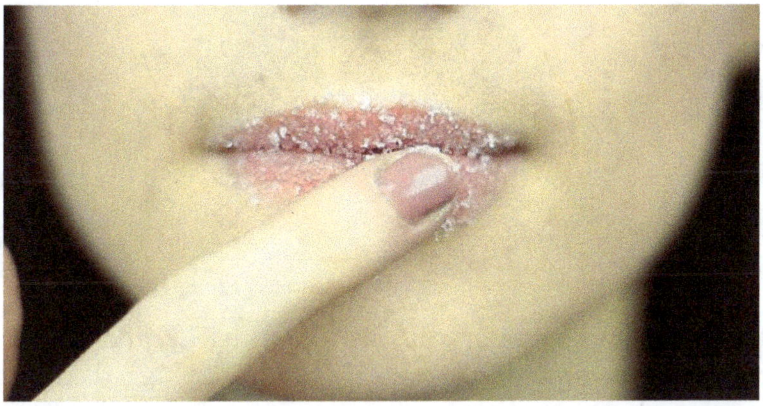

1. Exfoliate your lips. Whenever you're going to be wearing a bold lipstick look – or any lip product for that matter – it's a great idea to start out by exfoliating your lips. This will create a smooth base for your products, and help the colors glide on (and stay on) smoothly. Luckily, this isn't a difficult process.

- Make your own lip scrub with coconut oil or olive oil and sugar. Mix it up to form a paste, and then rub it on your lips using your finger or a soft toothbrush.

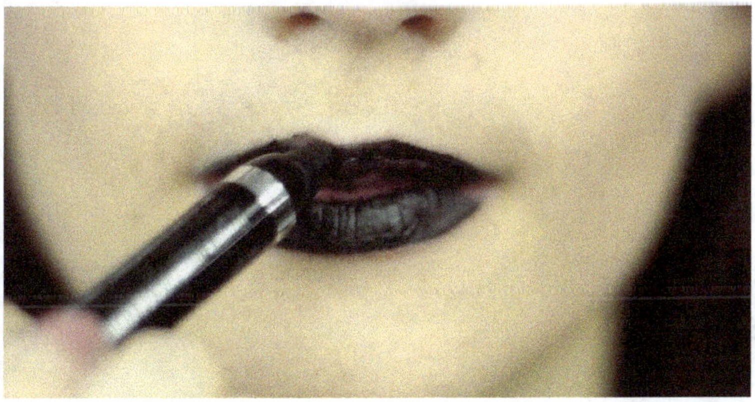

2. Apply opaque black lipstick. Black lipstick will be the base for your galaxy lips, for a very logical reason. The galaxy is made of all sorts of colors, from black to pink to blue to purple. By making the base black, you will be able to add on all those other colors and they will stand out beautifully against your pitch-black background. It would not work if you put down your lighter colors first.

- First, trace your lips with a black lip liner. This will help you create the perfect shape, while giving yourself a neat border to fill in later with your lipstick. Lip liner can also reduce the risk of your lipstick smudging outside the borders of your lips.
- Carefully fill in your lined lips with black lipstick.

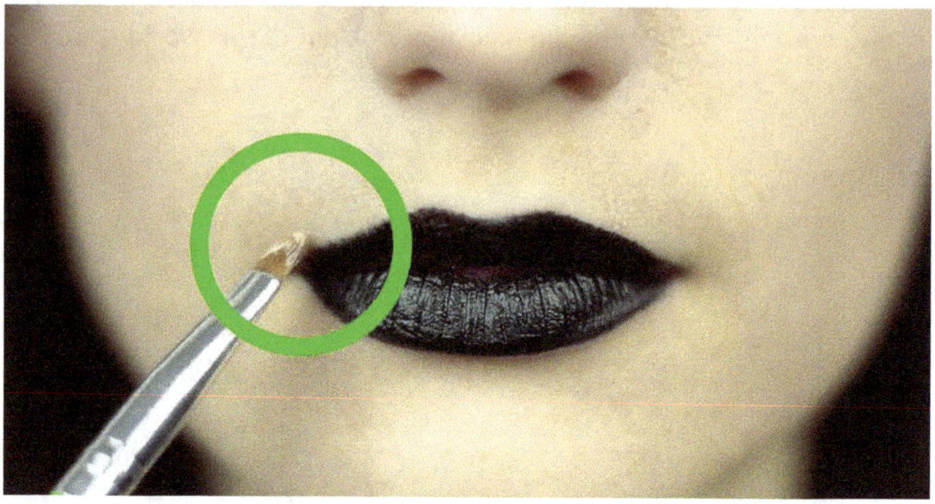

3. Clean up the border. Applying super dark lipstick can be tricky, and unfortunately one mistake sticks out like a sore thumb. However, don't worry if you notice a jagged edge or a bit of lipstick out of place. Once you've applied your lipstick, use a small concealer brush and concealer to clean up the perimeter of your lips. With just a few smooth strokes, your lips will look flawless.

Part 2

Creating Dimension

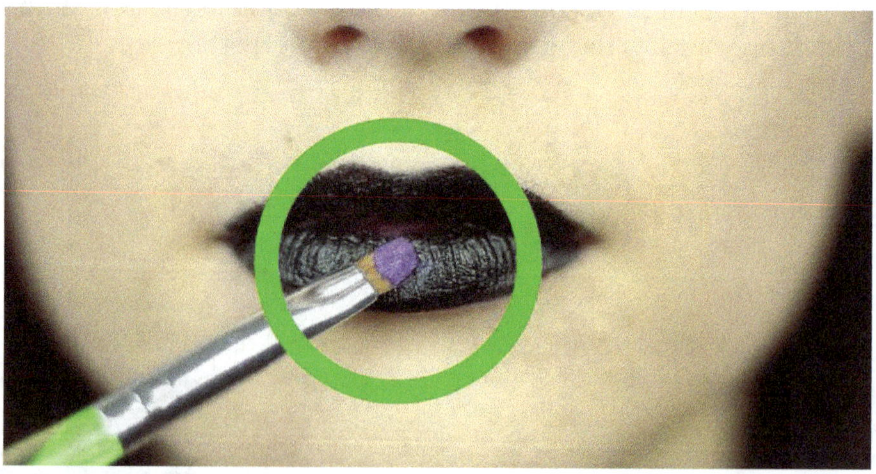

1. Apply purple liquid lipstick to your inner lips. Apply a bit of purple liquid lipstick along the inner rim of your lips, where the top and bottom lip touch. Paint a bit of the purple lipstick directly onto your lips, and then use a small fluffy brush to blend the color outwards. You want it to look almost sponge painted, with no stark edges between the purple and the black lipsticks.

- Continue applying purple lipstick and blending it out until you are satisfied with the look. It should look as if the purple seamlessly flows into the black.

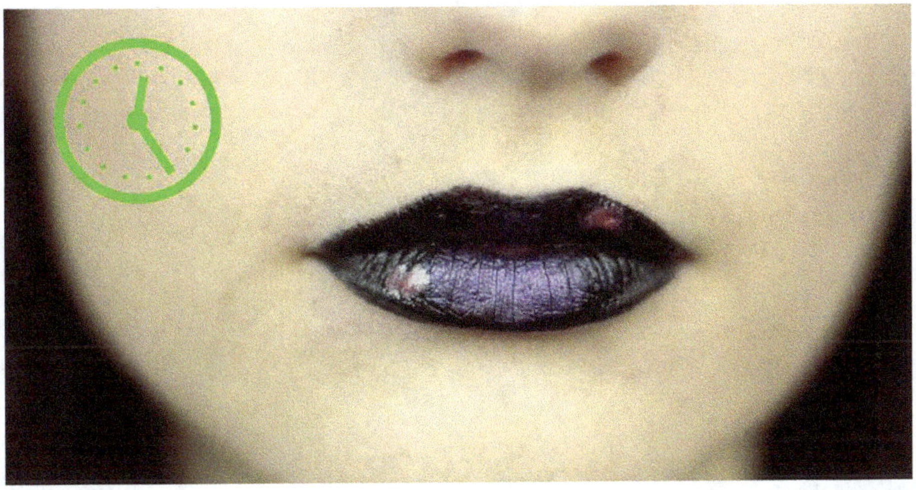

2. Use hot pink liquid lipstick to create spots. Apply a bit of pink liquid lipstick anywhere you want on your lips. For example, you can do one spot on the corner of your top lip and one on the opposite corner of your bottom lip. Let the pink lipstick sit on your lips for a moment, and then start blending it out with a small fluffy brush once it gets a bit tacky. These will look almost like pink shadows on your lips, mimicking the surreal colors in space.

- There are many different colors in space, and adding many colors on the black will make this look more realistic. The trick is to fully blend everything, so that the colors seem to blend into one.

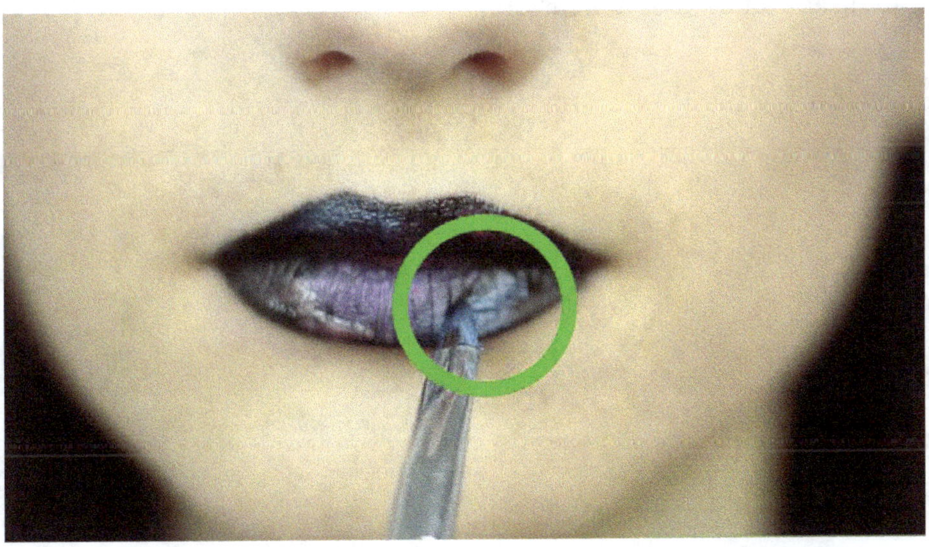

3. Create more "clouds" with blue liquid lipstick. Just like you applied the pink lipstick, apply a bit of dark or royal blue liquid lipstick. Then, blend the blue product out with a small brush. The final result should look like a beautiful, abstract blend of black, purple, pink, and blue – like the fantastical space photos you've certainly seen!

Part 3

Adding Stars

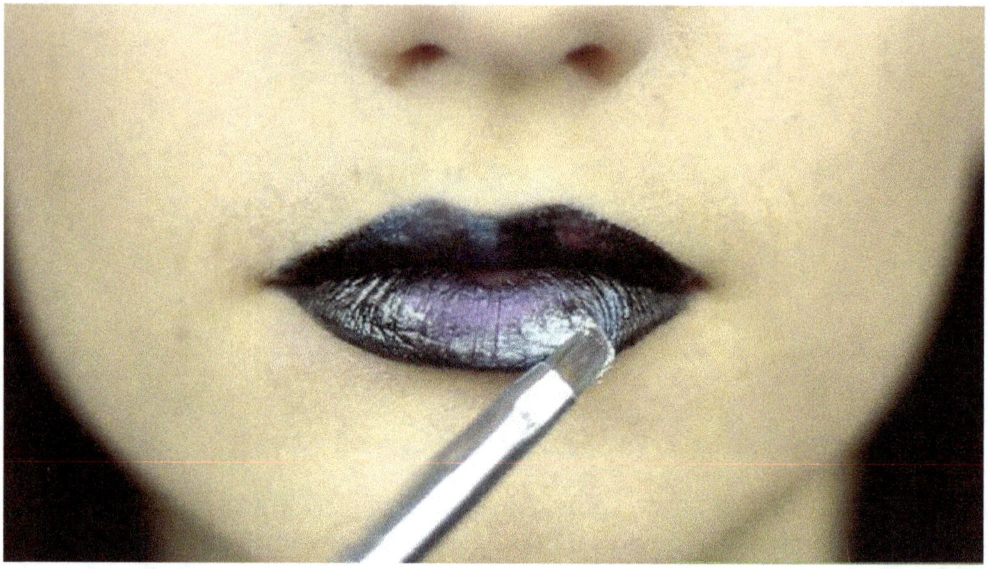

1. Apply a bit of white lipstick with a stippling brush. This is most effective when you apply it against the lighter pink areas of your lips. Gently stipple it on small sections of your lips – there is no exact science to applying it. Additionally, it'll start to lighten up places of your lips, as if by starlight!

- The light lipstick will create sections of your lips that are very light against the black base, adding an insane amount of dimension.

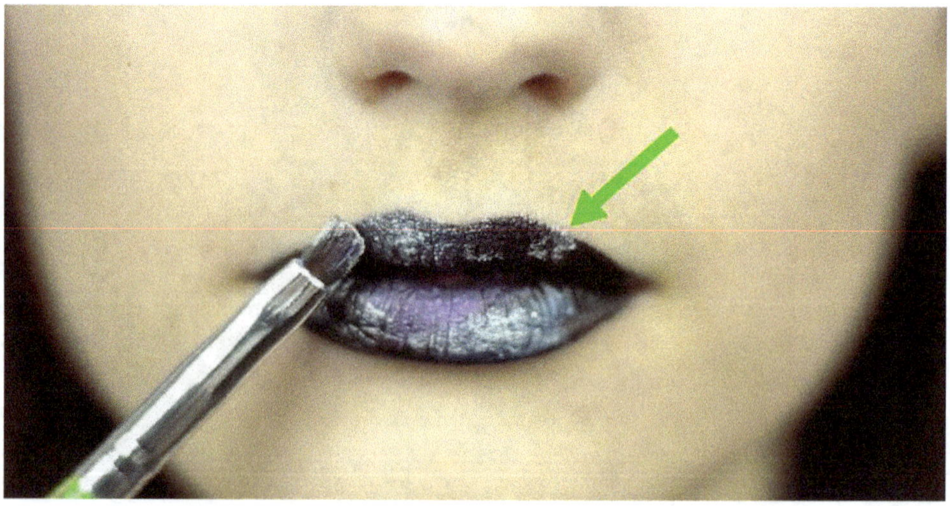

2. Create more starlight glow. Add a bit of light powder, or highlighter, to areas of your lips that you want to lighten up even more. Use a small powder brush, and remember that a little goes a long way! When it comes to creating the stars, you can be very creative. Lighten up your lips wherever you see fit!

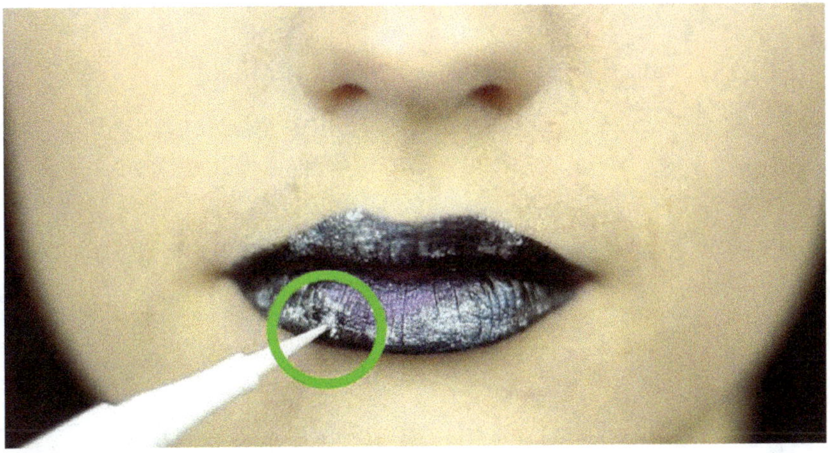

3. Draw your stars. Use a very tiny brush to paint tiny stars on your lips with the white liquid lipstick. You can paint one as an accent, or add several – it depends on both your personal preference and the size of your lips. Instead of creating your typical, five point stars, try creating more realistic stars. Create a plus sign, and then thicken out the center to create the body of the star. Have fun with this step! It's a very creative lip look, and it will never turn out the exact same way twice.

- You can also create clusters of tiny white dots to look like far away stars. You can also stipple a bit of white lipstick onto your lips and skip the blending – that can look a bit like the Milky Way!

How to Dye Lipstick

If your lipstick is boring and you want more color, this article is for you!

Method 1

In the Container

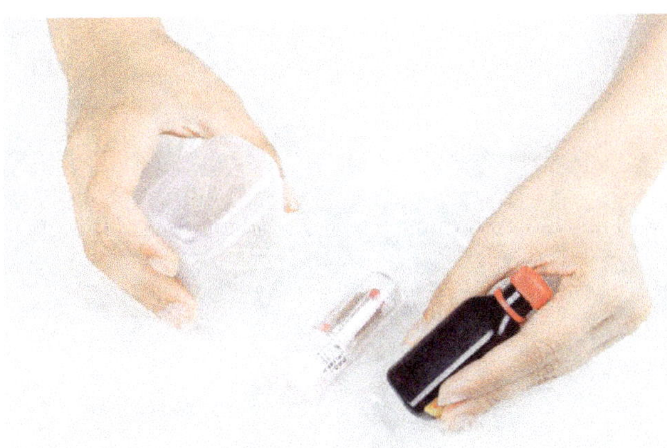

1. Gather the items listed in the You Will Need Section: lipstick (of your choice), food coloring, clean table, plastic gloves, toothpick.

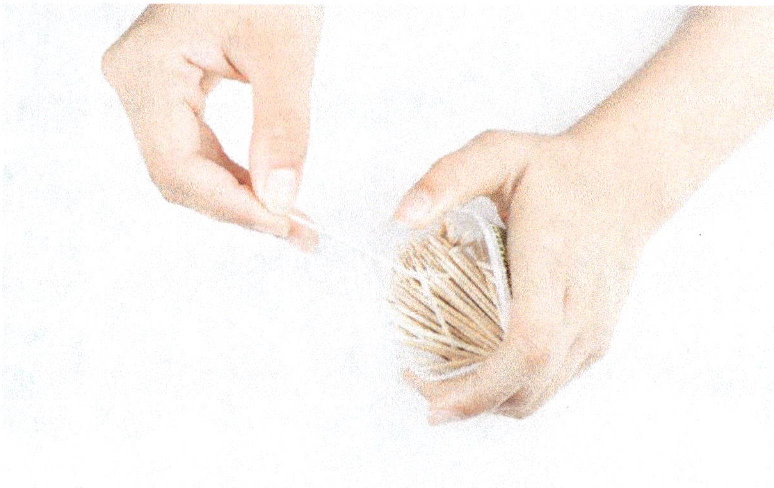

2. Grab a toothpick.

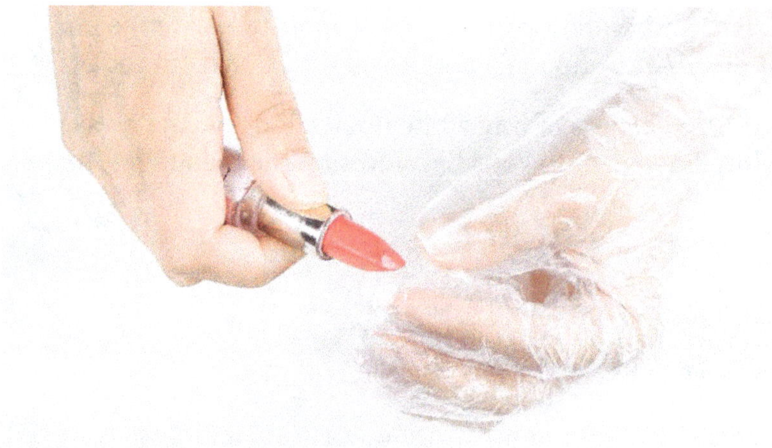

3. Hold the lipstick with your plastic gloves on.

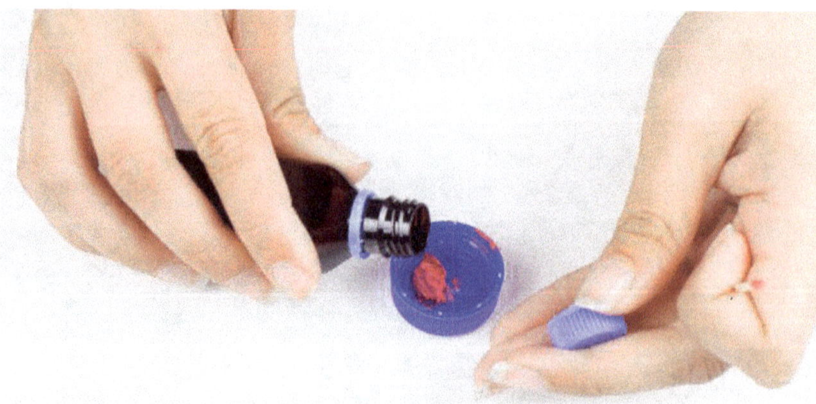

4. Squirt one drop of the dye into the lipstick.

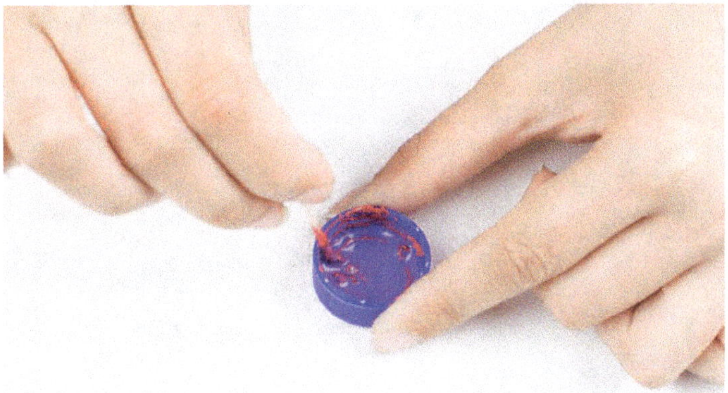

5. Use the toothpick to mix colors. This will be tricky as the lipstick is hard and in a tiny container.

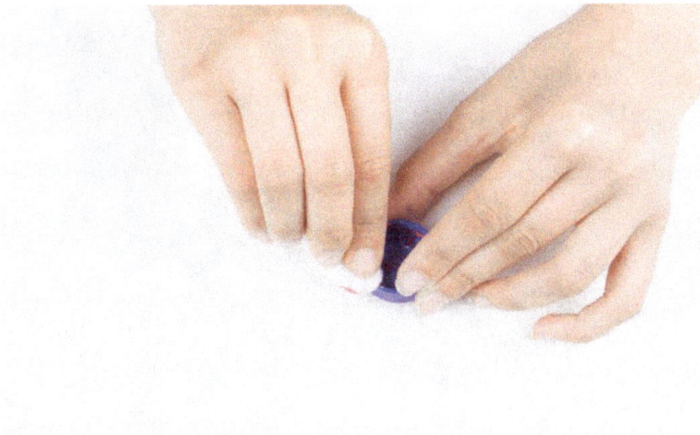

6. Smooth with a spoon if needed, use a paper towel to wipe the edges.

Method 2

In a Bowl

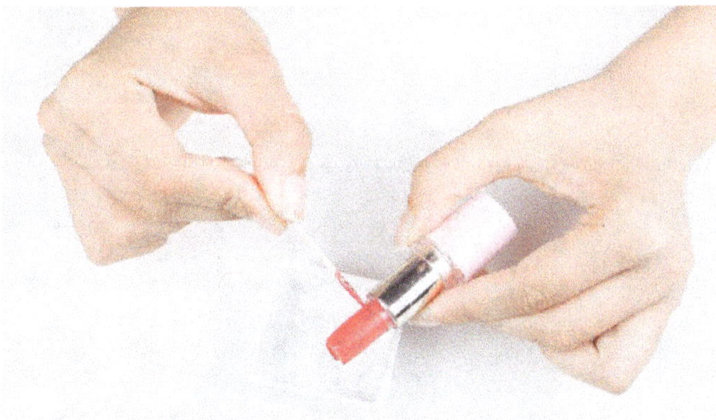

1. Grab your lipstick and use the toothpick to pick the lipstick product itself out of the tube.

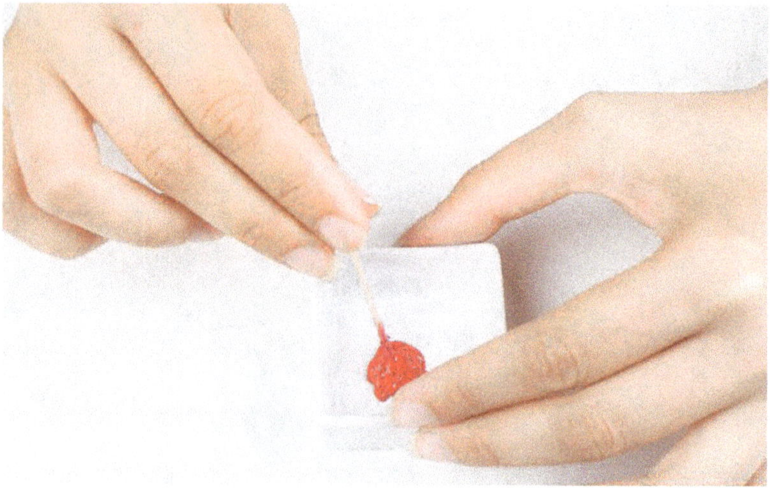

2. Put the product in the bowl.

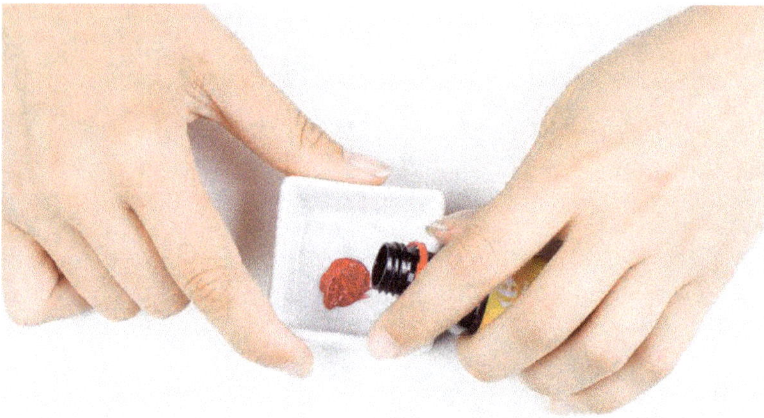

3. Put 1 drop of dye into the bowl for slightly brighter color, 2 for a little bit on the dark side.

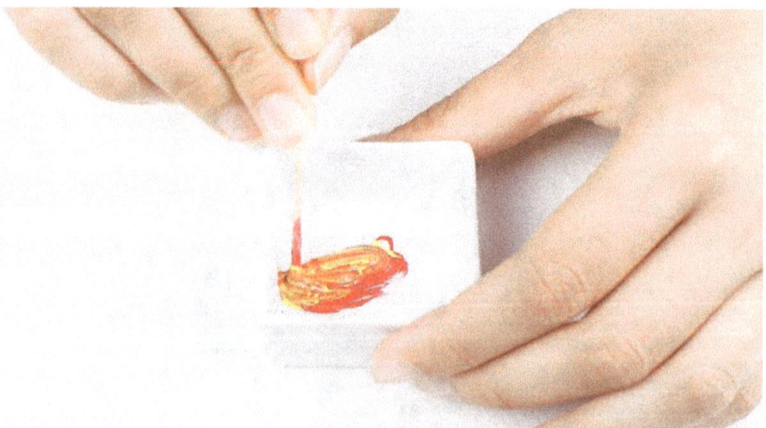

4. Mix for 2-3 minutes. This will be hard as lipstick is a fairly solid product.

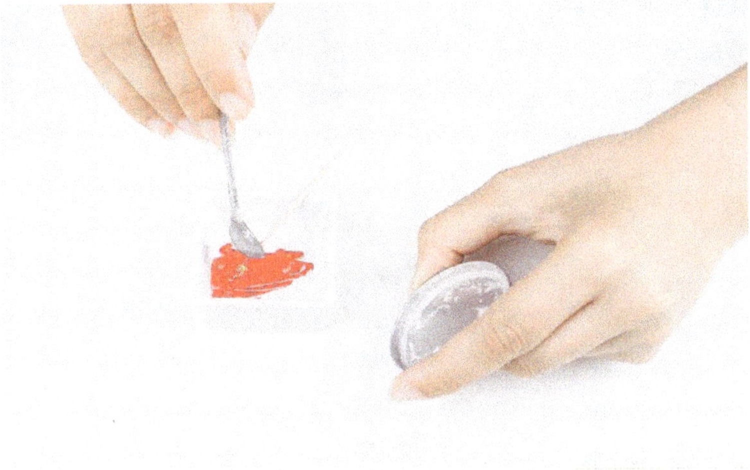

5. Pour or spoon back into container. This may prove virtually impossible.

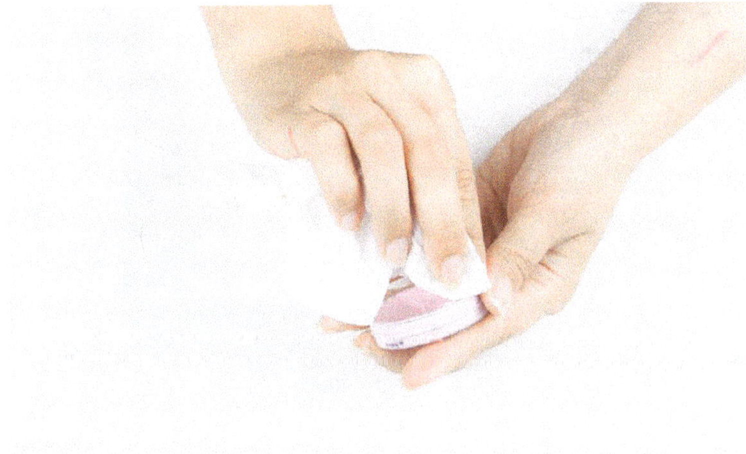

6. Use paper towel to wipe excess off rim.

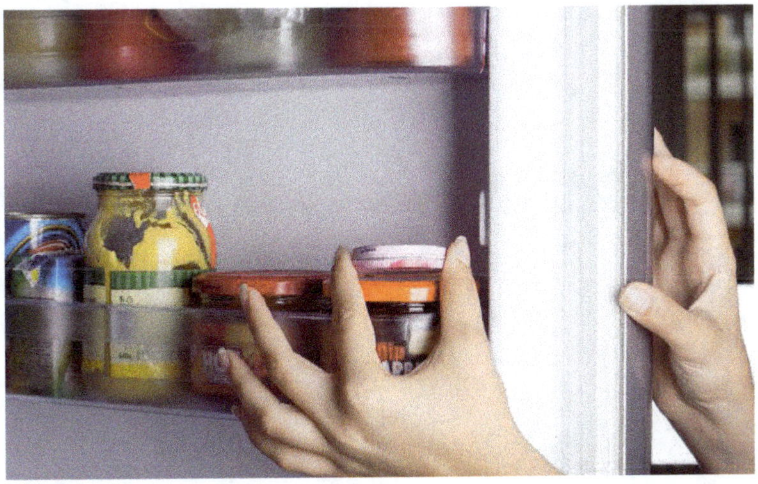

7. Place in fridge for 10- overnight. (Overnight for best results and don't put in warm places or freezing places.) and put lipstick cap on.

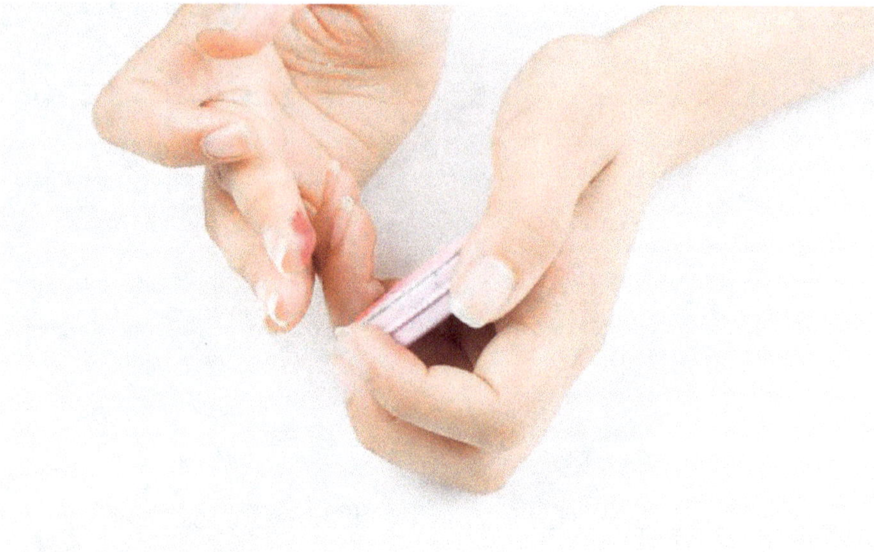

8. Get it out of the fridge and use!

Chapter 5 Makeup for Eyes

This chapter focuses on the cosmetics used for eye makeup. Some of the products used for eye make up are false eyelashes, curlers, mascara, kohl and eye shadows. In order to completely understand the application of makeup on the eye, it is important to understand the manner in which make up tools are used. The section below elaborates the modern techniques and looks created with a range of eye makeup products.

How to have Attractive Eyes

They say the eyes are windows to the soul, and they're often the first thing people notice about one another. Wearing makeup can make the eyes stand out and enhance their natural beauty, whether you prefer a attractive natural look or you want your eyes to look smoky and alluring. No matter what type of look you choose, make sure you take good care of your eyes so they look bright and beautiful.

Method 1

Creating an Attractive Natural Look

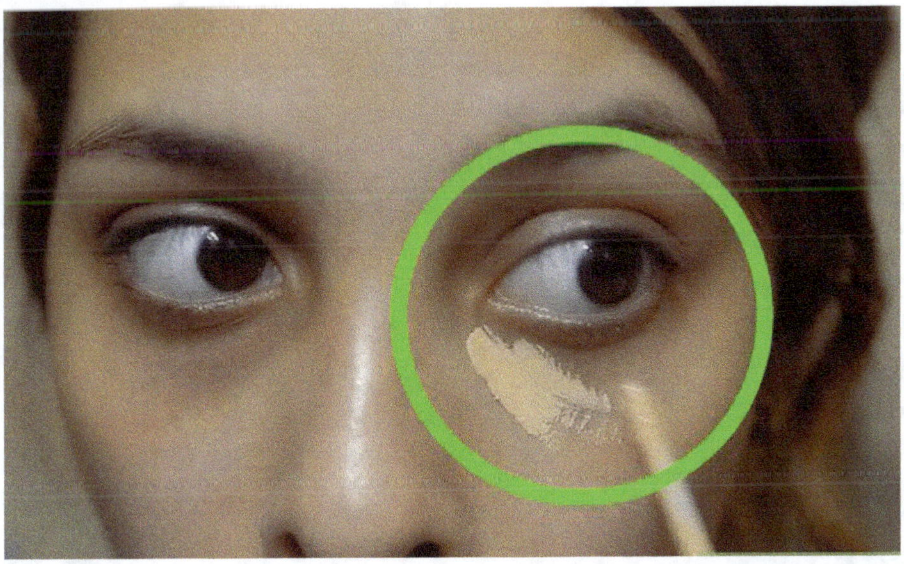

1. Start with concealer. Wearing an application of concealer can help your eyes stand out more. The concealer evens your skin tone around your eyes, providing a sort of blank canvass against which your eyes will look more striking. Choose a concealer that matches your skin tone, and lightly apply it around your eyes. Blend it in with your foundation to create an even palette.

- If you have dark circles under your eyes, you might want to go with a concealer that's a shade lighter than your natural skin tone.
- Apply it gently with your pinky finger, lightly dabbing and blending. Don't rub it in, since this can tear at the delicate skin around your eyes.

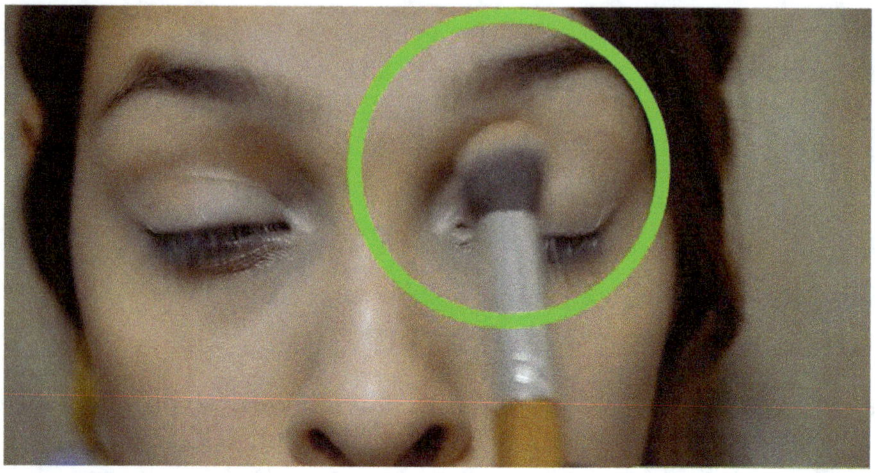

2. Apply a natural eye shadow. Since you're going for a natural look, choose a natural-hued pink, brown or gold shadow that's just a shade or two different from your natural skin tone. This will help your eyes pop without screaming "look at me!" The effect will be subtly attractive, almost like you're not wearing makeup at all.

- Use an eye shadow brush to apply the color to your lids, from one corner of your eye to the other.
- Blend lightly at the top of your lids up toward your brows so no distinct line is visible there. This will help the look appear more natural.

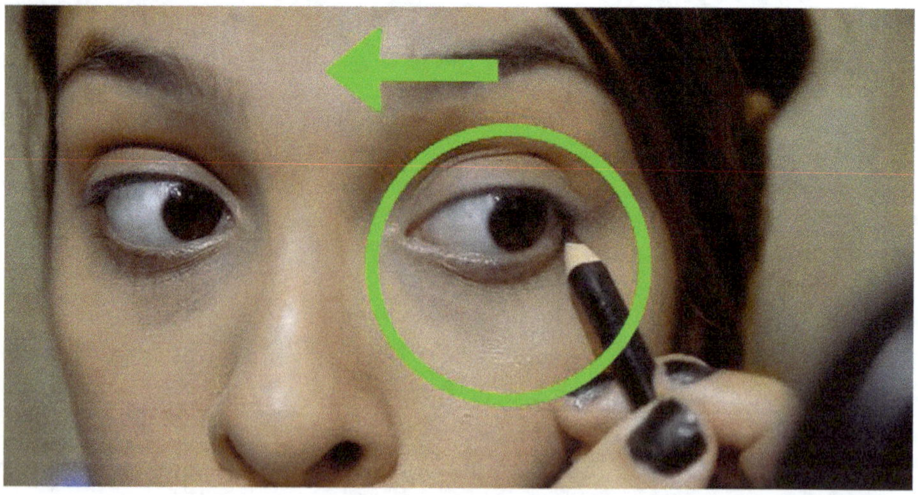

3. Apply light eyeliner. If you want look like you're barely wearing makeup, choose a liner that's just a few shades darker than your natural skin tone. Navy blue is also fine, but avoid using black, since it will create a much more striking look. Apply the liner on your upper and lower lids.

- Use a steady hands so that the liner goes on evenly. If you accidentally draw a wavy line, you can wipe it off and try again. Try to draw the line right up against your lashes.
- You can use a cream eyeshadow instead of regular eyeliner. Simply dip an eyeliner brush into your cream shadow and apply it on the upper and lower lids. This creates a much wider range of color choices.

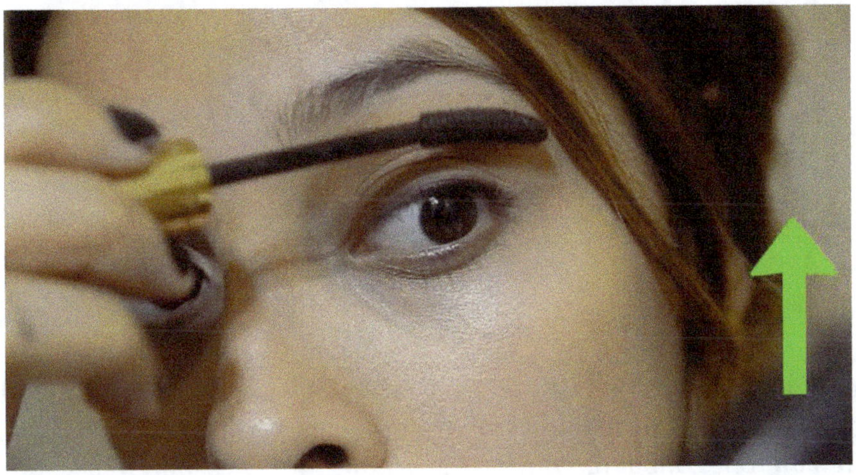

4. Don't forget your lashes. If you have short or thin lashes, curl them with an eyelash curler to help them stand out a little more. Otherwise, just apply mascara to your upper and lower lashes. Keep the application light so that your lashes don't clump.

- If your lashes clump, use a toothpick to gently separate them so you don't have to wipe it all off and start over.
- Avoid false eyelashes when you're going for a natural look. They can help your eyes stand out, but it's better to use them when the rest of your makeup is just as bold.

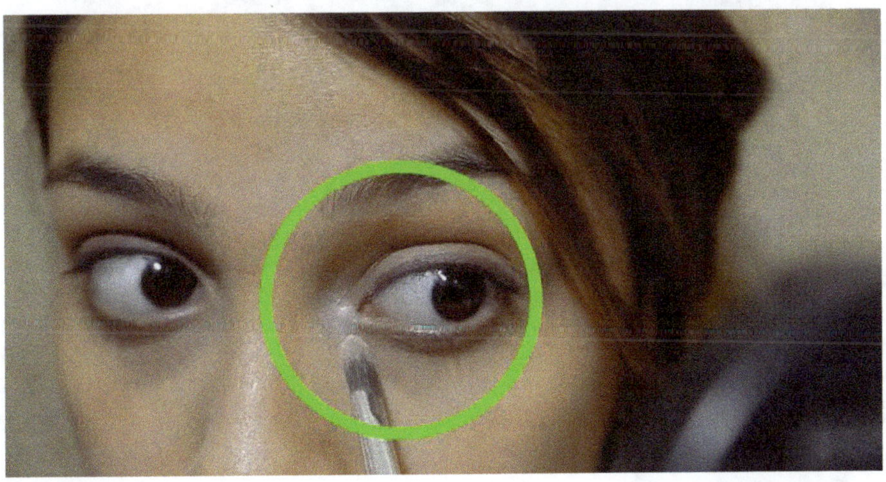

5. Try highlighter to brighten your eyes. Create a dewy, natural-looking glow by strategically applying highlighter around your eyes. Dab a little around the inner and outer corners of your eyes, as well as along your brow bone. Swipe more over the applies of your cheeks. The overall effect will be fresh, pretty and attractive.

Method 2

Creating a Smoky, Alluring Look

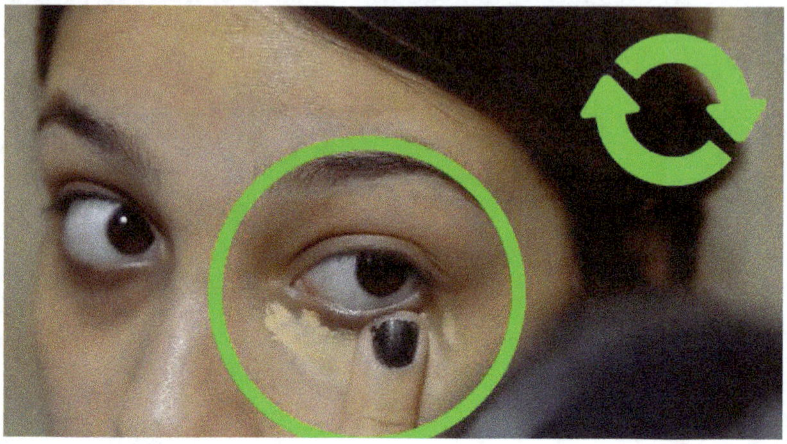

1. Start with concealer. Any time you want to bring focus to your eyes, using concealer is a good first step. Create an even palette against which your eyes will stand out even more by using a concealer that matches your skin tone. Dab it on under and around your eyes, and make sure to blend it well. Dab some over your lids as well, since it will serve as a base for your eye shadow to adhere to.

- If you have dark circles under your eyes, you may want to use a color that's a shade lighter than your regular skin tone.
- Blend it well with your fingertips to create a matte appearance. If your skin tends to get oily, use a little powder to set it.

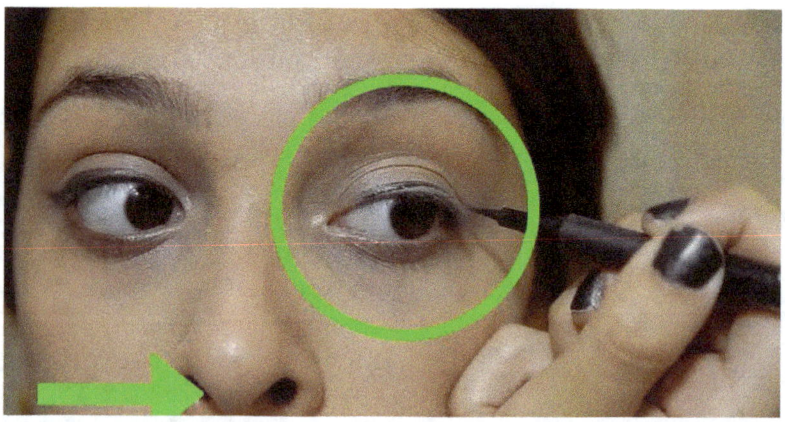

2. Line your eyes with dark eyeliner. Choose black, very dark brown or very dark grey to line your eyes. Create a thick line on your upper and lower lids, sweeping from the inner corners of your eyes to the outer corners.

- For a striking cat-eye look, continue the line past the outer corners of your eyes.
- Take a step back and look at your eyes. Make sure the lines are even and that your eyes look striking, but not raccoon-like.

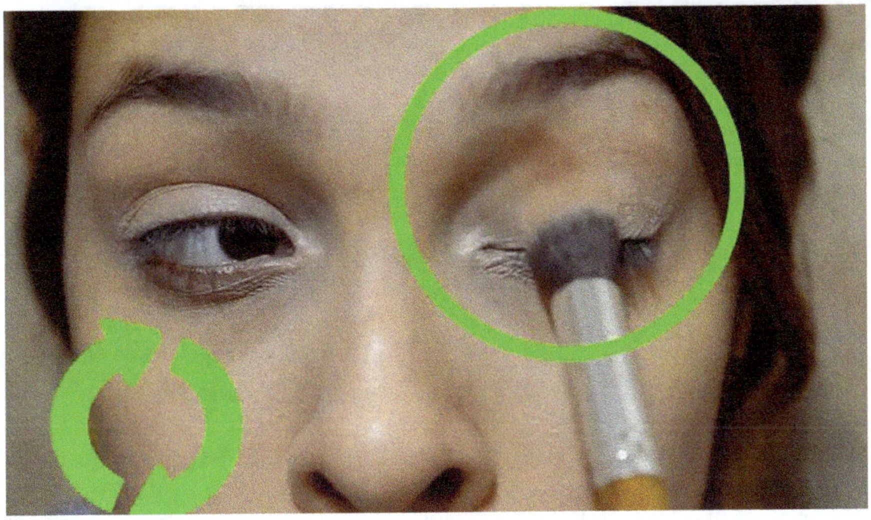

3. Apply a base shadow. Choose a medium brown or gray that will provide a base for the darker color you'll be applying to your lids. Apply it lightly from your upper lash line to the corners of your eyes, sweeping from the inside to the outside.

- Use a shadow color scheme that matches your skin tone. If you have a cool skin tone, choose a bluish-black or bluish gray; if you have a warm skin tone, choose dark brown or a black with some red mixed in.
- To figure out your skin tone, use jewelry to help you out. Which makes your skin seem to glow more: silver or gold? If it's silver, your skin tone is cool. If gold works better, it's warm.

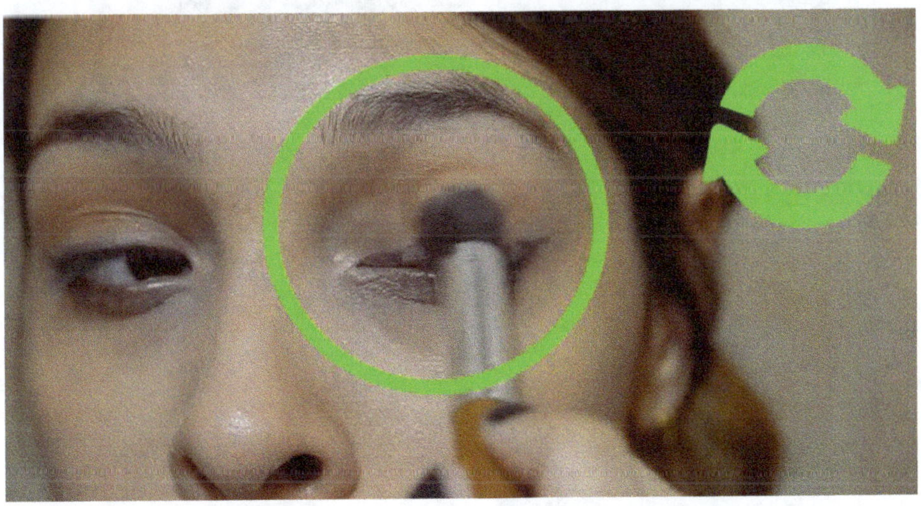

4. Apply dark shadow to your lids. Choose a dark, smokey grey or dark brown that looks striking against your skin tone. It should be in the same color family as the base shadow; you just want it to be several shades darker. Apply it to your lower lids, sweeping from the inner corner to the outer corner. Use your finger to blend it with the base shadow.

- Be careful to apply the shadow to your eyelid only. You don't want such a dark color ending up on other parts of your face.

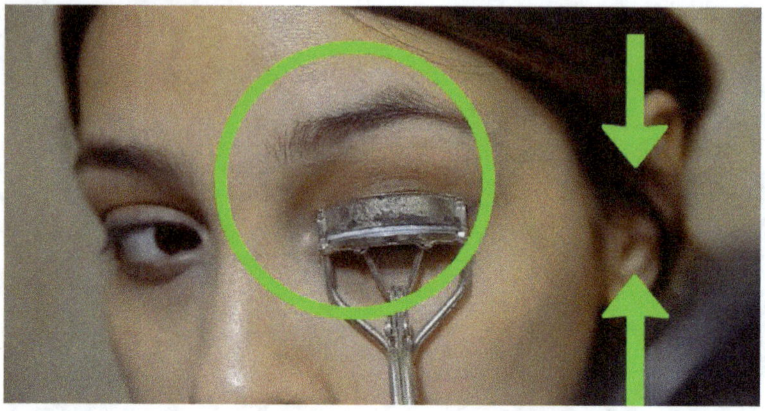

5. Play up your lashes. The smokey eye is not complete without a set of gorgeous lashes. Curl your lashes with an eyelash curler, then apply a coat of volumizing black mascara. For a truly attractive look, consider apply false eyelashes, which are becoming more and more popular as a way to create an attractive smokey eye.

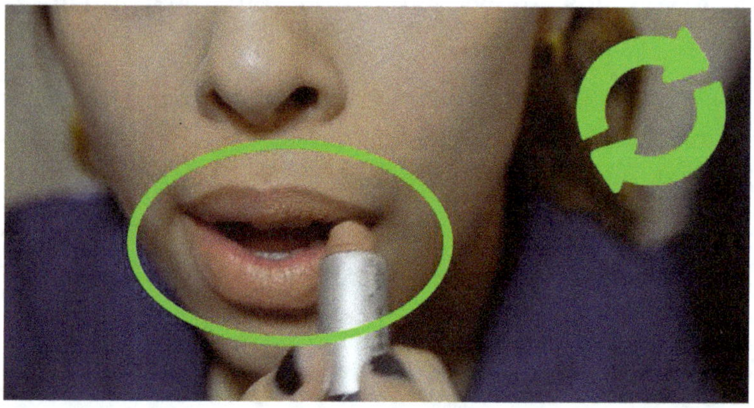

6. Contrast with a nude lip. With eyes this attractive, it's best to wear a nude lip instead of wearing an over-the-top cherry or berry color. Let your eyes stand out all the more as opposed to making them compete with a striking lip.

Method 3

Making Your Eyes Look Brighter

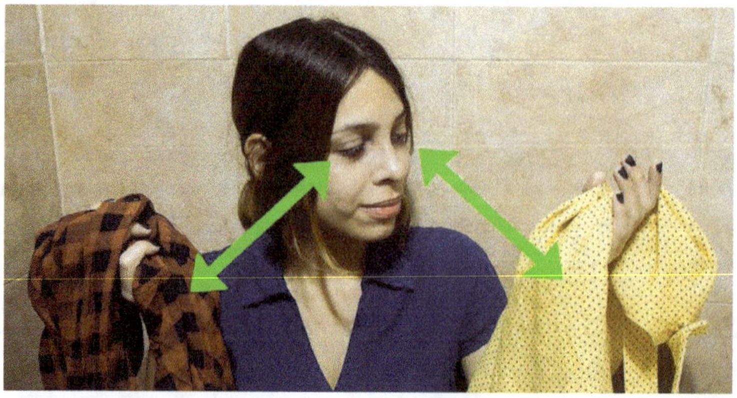

1. Wear colors that bring out your eyes. Have you ever had someone tell you that a certain color looks great with your eyes? The color of your clothes and jewelry can do a lot to make your eyes stand out. Figure out which items in your wardrobe enhance your features, and wear them when you want your eyes to look especially attractive.

- Try colors that are the opposite color of your eyes on the color wheel. For example, if you have green eyes, red will make them pop.
- Or choose colors that are in the same color family as your eyes to enhance them. For example, gold makes brown eyes look warm and inviting, and purple makes black eyes sparkle.

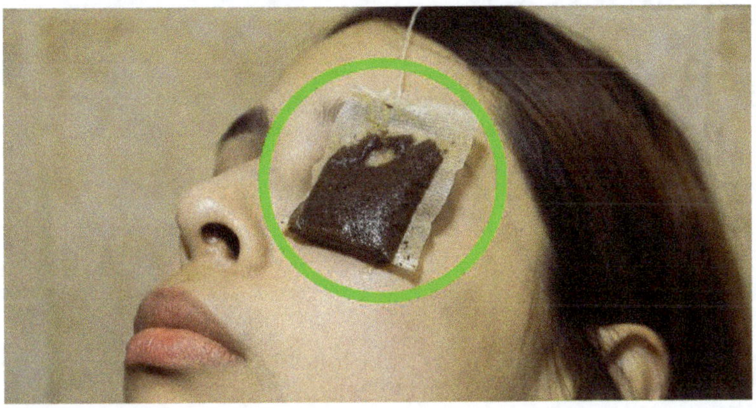

2. Deal with puffy eyes in the morning. When your eyes are puffy, they look smaller than normal, and you might appear to be tired or ill. If you tend to wake up with puffy eyes and dark circles, there are measures you can take to make your eyes look bright and pretty again.

- Put cold teabags or cucumbers on your eyes. It will help the puffiness go down.
- Try rubbing ice cubes wrapped in a dishtowel over your eyes for a few moments.
- Moisturize around your eyes to keep the skin supple.

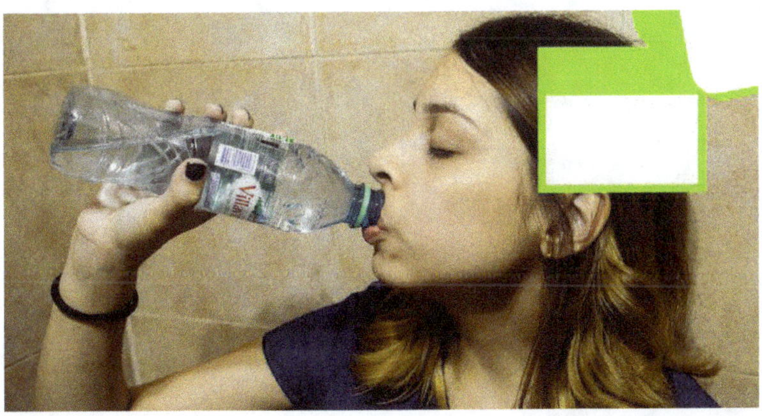

3. Drink plenty of water and eat a healthy diet. Your dietary habits have a huge effect on your eye appearance. First and foremost, stay hydrated so your eyes never look dry and irritated. You should also be eating plenty of vitamin-rich fruits and vegetables in order to keep your eyes healthy and bright. Carrots, sweet potatoes and mangoes, which are full of vitamin A, are especially good for your eyes.

- On the other hand, avoid drinking too much alcohol or coffee, since these beverages are dehydrating and can make your eyes look puffy.
- Same goes for very salty foods.

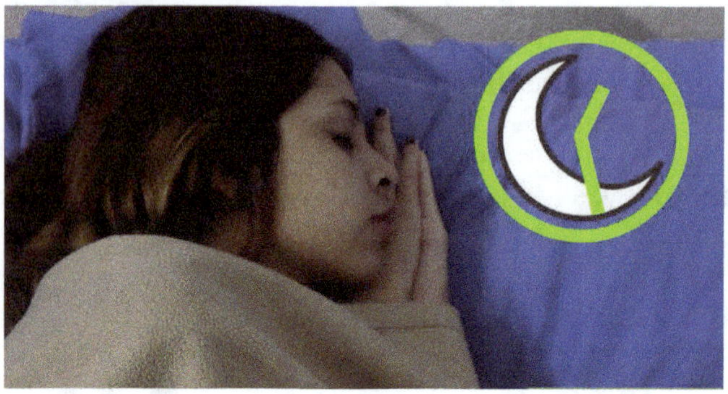

4. Sleep well to prevent under-eye circles. When it comes to having attractive eyes, nothing helps like beauty sleep. Aim to get eight hours of sleep every night so you wake up fresh and bright. Your body needs this time to renew itself, and when you don't get sleep, your eyes the first place to show your exhaustion.

- For the times when staying caught up on sleep is impossible, use eye drops to help your eyes feel fresh.
- If you're sleep-deprived, don't make matters worse by being dehydrated, too; remember to drink plenty of water to brighten your eyes.

How to Make Your Eyes Look Good without Makeup

You don't need tons of make up products to make your eyes stand out. Whether you are not allowed to wear makeup, have sensitive skin, or just prefer to go au naturale, this article will show you how to make your eyes look bright and beautiful without makeup.

Part 1

Making Your Eyes Pop

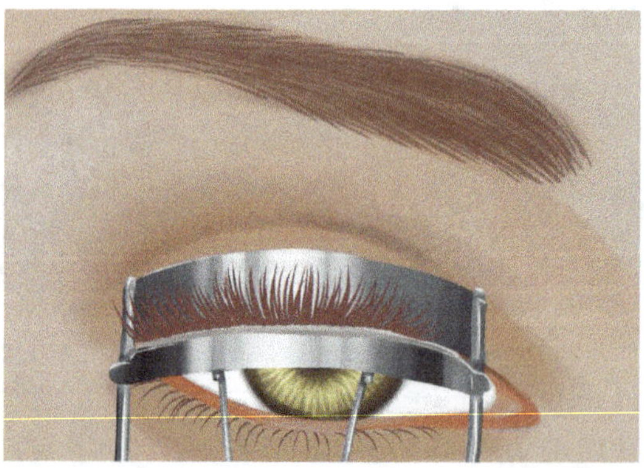

1. Curl your lashes. Even if you are wearing makeup, most makeup artists agree curling your

lashes is a must, because it makes your eyes look larger and more awake. Use an eyelash curler to first curl along the very base of your lashes (squeezing for 10 seconds), then the middle of your lashes and the ends. This will give your lashes a natural curl instead of just bending them up at one harsh angle. If an eyelash curler is out of the question, there are other ways to make your lashes stand out.

- Blow on the ends of your fingertips to warm them up, then gently press your lashes up. Hold for ten seconds, and repeat if necessary.
- Heat a spoon in a mug of warm water, then hold the edge of the spoon along the root of your eyelashes. The curved side of the spoon (the side that holds soup or cereal) should be facing out, away from you. Use your fingers to gently push your lashes up and against the edge of the spoon.
- Use a clean toothbrush to brush your lashes upward. Run the bristles under hot water to warm up the brush, wiping off excess moisture on a towel. Then brush the bristles up through your lashes, a starting near the root, and holding at the tips for ten seconds.

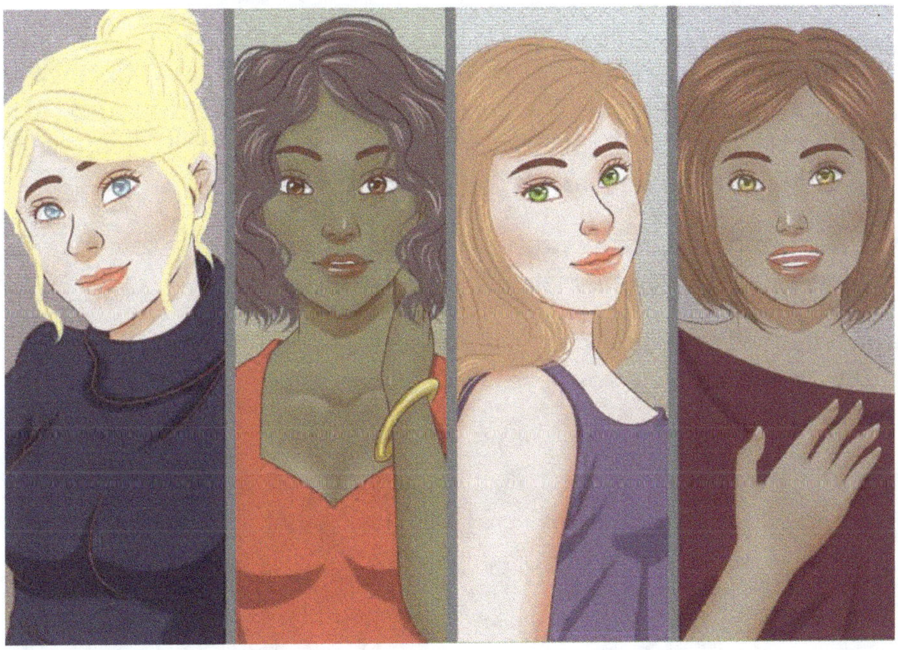

2. Wear colors that make your eyes pop. Figure out what shades really highlight your eye color and buy shirts and scarves in those colors. Think about what color you are wearing when people compliment your eyes, or try holding up a bunch of different colored fabrics to your eyes and have a friend tell you which ones look best.

- Blue eyes should start out with black and different shades of blue (darker blues will make your eyes look a deeper blue, lighter blues will lighten), purple, pinks, and light green.
- Brown eyes should start with oranges and red (or combinations like peach), shades of light brown, bold blues, lavender, gold, and moss green.
- Green eyes should try any shade of purple or green, black, navy, pale yellow, and deep

browns.

- Hazel eyes should try black, navy, and other dark neutrals, orange, burgundy, and lavender.

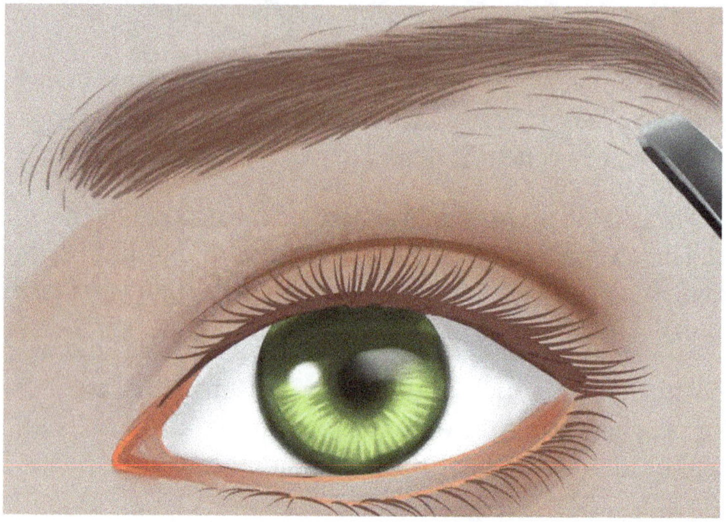

3. Keep your eyebrows on point. Your eyebrows frame your face and bring balance to your features. Stick with a strong, natural looking brow over over-plucked, pencil-thin lines. If you can have a professional salon shape your brows they will give you a template for how they should look and then you can do maintenance with a tweezer.

- Avoid waxing your brows, as the process damages the extremely sensitive skin around your eyes. Try plucking or threading instead.
- If you aren't allowed to tweeze your eyebrows, use a toothbrush to brush the hairs upwards slightly. This trick will make your eyes look bigger.

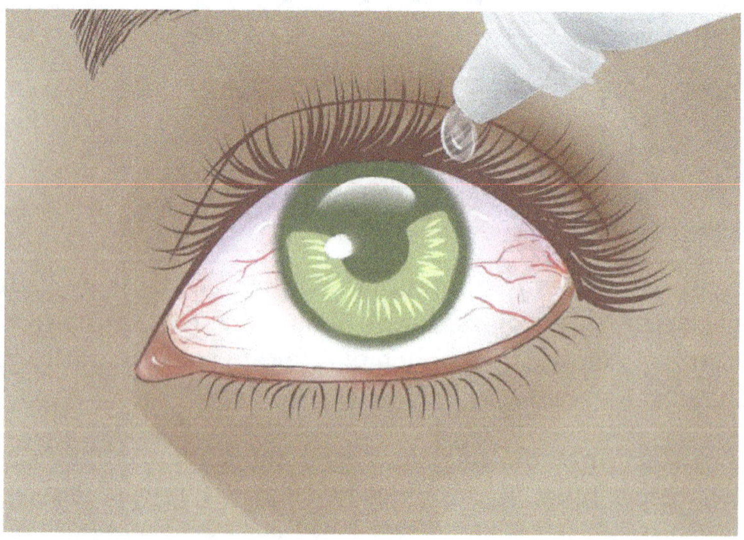

4. Use eyedrops if your eyes are bloodshot or tired-looking. A few squirts from hydrating eyedrops or eyedrops made to relieve redness will make your eyes look clear and awake.

- You can also use eyedrops to de-puff the skin around your eyes--just dab the liquid on the skin around your eyes.

Part 2

Caring for the Skin Around Your Eyes

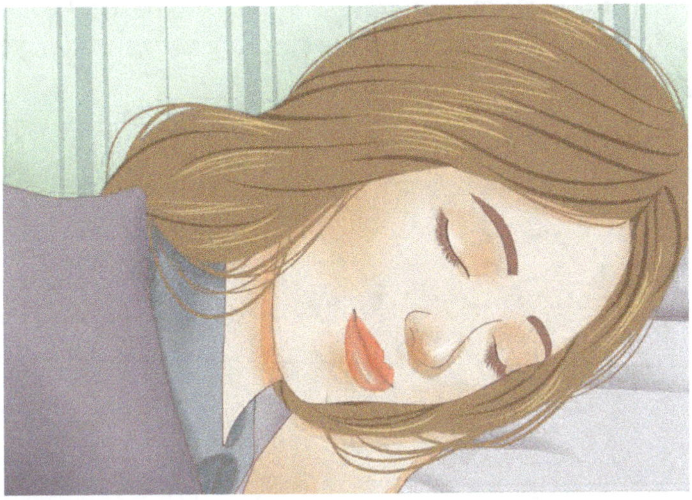

1. Get a good night's sleep to minimize puffiness and dark circles. The skin around your eyes is extra thin, which means it is extremely sensitive and will show the effects of a sleepless night. Lack of sleep can affect your circulatory system, making the blood vessels more visible through the paper-thin skin under your eyes.

- Sleep with your head propped up on two pillows, allowing the skin under your eyes to drain while you sleep and prevent puffiness.
- Dark circles can also result from allergies, genetics, or bone structure.
- To lessen puffiness, try sleeping propped up on two pillows, which can help drain excess fluid from your face overnight.

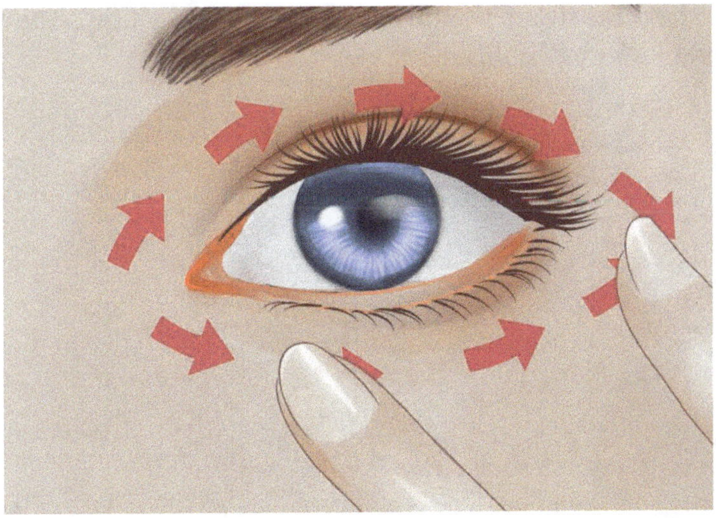

2. Massage the skin around your eyes to encourage drainage and reduce puffiness. Swollen-looking eyes are usually a result of excess fluid under the eyes. Gently massaging the skin around your eyes can help move the fluid out of your face and into larger lymph nodes where it can be processed efficiently.

- Gently tap and massage the skin around your eyes, using your ring finger (this is the weakest finger and will make sure you don't press or pull too hard). Work your way around your eye in a circle, starting at the outside corner, going down under your eye, and then over along the brow bone.
- Learn more extensive techniques for a full facial massage.

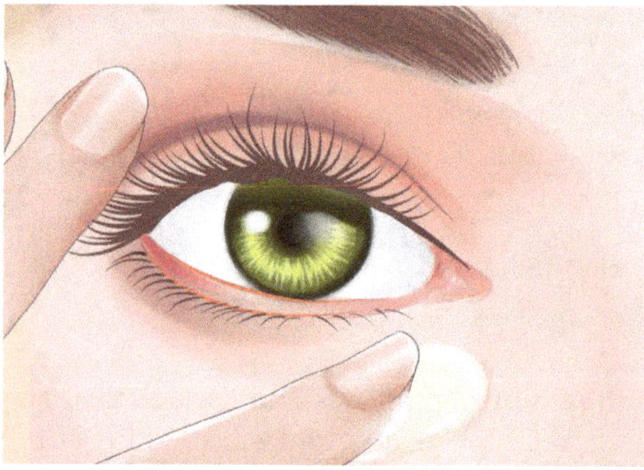

3. Invest in a good eye cream. You may need to experiment with a few different eye creams to find the right one, but you ultimately want something that is moisturizing and contains vitamin E. Beware of eye creams that are too rich, greasy, or waxy, as these can trap dead skin cells and lead to tiny white bumps, or milia, around your eyes.

- Look for creams that de-puff your skin (caffeine can help reduce puffiness) or contain gentle exfoliants.
- Older women should look for creams that reduce wrinkles and firm the skin around your eyes, which can begin to droop as you age. A cream that plumps the skin can help the area around your eyes look youthful.

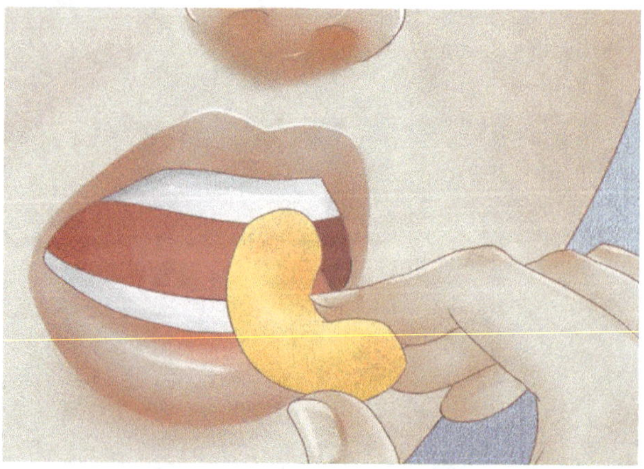

4. Take it easy on the salt. A diet high in salt, MSG, alcohol, or artificial sweeteners can damage the skin around your eyes or cause excessive puffiness. Too much salt can cause your body to retain water and appear bloated. Because the skin around your eyes is so delicate, this puffiness will be even more apparent around your eyes.

- Cut back on your salt intake to reduce puffiness, especially the day before a special event.

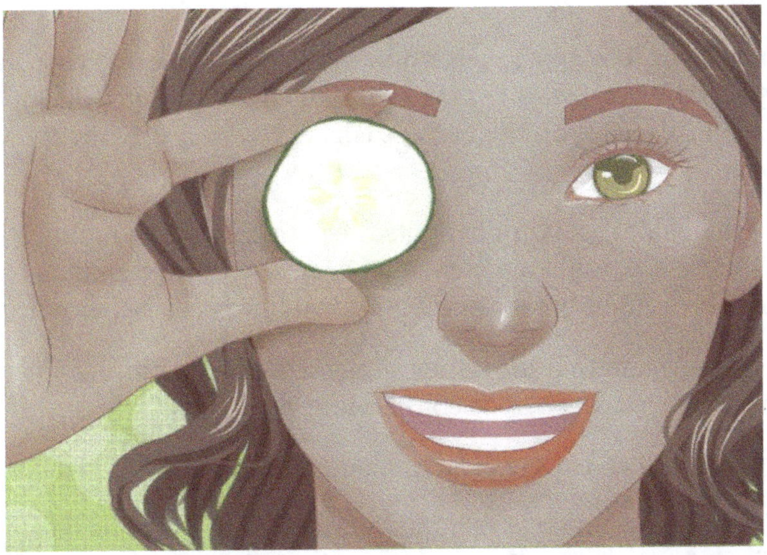

5. Pamper the skin around your eyes with household remedies. It's easy to de-puff and treat the delicate skin around your eyes with items you can find in your kitchen. That cucumbers on the eyes thing you've seen in the movies actually helps refresh the skin around your eyes. Either place two slices of chilled cucumber on your lids, or try plunging your face in a bowl of ice cubes and cucumber slices to brighten and de-puff your eyes.

- Try steeping two bags of black tea and, after allowing them to cool, place them over your eyes to reduce puffiness.

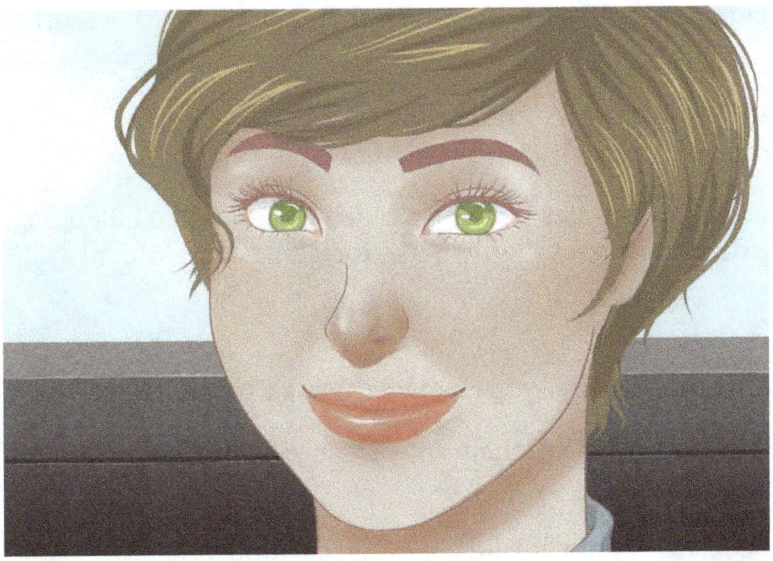

How to use False Eyelashes

Go for glamour with false eyelashes. Whether you apply a few singles to create a subtle change or full lashes for optimal drama, practice first'this is a tricky beauty enhancer.

Instructions

- STEP 1: Decide what look you're seeking. A full set of false eyelashes adds high drama to your evening appearance or returns the eyelashes that may have disappeared due to illness. Little clumps of fake lashes on the outside corners of your eyes create a subtle, sophisticated glamour.
- STEP 2: Choose a color that complements the occasion. For evening, stick to black (or dark brown if you have pale lashes), which adds drama without requiring mascara. In the daytime, go dark brown (light brown or blond if you have pale lashes) for a natural look.
- STEP 3: Check their length. Full lashes should follow the natural line of your own lashes. Trim them with sharp scissors to accommodate your needs.
- STEP 4: Begin with clean eyes, free of makeup or debris.
- STEP 5: Hold the lashes in your hand and apply a very thin line of glue or adhesive along the base; let it sit for 1 minute. Begin with a minimal amount of glue, adding more if needed.
- STEP 6: Look into a mirror, either on the wall or placed on a countertop. Apply the false lashes above your eyelashes, as close to your lash line as possible, following its natural curve.
- STEP 7: Adjust the lashes with your fingertips, tweezers or a toothpick.
- STEP 8: If you're using lash clumps, place them at the outside corners of your upper lashes (one or two per eye should suffice). Adjust their position with a toothpick, fingers or tweezers.
- STEP 9: Apply eye makeup. You may find your new lashes dramatic enough without mascara, so take a good look in the mirror first.
- STEP 10: Practice a few times before your debut. This is a challenging beauty trick to master, but a dress rehearsal should make for a smash opening.

Tips & Warnings

- Remove false eyelashes before you go to bed, using a warm compress or makeup remover.
- After wearing full lashes, soak them in eyelash-cleaning solution until the next time you wear them.
- Never pull the lashes from your lids, as you may pull your own lashes out or rip your

skin.

- Never apply glue directly to your eyelids; it may get into your eyes, or you may glue your eye shut.

Overall Things You'll Need

- Toothpicks
- Mascara
- False Eyelashes
- Liquid Eyeliners
- Eye Shadow Brushes
- Eyeliners
- Eye Shadow
- Eyelash Curlers

Eye liner

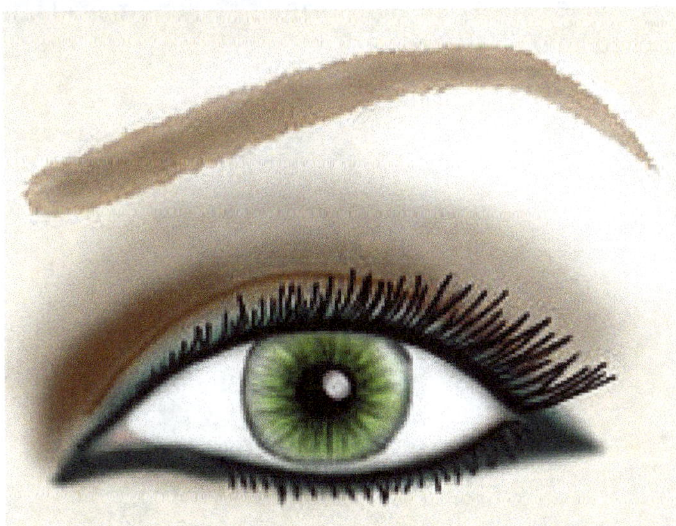

Dark teal eye liner along the rim of the eye

Eye liner or eyeliner is a cosmetic used to define the eyes. It is applied around the contours of the eye(s) to create a variety of aesthetic effects.

Modern usage

In the late twentieth and early twenty-first century, heavy eye liner use has been associated with

Gothic fashion and Punk fashion. Eye liner of varying degrees of thickness has also become associated with the emo subculture and various alternative lifestyles.

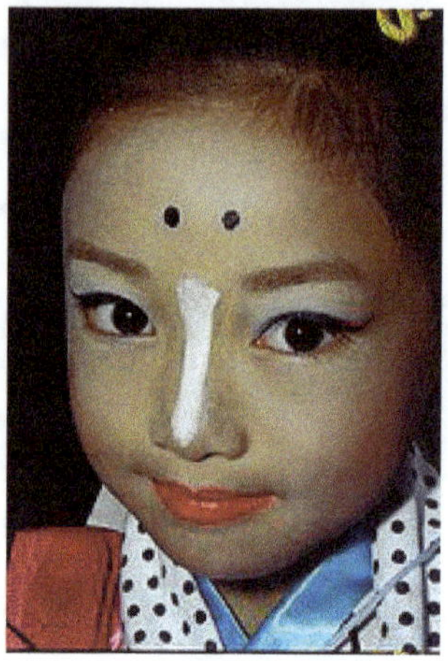

A girl wearing eye liner.

Eye liner is commonly used in a daily make-up routine to define the eye or create the look of a wider or smaller eye. Eye liner can be used as a tool to create various looks as well as highlighting different features of the eyes. Eye liner can be placed in various parts of the eye to create different looks with a winged eye liner or tight lined at the waterline. Eye liner can be drawn above upper lashes or below lower lashes or both, even on the water lines of your eyes. Its primary purpose is to make the lashes look lush, but it also draws attention to the eye and can enhance or even change the eye's shape. Eye liner is available in a wide range of hues, from the common black, brown and grey to more adventurous shades such as bright primary colors, pastels, frosty silvers and golds, white and even glitter-flecked colors.

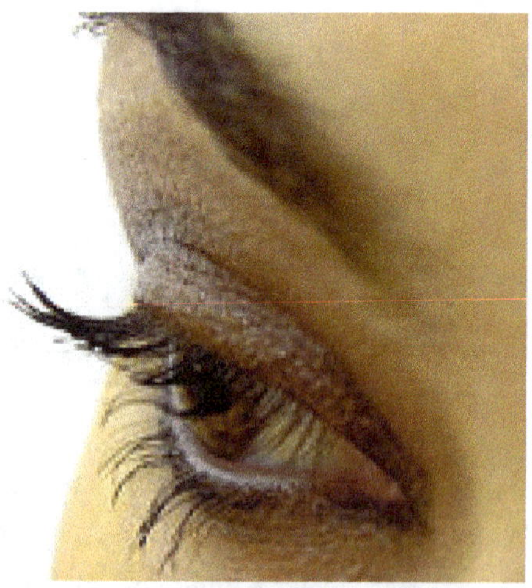

An eye with brown eye liner under the bottom lashes.

Eye liner can also be used for showing depression in photographs, such as the famous "Bleeding Mascara".

Different Modern Uses

Although many users of eye liner use it on a day-to-day basis for a simple definer of the eyes, there are others who use it for more than just an easy eye enlarger. There are many styles of eye liner. Most of them usually revolve around the winged eye liner, which is defining around your top eyelid shape and a line, about halfway toward the end of the eyebrow. It is usually connected to the defining around the top. However today there are some drastically toned eye liner.

Tight lining

Tight lining is the use of eye liner tight against the waterline under the lashes of the upper lid, and above the lashes of the lower lid. Due to the proximity to the membranes, and the surface of the eye itself, waterproof eye liner is preferred. Tight lining is a technique which makes the eyelashes appear to start farther back on the eyelid, thus making them look longer. Gel eye liner and a small angled brush may be used to create this look.

Types

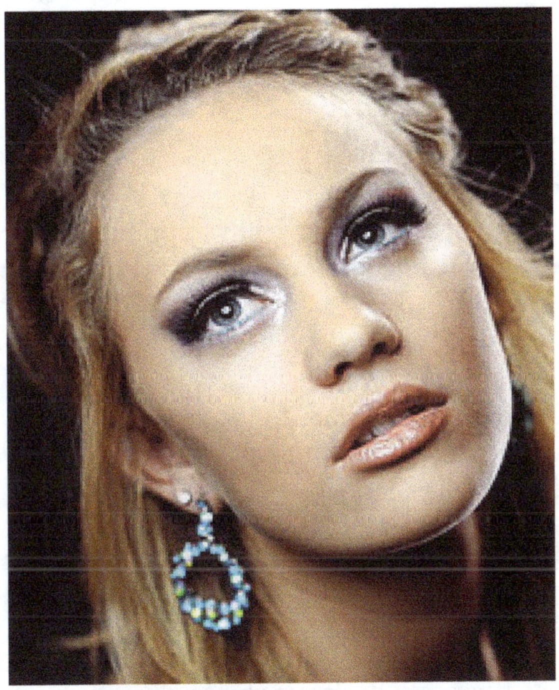

Woman with turquoise eye liner

Depending on its texture, eye liner can be softly smudged or clearly defined. There are five main types of eye liner available on the market: each produces a different effect.

- *Liquid eye liner* is an opaque liquid that usually comes in a small bottle and is applied usually with a small brush with a sharp tip. It creates a sharp, precise line. Because liquid eye liner gives a much heavier appearance, it is often only applied to the upper lash-line, however nowadays it is used in all types of new ways.
- *Powder-based eye pencil* is eye liner in a wood pencil. It is generally available in dark matter shades.
- *Wax-based eye pencils* are softer pencils and contain waxes that ease application. They

come in a wide variety of intense colours as well as paler shades such as white or beige. Wax-based eye liners can also come in a cone or a compact with brush applicator.

- *Kohl* eye liner is a soft powder available in dark matte shades. It is most often used in black to outline the eyes. It comes in pencil, pressed powder, or loose powder form. This type of eye liner is more likely to smudge.
- *Gel eye liner*, which is a softer gel liner, that can be easily applied with an eye liner brush. It can be precisely applied and is much softer than Kohl.

Chemical composition

Traditional wax-based eye liners are made from about 20 components. About 50% by weight are waxes (e.g., Japan wax, fats, or related soft materials that easily glide on to the skin. Typical pigments include black iron oxides, as well as smaller amounts of titanium dioxide and Prussian blue.

How to Apply Eyeliner

Shape and define your eyes with eyeliner after you've applied eye shadow and before applying mascara. Whether you choose a soft line or a dramatic stroke, eyeliner draws attention.

Instructions

- STEP 1: Choose an eyeliner appropriate for your eye color. Brown, navy and charcoal accent light eyes well, while brown and plum shades flatter brown eyes. Make sure your liner complements the color of your shadow.
- STEP 2: Consider the type of look you're after. Pencil eyeliner gives your eyes soft definition, while liquid versions offer precision and drama. You can also moisten dark eye shadow and apply it with a small, flat brush.
- STEP 3: Prepare a cake liner or a dark eye shadow by applying a small amount of water to your brush. Or, if you're using a pencil eyeliner, ensure that you've sharpened the pencil adequately.
- STEP 4: Move the wet brush gently through your cake liner or dark shadow. Hold the brush or pencil as you would hold a pen.
- STEP 5: Tilt your head back slightly and bring your eyes to a half-open state. This creates a good angle for application, while allowing you to see what you're doing.
- STEP 6: Draw a line across the upper lid just above the lashes, from the inside corner to the outside corner of the eye. If you're using liquid liner, allow it to dry before opening your eyes all the way, or the color may transfer into the crease of your eye.

- STEP 7: If you used a brush or a pencil, soften the look by gently smudging the line with your brush, a cotton swab or your finger.
- STEP 8: Line the lower lids. Moving from the outside edge inward, draw a line on the outer two-thirds of the lid or more, depending on the look you're going for. Your line should be slightly thicker at the outside corner, becoming thinner as it moves in toward your nose. Using your brush or pencil, lightly stroke the area. If using a liquid liner, apply it in one smooth stroke. Apply less color so your eyes don't appear raccoonlike.

Tips & Warnings

- You may find eyeliner, particularly the liquid version, difficult and messy the first few times. Practice and have patience.
- Wash brushes regularly with makeup remover or a mild gel shampoo.
- Lining the inside of the lower lid is not recommended'it may cause eye infections, and it greatly increases the risk of getting makeup in your eye.

Overall Things You'll Need

- Eyeliners
- Thin Eye Shadow Brush
- Liquid Eyeliners

Eye shadow

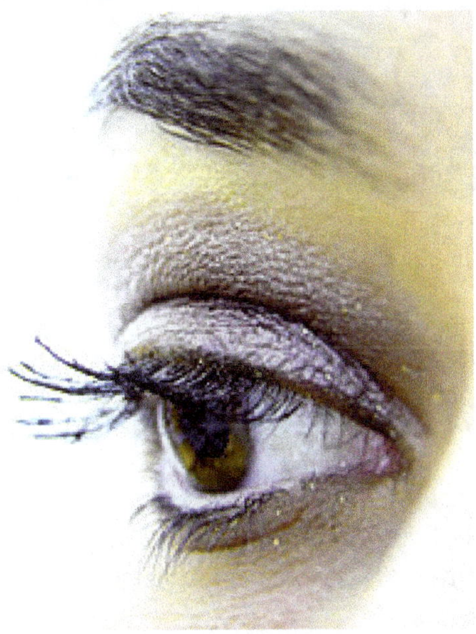

An eye with heavy purple eye shadow

Eye shadow is a cosmetic that is applied on the eyelids and under the eyebrows. It is commonly used to make the wearer's eyes stand out or look more attractive.

Eye shadow can add depth and dimension to one's eyes, complement the eye color, make one's eyes appear larger, or simply draw attention to the eyes. Eye shadow comes in many different colors and textures. It is usually made from a powder and mica, but can also be found in liquid, pencil, cream or mousse form.

Civilizations across the world use eye shadow predominantly on females but also occasionally on males. In Western society, it is seen as a feminine cosmetic, even when used by men. In Gothic fashion, black or similarly dark-colored eye shadow and other types of eye makeup are popular among both sexes.

Many people use eye shadow simply to improve their appearance, but it is also commonly used in theatre and other plays, to create a memorable look, with bright, bold colors. Depending on skin tone and experience, the effect of eye shadow usually brings out glamour and gains attention. The use of eye shadow attempts to replicate the natural eye shadow that some women exhibit due to a natural contrasting pigmentation on their eyelids. Natural eye shadow can range anywhere from a glossy shine to one's eyelids, to a pinkish tone, or even a silver look.

Use

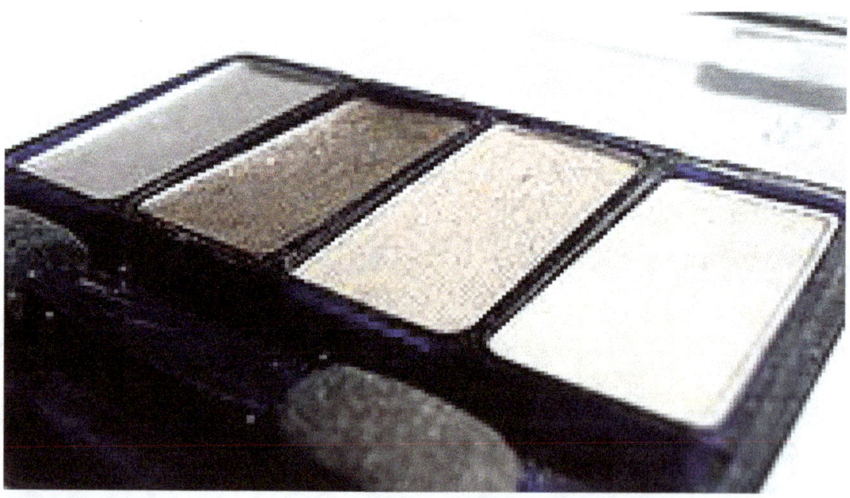

A powder eye shadow palette with brown shades for normal day wear; the two center colors are sparkly while the silver and white shades are for creating shadows and highlights.

Eye shadow can be applied in a wide variety of ways depending upon the desired look and formulation. Typically application is done using fingers or brushes. The most important aspect of applying eye shadow, and makeup in general, is blending well. However, you must not forget to include a primer to limit the chances of creases in your eye shadow later.

To remove eye shadow, a commercial eye makeup remover can be utilized, though a rich face wash will usually remove all traces of color. Generally it is easy to remove, and simple water and soap can be used. Eye shadow, eyeliner, and mascara may also be removed using baby oil. There are also makeup wipes that can be used.

How to Apply Eye Shadow

Sweep a touch of shadow over your lids to accent eyes. You can define them, add drama, and make them stand out in a few quick steps.

Application on Entire Lid

Instructions

- STEP 1: Prime the eyelids by dusting them with a small amount of loose powder.
- STEP 2: Select a light base shadow. Using a shadow brush, sweep it across your entire lid, from brow to lash line.
- STEP 3: Use a medium-toned shade to cover your lower lids.
- STEP 4: Contour the crease of your eyelid with a dark shade, using a smaller eye shadow brush. This color can also work as an eyeliner.
- STEP 5: Blend shadow by stroking the lid gently with an eye shadow brush. Don't use your finger'you could wipe off the shadow entirely.
- STEP 6: Use a cosmetic puff and a little pressed powder to tone down heavy shadow. Shake any excess powder off the puff, then press it gently on your lid.

Eye Shadow to Line the Eyes

Instructions

- STEP 1: Choose a medium or dark shadow color to line your eyes.
- STEP 2: Use a small, flat, angled brush for the application.
- STEP 3: Stroke the brush over the eye shadow.
- STEP 4: Start at the inside edge of your upper lid. Angle the brush so that the longest tip follows the shorter end as the brush moves across your lash line. Bring the brush to the outer corner of the eye.
- STEP 5: Create a more dramatic line by wetting the brush before stroking it through the shadow. Mist a small amount of water onto the brush, or dab it into a few drops of water and proceed with the line. The shadow may feel wet as you draw your line, but it will dry quickly.

Overall Things You'll Need

- Thin Eye Shadow Brush
- Makeup Kits Puff

- light, medium and dark eye shadow shades
- Face Powder

Overall Tips & Warnings

- Don't share eye makeup or tools'you can unknowingly transfer eye infections such as pink-eye (conjunctivitis).
- If you get shadow in your eyes, flush them gently with tepid water.

Topics Addressed

- How to put on eye shadow
- How to use eye shadow
- Choose eye shadow
- Apply makeup
- Use eye makeup

How to Apply Foil Eyeshadow

Foil eye shadow is eyeshadow that's wetted before application to create a shiny, metallic look. It can be great for events like New Year's Eve parties. To apply foil eyeshadow, you must first prepare the pigment. Then, apply your regular eye shadow as you normally would and then top it off with the foil eyeshadow. It's a good idea to keep your other makeup minimal, as foil eyeshadow can be quite dramatic.

Part 1

Creating Your Foil Pigment

1. Gather your materials. Before you begin, you should have all your materials ready. You should have all your regular makeup and eyeshadow supplies. In addition to this, you'll need some supplies specifically used for foil eyeshadow.

- You will need pigmented eyeshadow in a color of your choice.
- You will need a medium for mixing the eyeshadow. You can use primer water or a makeup spray specifically designed for misting foil eyeshadow.
- You need to find a flat surface to work on.
- You will need two eyeshadow brushes. Make sure at least one is flat and stiff.

2. Mist your pigment. Open your makeup pigment. Shake out as much pigment as you think you

will use into the lid. Remember, you can always add more later if you want another layer. Shake out a few drops of your mixing medium.

3. Mix the pigment. Take your makeup brush and stir the pigment. You want to get the pigment to the consistency of paint. If necessary, add more of your mixing agent or pigment to get the right texture.

4. Apply your regular eye makeup. Foil makeup always goes over your regular look. Before applying the foil makeup, apply your eye makeup as you normally would. However, you may not need to apply as much eyeshadow as you normally would. Most of your lid will be covered by the foil.

- Foil eyeshadow can also be added at the end of the day, before you go out. You can simply apply a layer of foil eyeshadow over your regular everyday look. This can add some flare to your makeup for a night out.

Part 2

Applying the Pigment

1. Add the pigment to your brush. Use the flat, stiff eyeshadow brush here. Dab it in the foil pigment. You want your brush to be damp, but not soaking wet. After wetting the brush, tap it a few times on the edge of the lid to shake off any loose bits of pigment.

2. Dab the foil shadow onto the center of your lid. Start at the very center of the eyelid. You apply foil shadow using light, dabbing motions. Move from one end of the eye to the other, gently dabbing on the makeup.

- Be very delicate with your dabbing. You don't want to smear the foil makeup. It may take awhile to get all the makeup on neatly.

3. Repeat until you get the right effect. You may only want a light dusting of foil makeup, in which case one or two layers will be enough. However, if you want something more dramatic, do three or four layers. Keep repeating the process of filling your brush and gently dabbing on the makeup until your makeup is as dramatic as you want it.

- If you want a very dramatic look, you may need to make more foil pigment at one point. Repeat the same process you used the first time to get more pigment for your eyes.

4. Blend out the foil eye shadow when you're done. Take a clean eyeshadow brush. Gently dust the outline of the foil makeup so it blends naturally into your existing eyeshadow. If you want to add in any additional colors of eye shadow, you can do so at this point.

- Make sure to wait until your foil makeup has dried completely to blend out the makeup.

Part 3

Creating Your Look Effectively

1. Feel free to use your fingers, if necessary. A brush usually applies makeup the neatest, and fingers are not generally recommended. However, foil makeup can sometimes dry while on a brush

as the fibers absorb it. If your makeup is drying on the brush while you're attempting to apply it, simply apply it with your fingers.

- Many people find their ring fingers work best for applying foil eyeshadow.

2. Top off other colors with foils. Never place other colors over foils. You can add additional colors surrounding the foils after applying the foil shadow, but anything applied over foil eyeshadow will not show up well. Foil is meant to be applied over existing eyeshadow and makeup.

3. Apply a thicker layer of foil. Foil eyeshadow is usually used as part of a more dramatic look. Therefore, thicker is generally better. Keep applying layers until your full lid is covered. If your eyelid is exposed, your eyeshadow will look patchy.

4. Keep your other makeup minimal. When applying something as dramatic as foil eyeshadow, you do not need a lot of heavy makeup. Use a light layer of foundation, concealer, lipstick, and other makeup products. By sticking a more natural look elsewhere, you won't take any attention away from your dramatic eyes.

Mascara

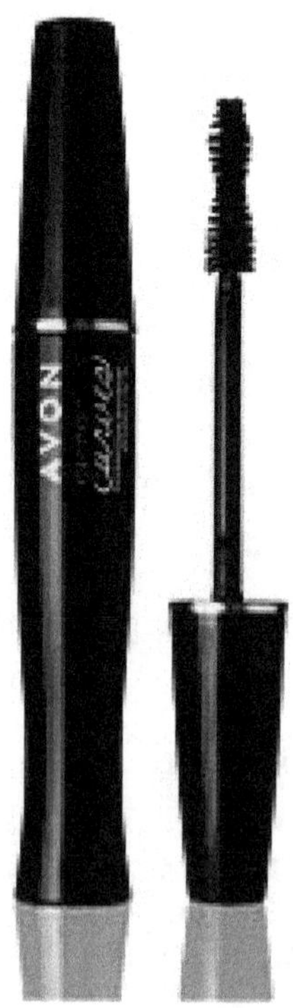

A mascara tube and a wand applicator

Mascara is a cosmetic commonly used to enhance the eyelashes. It may darken, thicken, lengthen, and/or define the eyelashes. Normally in one of three forms—liquid, cake, or cream—the modern mascara product has various formulas; however, most contain the same basic components of pigments, oils, waxes, and preservatives.

Ingredients

The increased demand for mascara led to the development of the many formulas seen in the current market. Despite the many variations, all formulas contain the same basic elements: pigmentation, oils, and waxes.

The pigmentation for black mascara is similar to the pigmentation used by the Egyptians and Victorian women. Carbon black, instead of soot or ash, is used. Tar and coal derivatives are strictly prohibited by the FDA. Brown mascaras typically colored by use of iron oxides though the specific compounds are unique to each brand. In some mascaras, an additional pigment of ultramarine blue is added.

There is a great deal more leeway and variety among the oils used. Different mineral oils, linseed oil, castor oil, eucalyptus oil, lanolin, and oil of turpentine can be found most frequently among the many formulas. Sesame oil is also commonly used.

Waxes usually found in mascara are paraffin wax, carnauba wax, and beeswax.

The desired effects of the mascara account for most variations of ingredients. The most basic effect considered is whether the mascara will be water-resistant or not. Water-resistant mascaras have basis in substances that rebuff water, like dodecane. Non water-resistant mascaras have base ingredients that are water-soluble. Mascaras designed to lengthen or curl the eyelashes often contain nylon or rayon microfibers. Additionally, ceresin, gum tragacanth, and methyl cellulose are regular ingredients added to act as stiffeners.

Manufacture

Which ingredients are chosen also relies on how the mascara is manufactured. Today, there are two main methods of production. The first is referred to as anhydrous. In this method all waxes, oils, and pigments are mixed, heated, and agitated simultaneously in formulated ratios. The result is a semi-solid substance that is ready to be placed in tubes, packaged, shipped and sold. The other method used is termed emulsion. The emulsion method also results in a semi-solid substance, but its procedure greatly differs. In the emulsion method, water and thickeners are first combined. Separately, waxes and emulsifiers are mixed and heated. Pigment is then added individually to both mixtures. Finally all is combined in a homogenizer, which acts as a high-speed agitator in order to thoroughly mix the oils, water, waxes, and emulsifiers—ingredients that naturally repulse each other.

How to Choose the Right Mascara

Instructions

- STEP 1: Decide whether you would prefer to use waterproof or water-soluble mascara. Water-soluble is easier to remove without eye makeup remover, thus minimizing the amount of rubbing around the eyes, which can lead to saggy skin. Waterproof mascara is a better choice for athletes, especially swimmers.

- STEP 2: Choose a mascara color according to your hair color; brunettes should use black to bring out their eyes, but brown mascara will have a more natural effect on fair-haired women.
- STEP 3: Avoid choosing colored mascara if it is to be worn with a conservative outfit or in the workplace. However, if you're planning to wear it for a fun evening out, feel free to get creative with different colors.
- STEP 4: Choose the type of mascara brush according to your preference. A straight brush is good for coating the hard-to-reach corner lashes, while a curved brush makes it easier to coat more of your lashes at once.

Tips & Warnings

- If the mascara you choose is already dried out upon purchase, return it and request a refund.
- Some beauty consultants suggest replacing your mascara tube every three months.

Overall Things You'll Need

- Mascara
- Waterproof Mascaras
- Mirrors

How to Apply Mascara

Mascara'one of the most popular beauty items'defines and brings color to the lashes, and highlights and dramatizes eyes. Different formulas can enhance your lashes in different ways.

Instructions

- STEP 1: Consider the types of mascara and select one appropriate for your lashes and the occasion. You have a choice of lengthening, thickening, long-wearing, conditioning and waterproof formulas, among others. For day, you might decide to add length, while a night on the town may require a long-wearing or thickening formula.
- STEP 2: Select a color. If you have blond or red lashes, opt for brown mascara. Darker-lashed women can consider brown for a casual look, and black or brown- black for more pronounced or dramatic lashes.
- STEP 3: Curl your lashes with an eyelash curler, if desired, and apply all other eye makeup prior to your mascara.
- STEP 4: Remove the wand from the tube in one pull. Pumping the mascara will push air into the tube, potentially drying out the formula and introducing bacteria into it.

- STEP 5: Begin with the underside of your upper lashes, moving the brush slowly upward toward the tips of your lashes. Always hold the wand parallel to your eyelid. Roll the brush slowly on the upward stroke to promote separation of the lashes.
- STEP 6: Allow the first coat of mascara to dry before applying the second coat in the same manner.
- STEP 7: Use an eyelash comb to separate the wet lashes. Also blot the lashes with tissue paper if necessary to remove excess mascara.
- STEP 8: Use less mascara for the lower lashes. Begin where the lashes meet the rim of the lower eyelid, and gently stroke downward.
- STEP 9: Remove any stray mascara around the eye with a cotton swab dipped in a small amount of eye makeup remover.

Tips & Warnings

- Contact lens wearers should stick to waterproof mascara formulas, as they break down more slowly, minimizing the chance of any flakes getting into the eyes.
- Always remove eye makeup thoroughly before going to bed. This will keep lashes healthier and prevent any mascara from getting into your eyes during the night.
- Apply mascara after eye shadow and eyeliner.

Overall Things You'll Need

- Eyelash Comb
- Waterproof Mascaras
- Facial Tissues
- Cotton Swabs
- Mascara
- Eye Makeup Removers
- Eyelash Curlers

How to Apply Goth Mascara

You got the clothes, you have the hair, and all the other makeup, but you just can't seem to figure out how to apply Gothic mascara. Don't worry, we'll have your lashes looking gorgeously Gothic in no time!

Steps

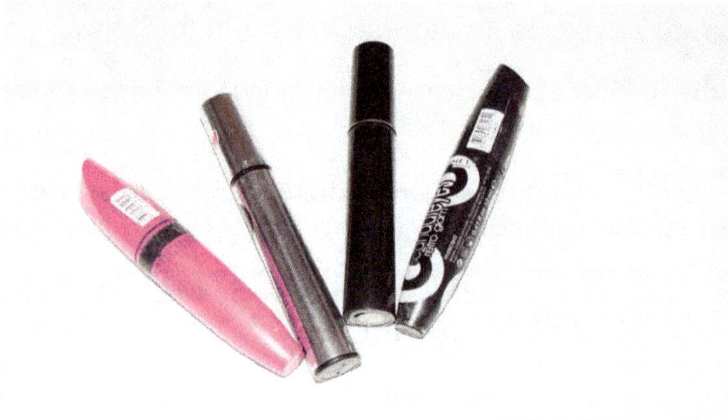

1. Buy two or three different types of black mascara (Lengthening, volumizing, non-clumping, et cetera) and an eyelash curler.

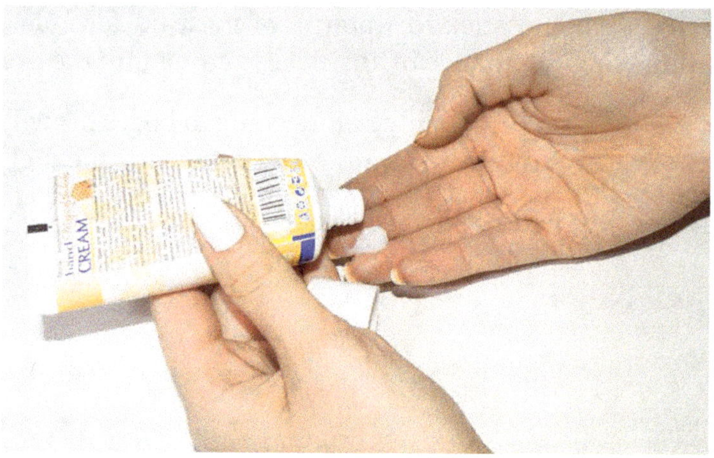

2. Clean and moisturize your face.

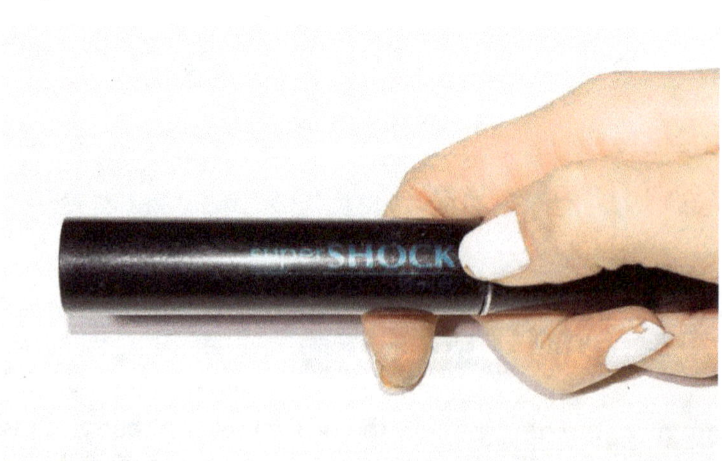

3. Apply the volumizing mascara to your top lashes first. Let them dry (careful not to blink!) and then apply an additional coat.

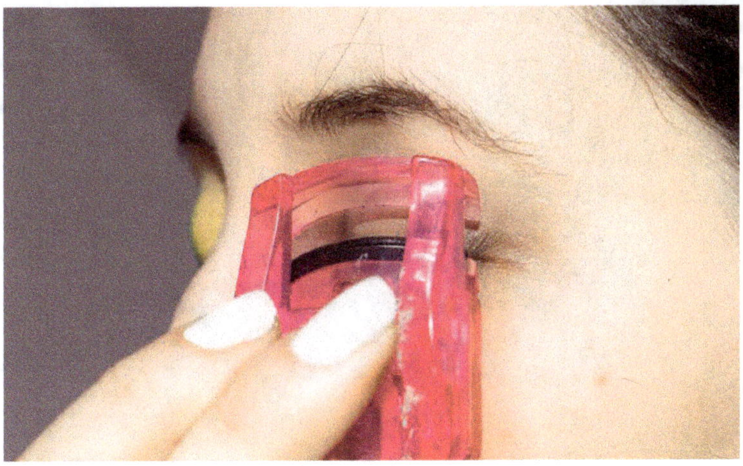

4. Curl your lashes with the eyelash curler. Position the clamp where you want the lashes to start curling and hold for fifteen (15) seconds.

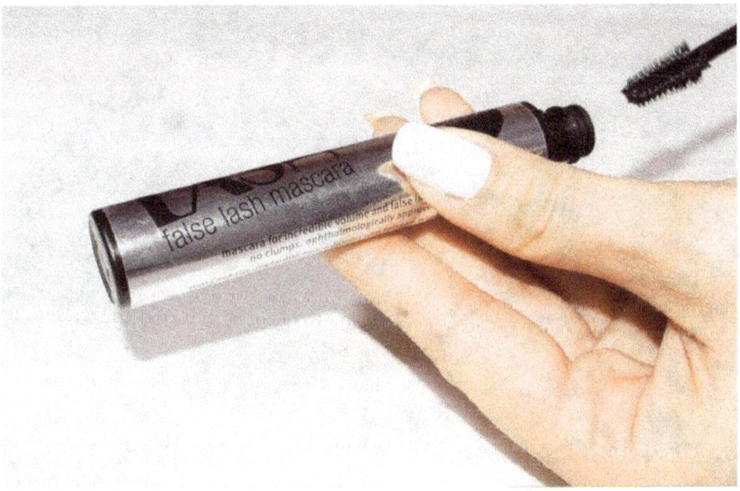

5. Apply the lengthening mascara to your top lashes. Let them dry (again, try not to blink).

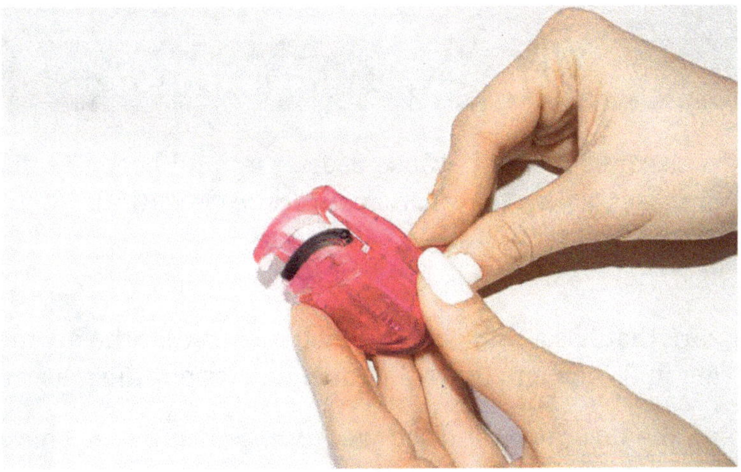

6. Curl your lashes one more time. Try to get the clamp in the same spot as last time.

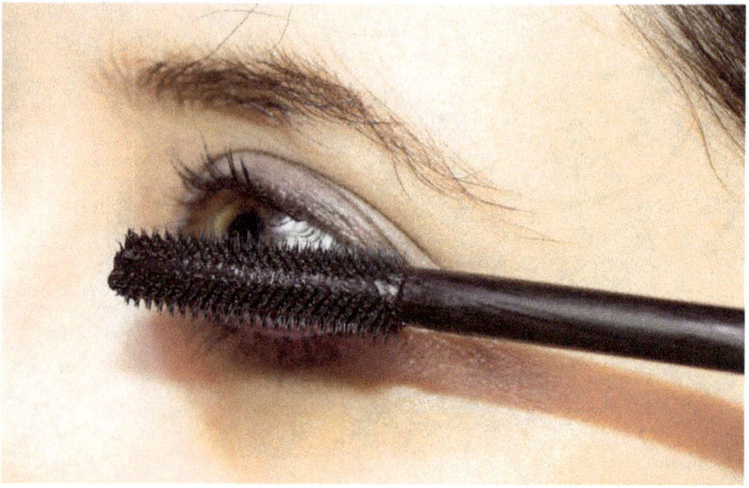

7. Apply another coat of mascara.

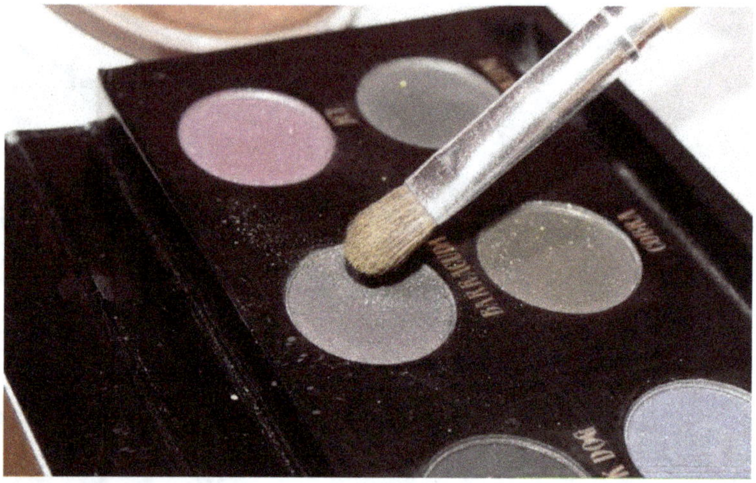

8. Apply the rest of your makeup.

How to Make your Mascara Last Longer

Sick of replacing your mascara so often because it dries up and becomes difficult to use? Follow these steps to keep your mascara easy to use and your lashes beautiful.

Instructions

STEP 1: Choose a mascara that has a thin brush, which means that the opening to the tube will be small and less air will get in. When air enters the tube, it dries out the mascara.

STEP 2: Avoid pumping the mascara wand too vigorously during use. This allows air to get into the tube.

STEP 3: Add one drop of water to the tube of dry mascara if necessary. It's not a great idea, but in an emergency, you will be able to get more out of the tube by using this trick.

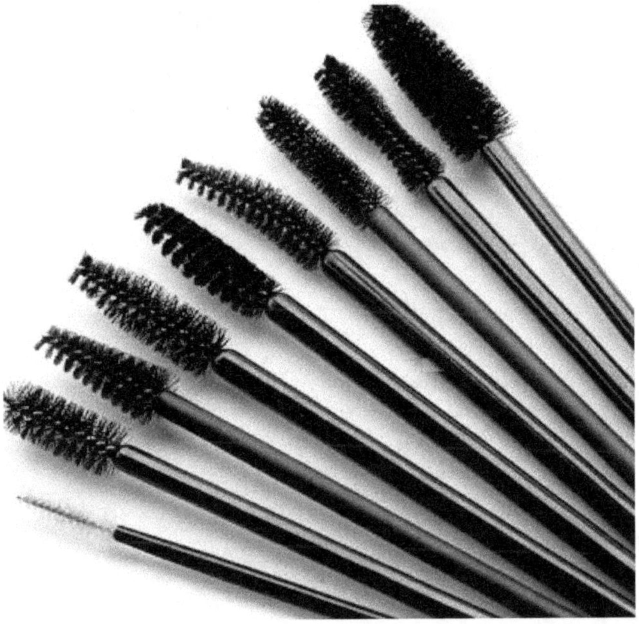

Tips & Warnings

- Make sure you only use the water trick on water-soluble mascaras, not waterproof mascaras.
- If you've had your mascara longer than 3 months, it is probably a good idea to replace it and start using these tricks with a new tube.

Overall Things You'll Need

- Mascara
- Waterproof Mascaras
- Mirrors Distilled Waters

How to Apply Eye Makeup

Clean your face and remove previous eye makeup. Skip the moisturizer, unless you have around 10 minutes to let it soak into your skin properly, but consider applying primer and concealer. Use a brush to apply eyeshadow to the lid, crease, and brow bone. Blend everything in, then apply liquid or pencil eyeliner to your upper lid. Curl your lashes with an eyelash curler, then apply mascara.

Eye Makeup Chart

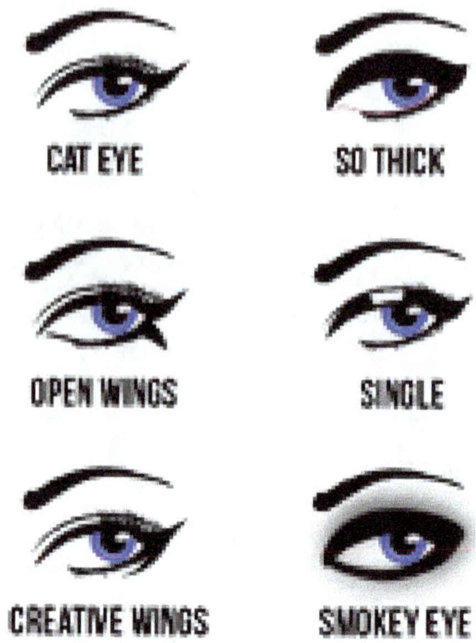

Makeup Chart

Method 1

Basic Technique

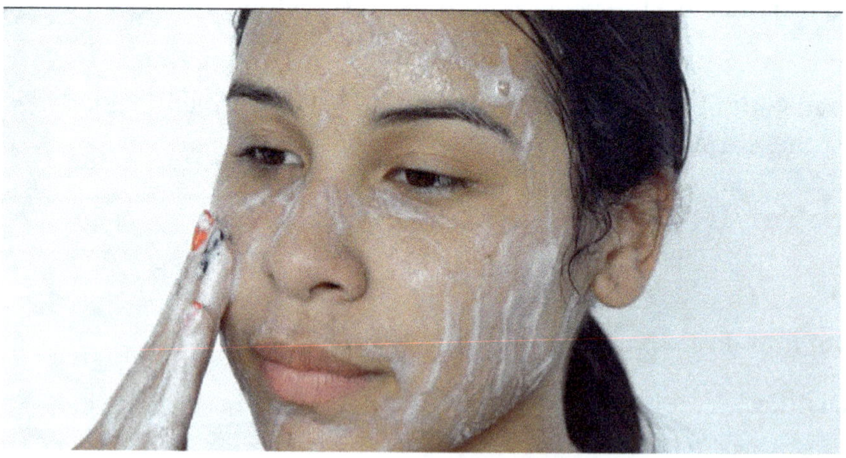

1. Start with a clean slate. Wash your whole face with a gentle cleanser or makeup wipe before you begin, paying particular attention to any leftover mascara or eyeliner. If you're having trouble removing residual eye makeup, try using cold water or regular lotion on a cotton swab. If you have dry skin around your eyes or suffer from eczema, rub a little moisturizer underneath your eyes, as well as between the outer corners of your eyes and your temples. Don't put moisturizer on your eyelids - this will make them greasy, and the makeup you apply will run off.

- Apply primer to your eyelids(optional). Primer or base smooths out your skin and gives the makeup something to stick to. If you do choose to use primer, apply it all over your eyelid and up to the brow bone.

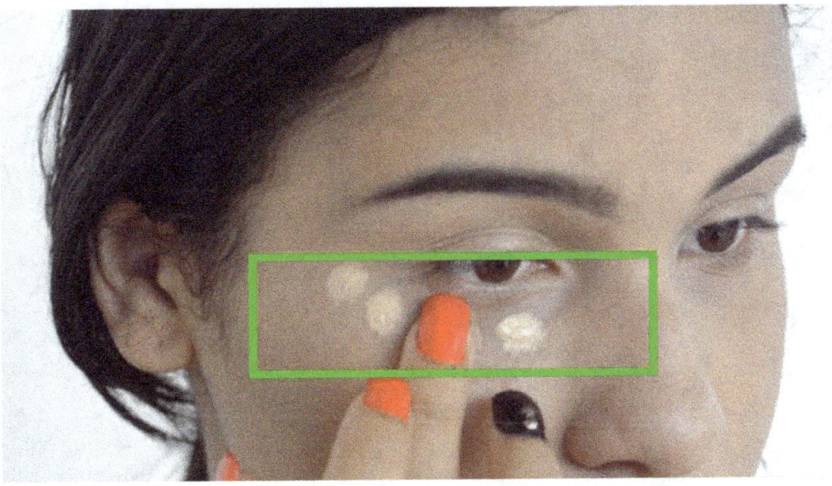

2. Even out the skin tone around your eyes. Apply concealer to dark under-eye circles and to the area where your inner eye meets your nose. (Shop for concealer somewhere that allows you to test samples and swipe them across your inner wrists - buy the one that covers up the veins best.) Use your fingers or a concealer brush to blend the makeup outward to your cheekbones and nose. Set the concealer by brushing a loose, flesh-toned powder over it; apply some powder to your eyelids, as well.

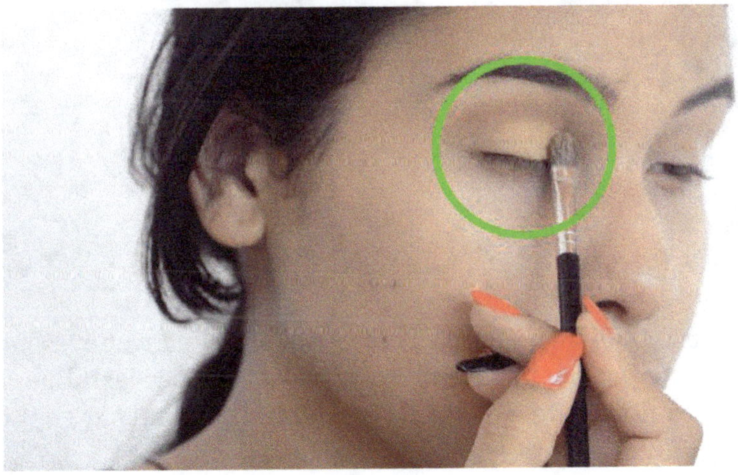

3. Apply eyeshadow. You can use one color, or several. Here's a basic three-color plan.

- Apply a medium color on your eyelid. Your eyelid is the area running from your eyelashes to your crease (the slight dip between your eyelid and your brow bone). Pick a medium pink, light brown or any other middle-of-the-road hue for this area.
- Apply a light color on your brow bone. Most people have an area of their brow bone that sits beneath the eyebrows proper. Highlight this area and make more light bounce off of it by brushing on a pearly off-white, light gold or other delicate color that matches your eyelid color in tone.
- Apply a dark color on your crease. Use light, little strokes to deposit little bits of darker powder on the crease of your eye. Go from the outer corner of your crease and follow the

arch about 2/3 of the way in toward the inner corner of the eye. Try a violet, brown or other dark color that matches up with the first two colors you used.

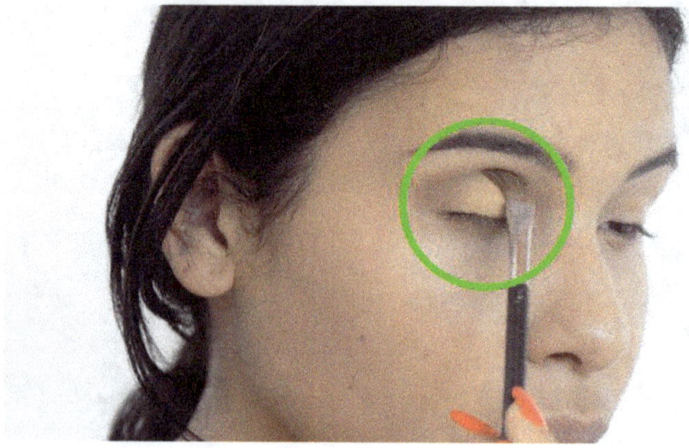

4. Blend the colors. If you applied more than one color of eyeshadow, use your fingers or a fluffy, tapered blending brush to mix the colors a bit. This will create a more natural, cohesive look.

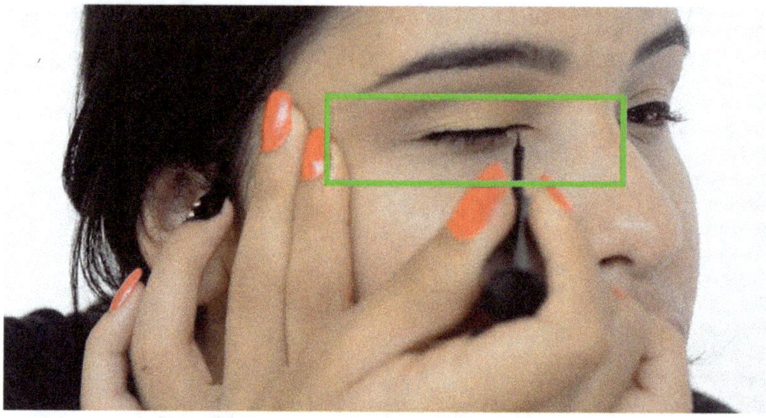

5. Apply eyeliner. You can use liquid eyeliner, a liner pencil, or even wet eyeshadow on an angled brush to line your eyes. Whatever you pick, move across your upper lash line in tiny, controlled strokes as if you're drawing a dotted line. Go back and fill in the blanks with more small strokes. For more drama, line your lower lashes as well.

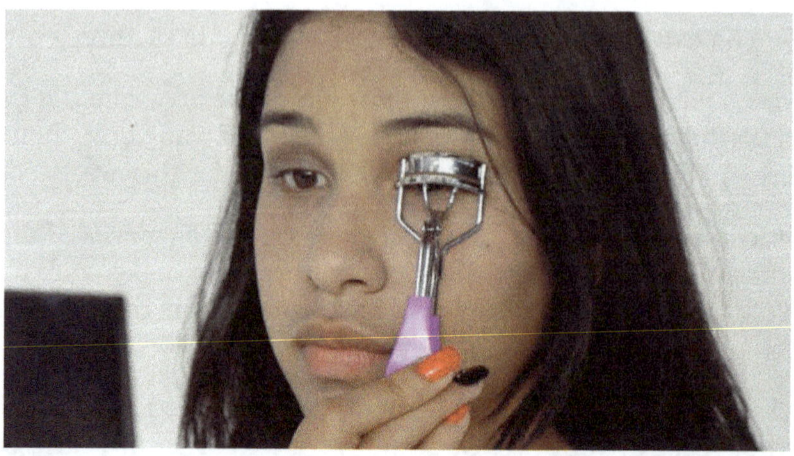

6. Curl your lashes. Use an eyelash curler to grip your upper lashes. Hold the clamp for about five seconds. Accessing your lashes is easiest if you half-close your eyes. Remember, always curl before you apply mascara, never after.

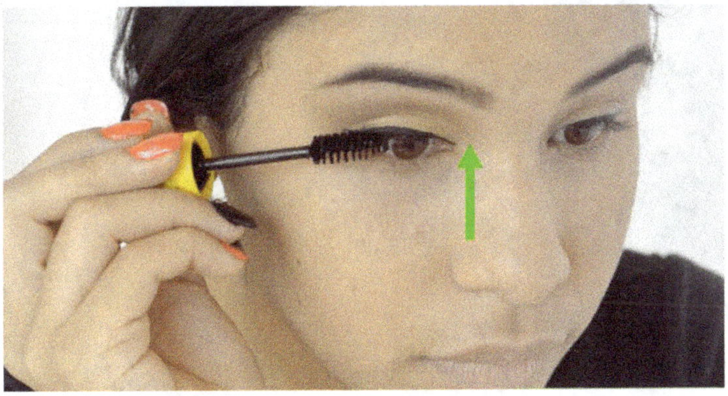

7. Apply mascara. You can apply a little or a lot, and there are many different brands and formulas for volume, length and definition. Find a product you're happy with. Start at the base of your upper lashes and slowly sweep upward. For a more dramatic effect, apply mascara to the lower lashes as well. If you want to apply multiple coats, do it while the first coats of mascara are still wet - applying a new coat to dry mascara will result in clumps.

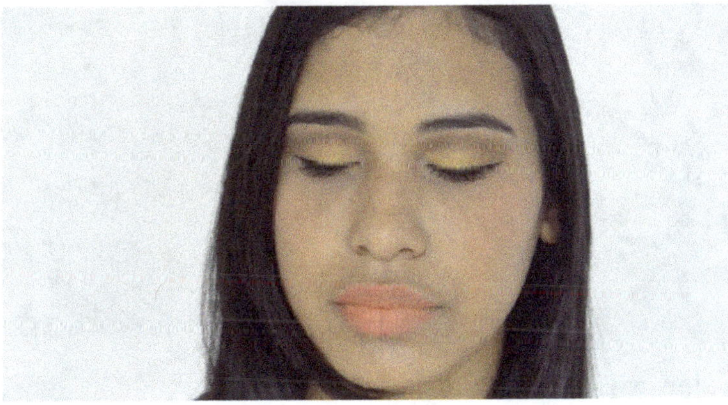

Method 2

Specific Techniques

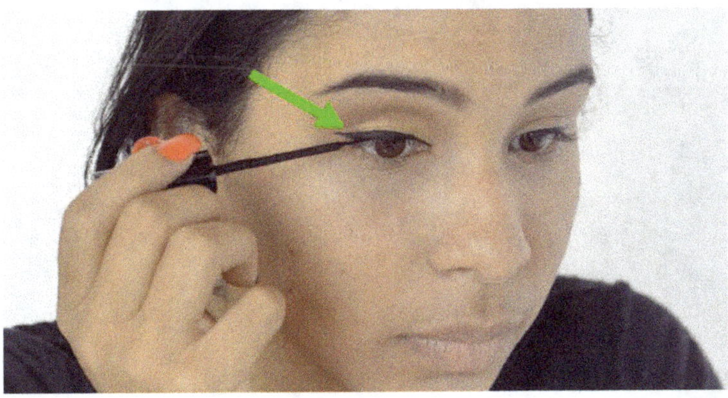

1. Work on specific techniques for applying eyeliner.

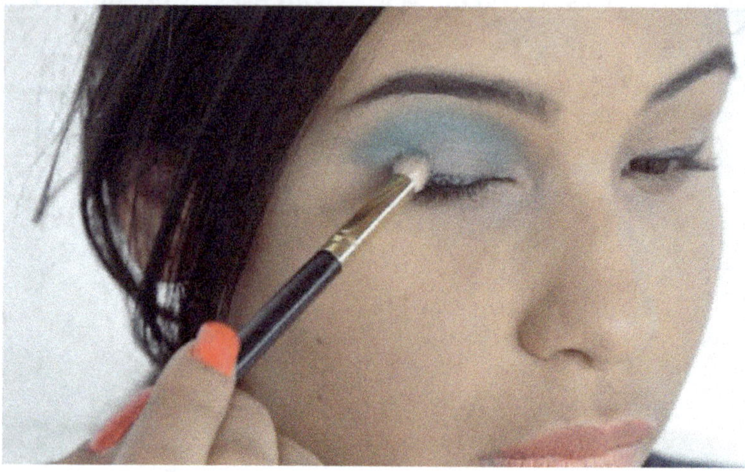

2. Learn more tricks and tips about applying eyeshadow.

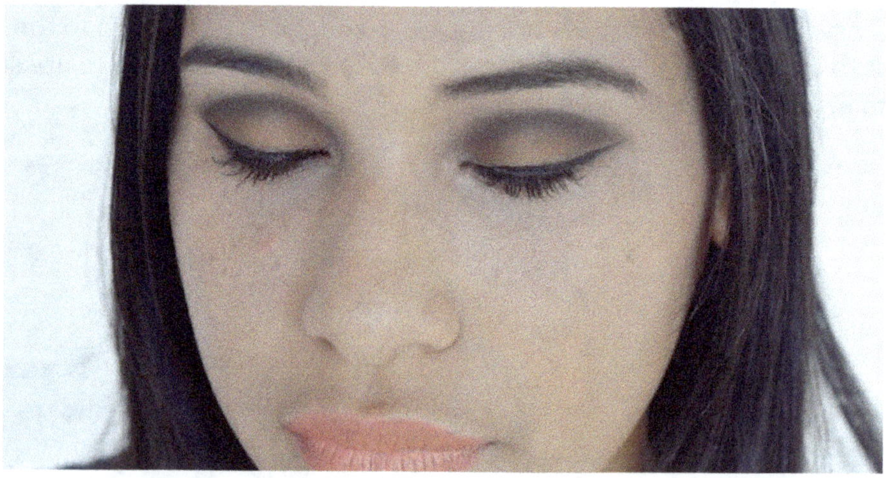

3. Apply smoky eyeshadow without eyeliner.

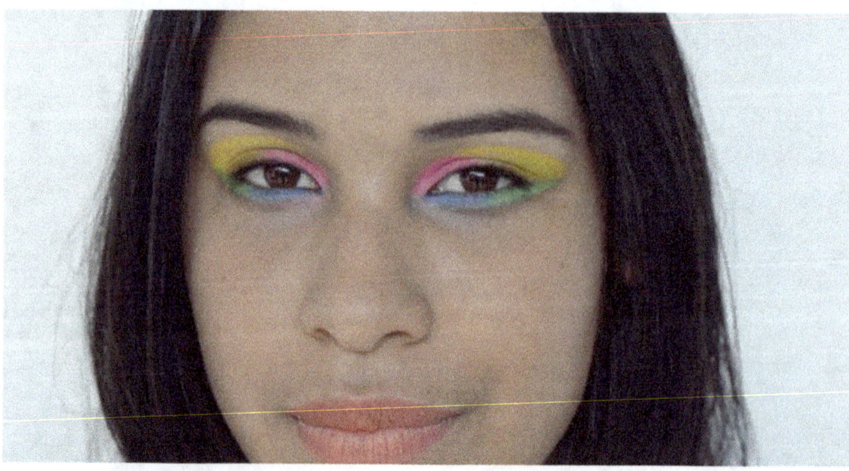

4. Try a bright, rainbow-eye look.

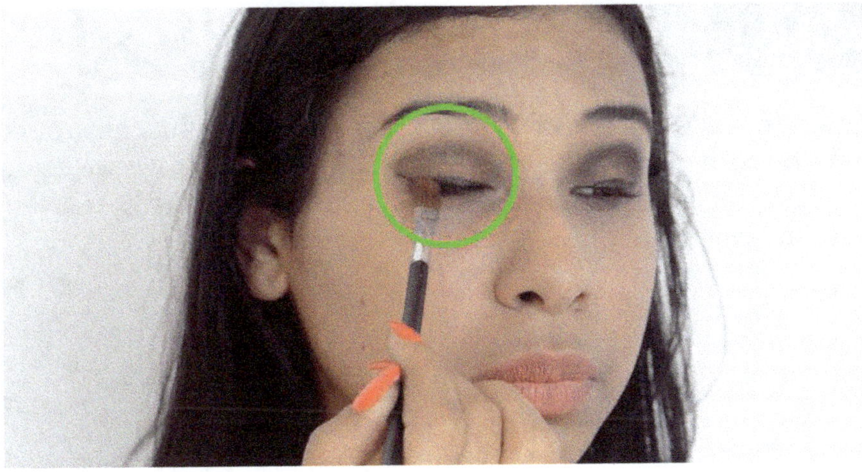

5. Add glitter to your eyeshadow and eyeliner.

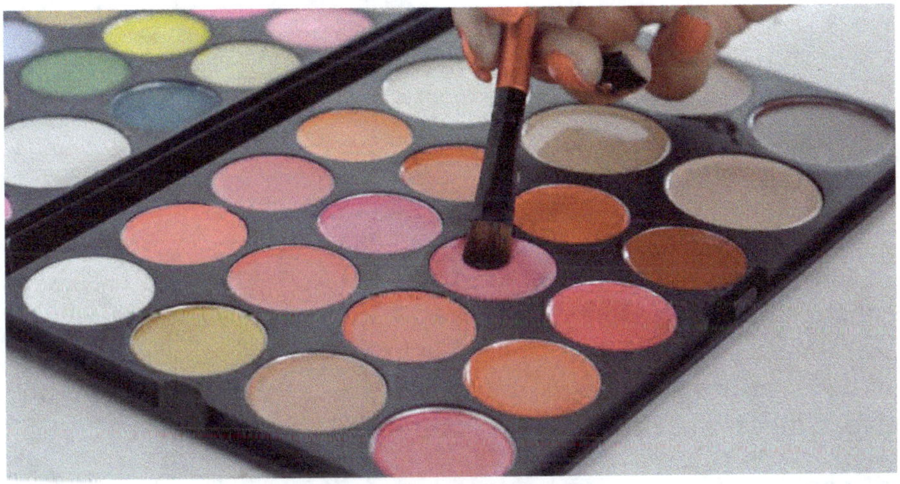

6. Learn how to apply eye makeup on a creaseless eye.

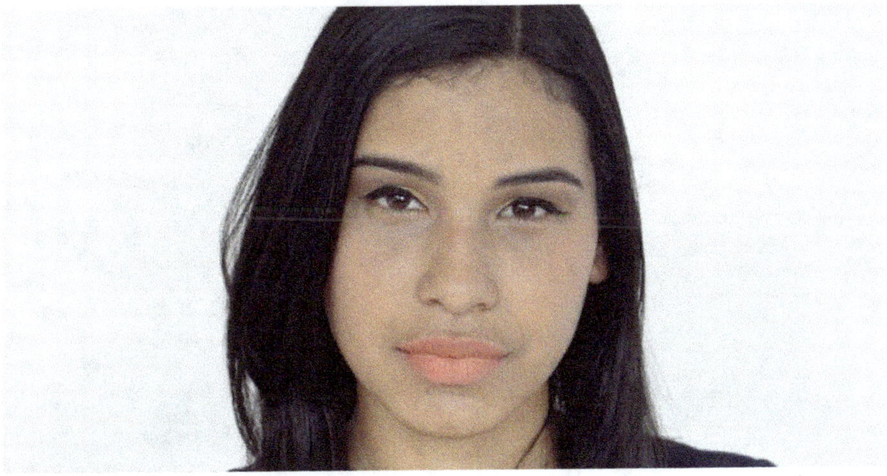

7. Use eye makeup to accentuate your eyes and make them look bigger.

How to Make Eyes Look Bigger

There are lots of ways to make eyes look bigger. Avoid applying eyeliner all around your eyes. Extend it beyond the outer corners of your eyes instead. Keep your eyebrows well groomed. Lengthen your lashes by curling them, wearing mascara, or using false lashes. Lastly, treat any eye problems, such as puffiness or under-eye circles.

Method 1

Using Makeup

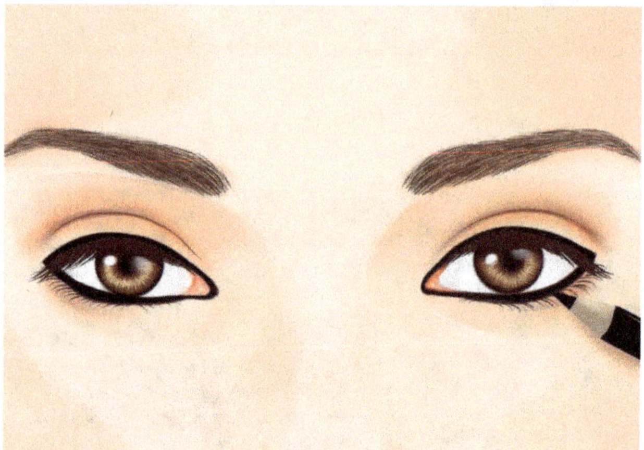

1. Don't apply eyeliner all the way around your eyes. Doing so will cause your eyes to look smaller, as they will appear fenced or ringed in by the circle line. This also means avoiding the smoky eye look). This is not necessarily a bad thing––small eyes can still look mysterious and dramatic, but if you're looking for a bigger eye effect, that's not the effect that you want.

- When you apply eyeliner on your lower lashes, do it just *below* the lash line, not inside the rim. In particular, don't let the line come all the way to the inner corner of your eye.

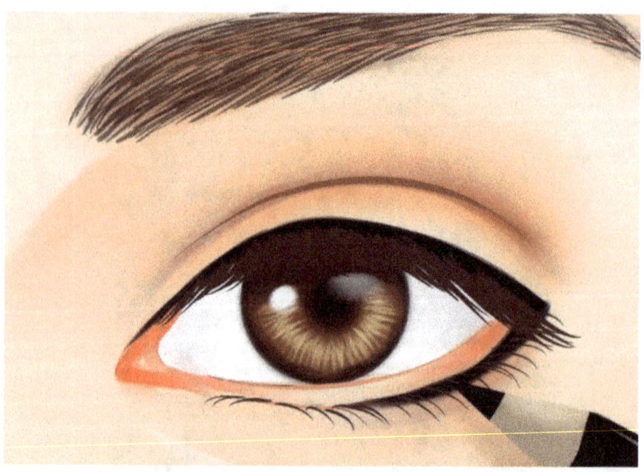

- You might also want to line your wet line with white or other light color. It makes eyes look noticeably bigger, but be careful, as overdoing it will look awkward.

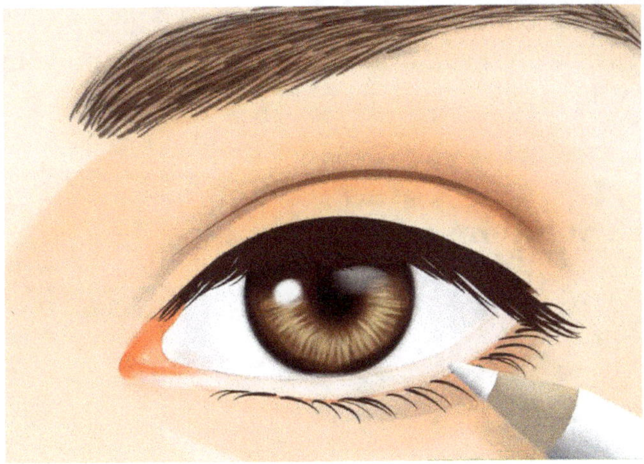

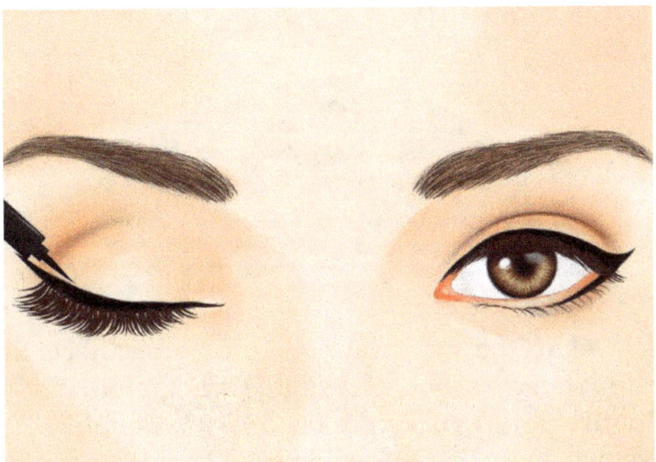

2. Extend the eyeliner beyond the outer corners of your eyes. This line should move upwards a little as well, mimicking a very long eyelash. This technique will make your eyes appear wider, but is a tricky technique to do well. If the eyeliner isn't applied symmetrically, it can make your eyes look lopsided, so try doing this with a mirror or ask a friend to help initially.

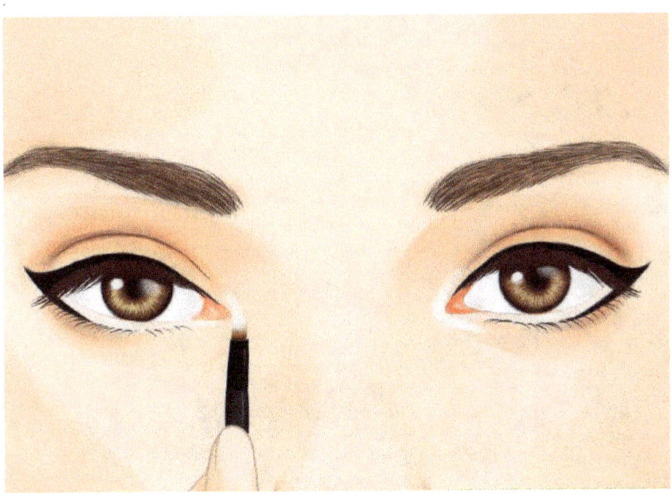

3. Add white eyeshadow or eyeliner to the inner corner of your eyes. This technique helps to bring

more light into your eyes and produces the effect of larger-looking eyes. Use soft white though; a harsh white will look theatrical. You can also use the white liner on your lower waterline, which extends the white part of your eye.

Method 2

Eyebrow and Eyelash Solutions

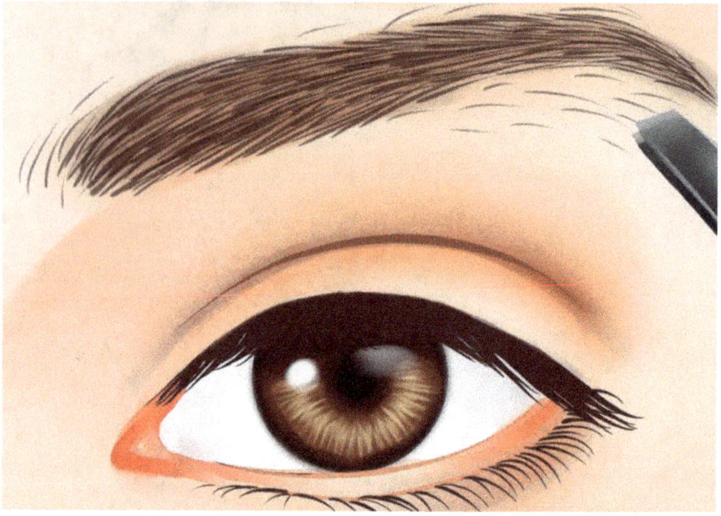

1. Groom your eyebrows. In much the same way a picture frame affects the way the picture looks, your eyebrows affect the way your eyes look. The simple act of removing stray hairs can make your eyes more noticeable. However, don't make the mistake of assuming that the thinner your eyebrows, the bigger your eyes will look. Read How to Shape Eyebrows for more advice.

2. Make your eyelashes look longer. There are several ways to go about doing this:

- Curl your upper eyelashes with an eyelash curler.

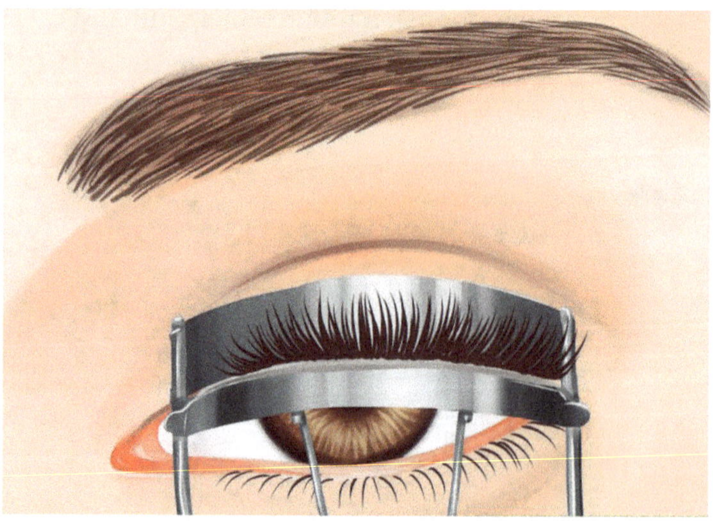

- Apply mascara.

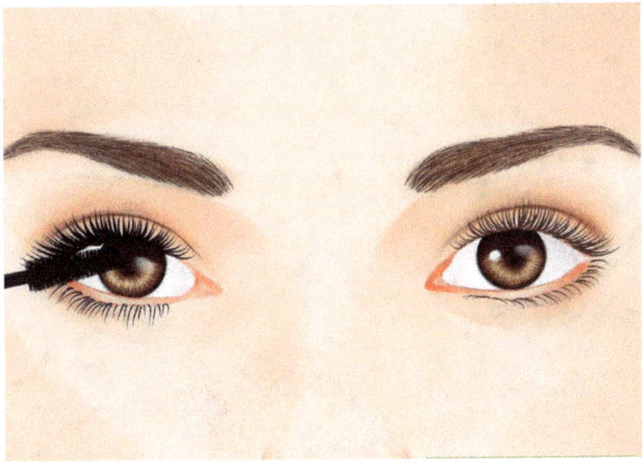

- Apply false eyelashes.

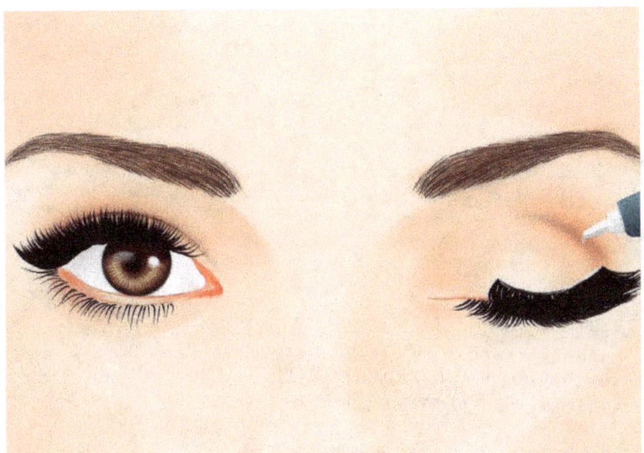

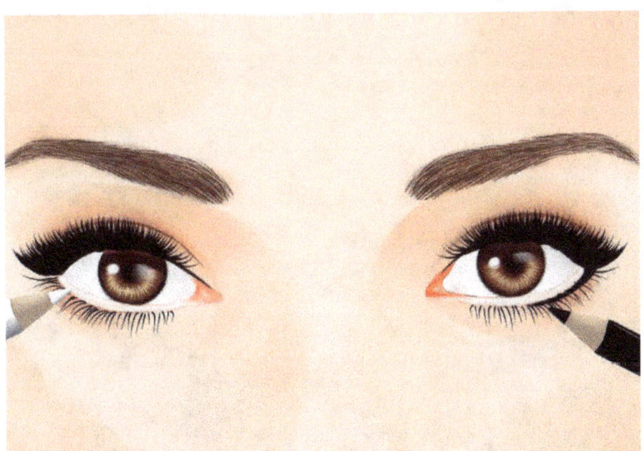

3. Shape your eyes. Apply white eyeliner to your waterline, or apply black eyeliner from the outer corner to the middle, not the whole way.

- Curl your lashes.
- Apply lighter eye shadows like cream, beige, white etc.

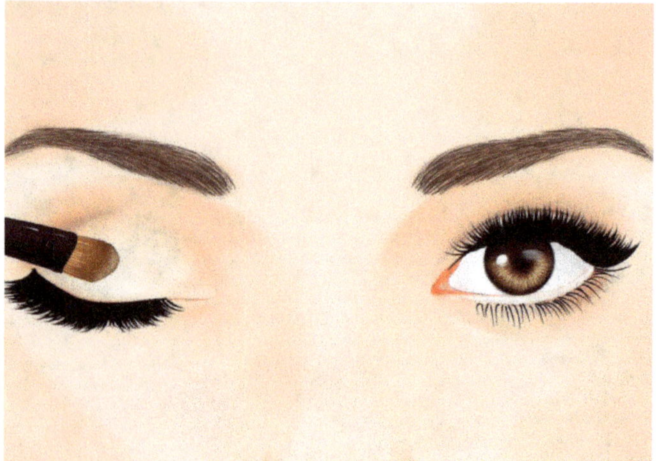

- Apply a thin line of eyeliner on the top of your eyelid and wing it out.

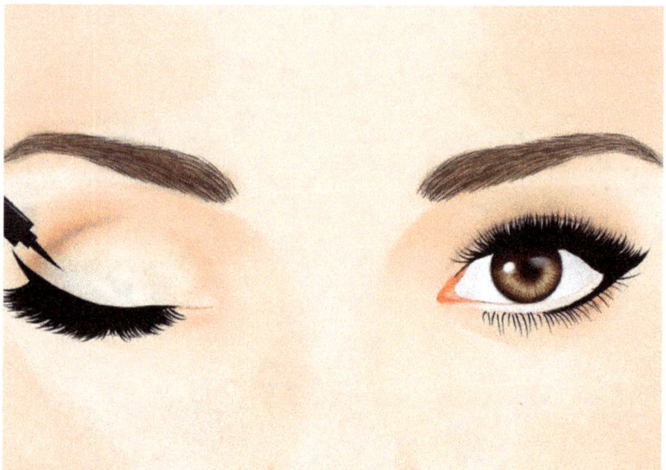

Method 3

Treating Eye Problems

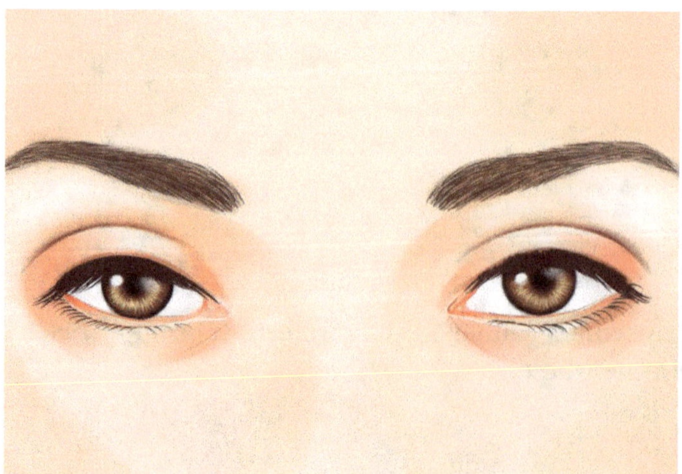

1. Reduce any puffiness in your eyes. Swelling in the skin on and around your eyes can make them look smaller. Try these steps to reduce puffiness:

- Get plenty of sleep.
- Wash your face with cool water.
- Place cold, used teabags over your eyes. The tannins in the tea act as an astringent, tightening the skin.
- Reduce your salt intake. Too much salt leads to water retention, which leads to eye puffiness.
- Exercise to increase circulation, which in turn reduces water retention.

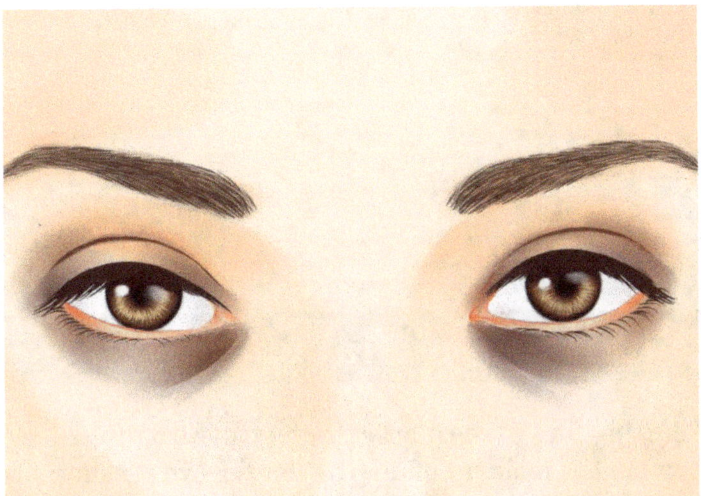

2. Get rid of dark circles under your eyes. This won't necessarily make your eyes look bigger, but dark circles will detract from even the biggest, most beautiful eyes.

- Stay healthy. This means getting plenty of sleep, eating a balanced, healthy diet and minimizing the intake of salt in your diet.

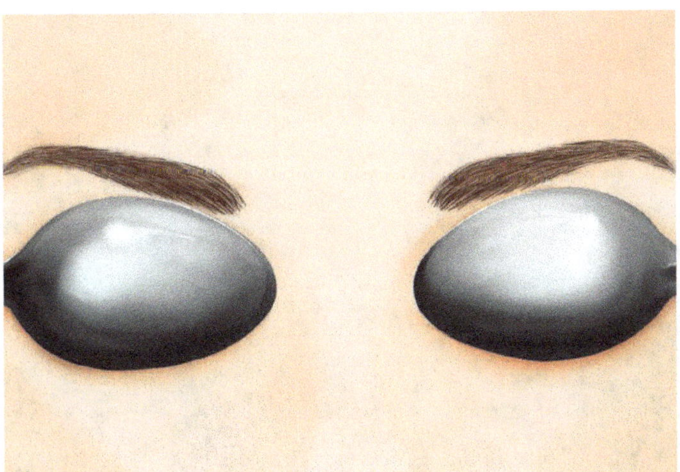

3. Try applying cold spoons. Before you go to bed, place two spoons in the freezer overnight. Wake up, rub the sleep out of your eyes, and place the two spoons over each of your eyes for about 1 minute. This method helps your eyes to appear bigger and brighter throughout the day. (Plus, it helps to reduce the appearance of under-eye circles.)

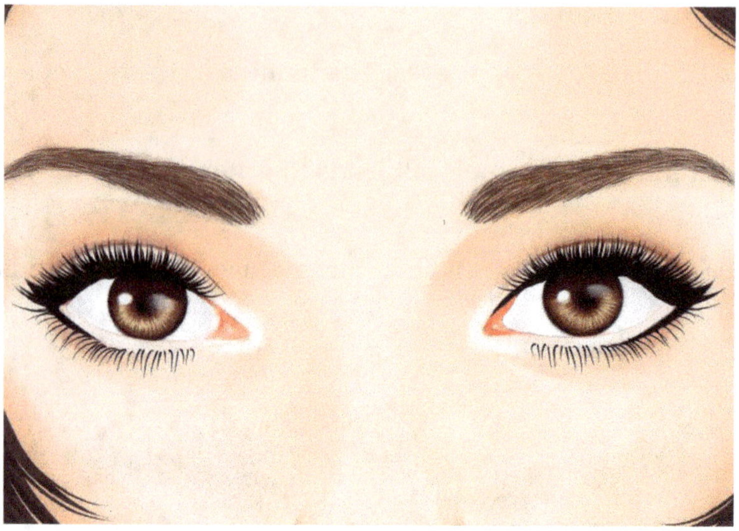

How to use Different Eye Makeup Brushes

There are so many makeup brushes in the market that it can be hard to decide which to use. As eye makeup is the most complicated makeup of all, the list for eye makeup brushes is never ending. Once you know the essential and basic brushes for eye makeup, you can hone your skills in putting them to good use.

Method 1

Using a Flat Eyeshadow Brush

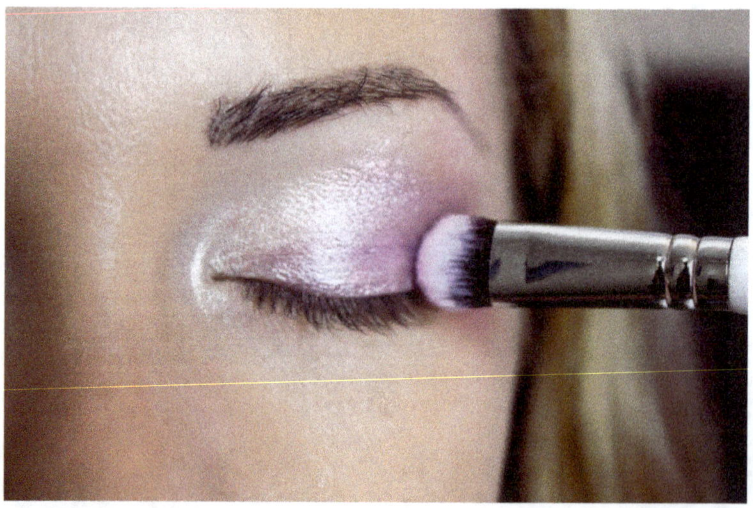

1. Use a flat eyeshadow brush for basic applications. This is the basic brush for applying your eye makeup. It can be used either wet or dry depending upon your eye look.

2. Prime your eyes (you can even use your fingers for this).

3. Take a clean flat eyeshadow brush and rub it over your eyeshadow in a zig zag fashion. In this way, the brush picks up more product.

4. Use this brush to apply your eye shadow on the eye lid by tapping it on your lid area. This gives a wash of the color of your eye makeup.

5. Add more shadow on the lids, if required.

Method 2

Using a Crease Line Brush

1. Use a crease line brush to add depth to your eye makeup.

2. Crease line brushes are of two types: thin and a little pointed/ fluffy and pointed to add color to the crease line.

3. Pick a darker color for adding to your crease of the eyes. (In between the brow bone and eye lids.)

4. Tap the tip of the crease line brush on the eye shadow that you want for your crease.

5. Sweep the brush over the crease line and blend any hard lines above your eye lids (Softer color can help to blend the hard lines).

6. Use the brush in an anti-clockwise motion from the outer corner to the inside for more blending.

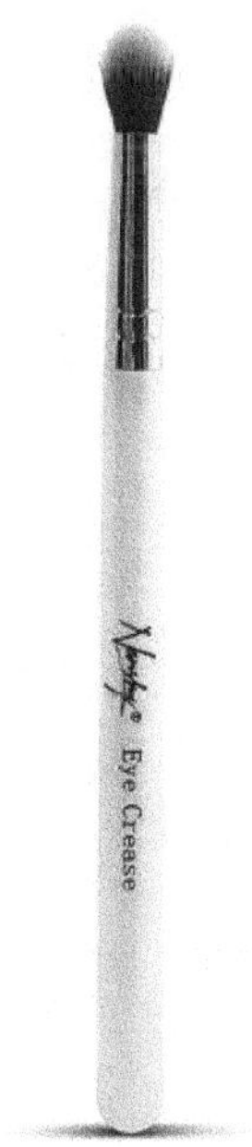

Method 3

Using a Blending Brush

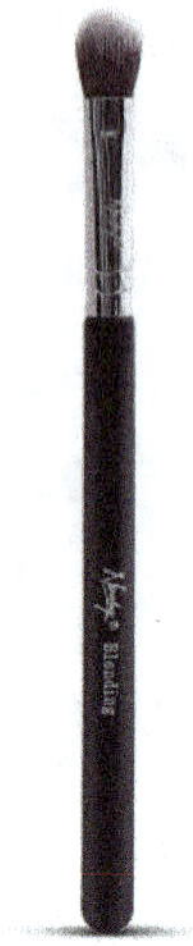

1. Pick a blending brush for blending the eye shadow.

   - Blending brushes come in various sizes. They can be used as per your requirement.

2. Smudge the liner/ kohl along the lash line and on the outer-V of the eyes. Generally, a darker color is smudged on the outer-V and the crease line of the eyes.

3. Blend the hard lines across the lids after applying the eye-shadow using this brush.

Method 4

Using an Angled Brush

1. Use an angled brush to highlight the brow bone.

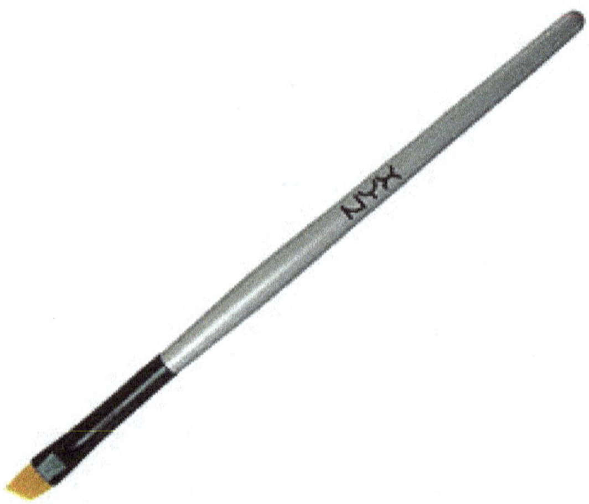

2. Take some color on this brush and sweep it across your brow bone.

- The angled brush is also used for applying liners (generally for cat eye liner).

Method 5

Using a Line Brush

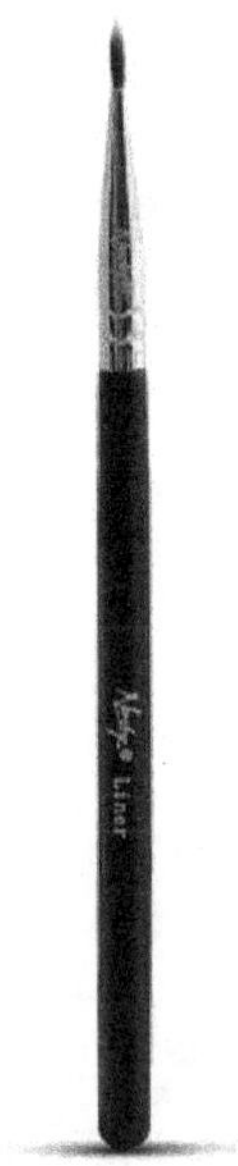

1. Use the line brush for precision. It's a thin, precise and pointy brush.

2. Take some liquid or gel-liner and experiment your looks with this brush. You can do cat eyes, normal/ basic liner, etc.

- This brush is also used for applying color to your lower lash line or water line.

How to Tweeze your Eyebrows

Tweezing your eyebrows is one of the most dramatic way to change your face without makeup or surgery. It can make your eyes look larger and give your face a clean, polished look.

Instructions

- STEP 1: Sit near a window to get the best light.
- STEP 2: Wash the area thoroughly so it's not oily.
- STEP 3: Decide what shape you want for your eyebrows. Styles change; it may help to flip through fashion magazines for ideas.

- STEP 4: Draw in a brow line on your eyebrow with a brow pencil to serve as a guide. Follow the brow's natural line when tweezing eyebrows by conforming to the curve of your upper eyelid.
- STEP 5: Pull the skin at the outer end of the eyebrow taut against the brow bone, and use the brow bone as an additional guide.
- STEP 6: Use a pair of angled eyebrow tweezers to remove the hairs below the brow; never shape your brow by plucking above it. Pluck only one hair at a time.
- STEP 7: Start tweezing your eyebrows in the middle of the eyebrow and tweeze toward the outer end; then go back to the middle and tweeze toward the nose. Your brows should extend a little beyond each corner of your eye.
- STEP 8: Use a cotton ball or pad soaked in pure tea tree oil or witch hazel to soothe your tweezed brows.

Tips & Warnings

- Consider having your brows waxed professionally to get exactly the shape you want. You can then tweeze the strays as they grow in.
- Habitual tweezing of your eyebrows may make some hairs stop growing permanently, so pluck with caution.
- There are tweezers on the market that are specially designed for tweezing eyebrows. They cost a bit more but make the experience less painful.

Overall Things You'll Need

- Pure Tea Tree Oils
- Eyebrow Tweezers
- Fashion Magazines
- Witch Hazel
- Cotton Swabs

How to do Makeup for Green Eyes

Green eyes are rare and beautiful. They deserve to be enhanced. Makeup is a great way to bring attention to eyes, but there are certain colors that really make green eyes pop. This article will give you a few tips on how you can bring out the sparkle in your green eyes.

Method 1

Choosing Eyeshadow Colors

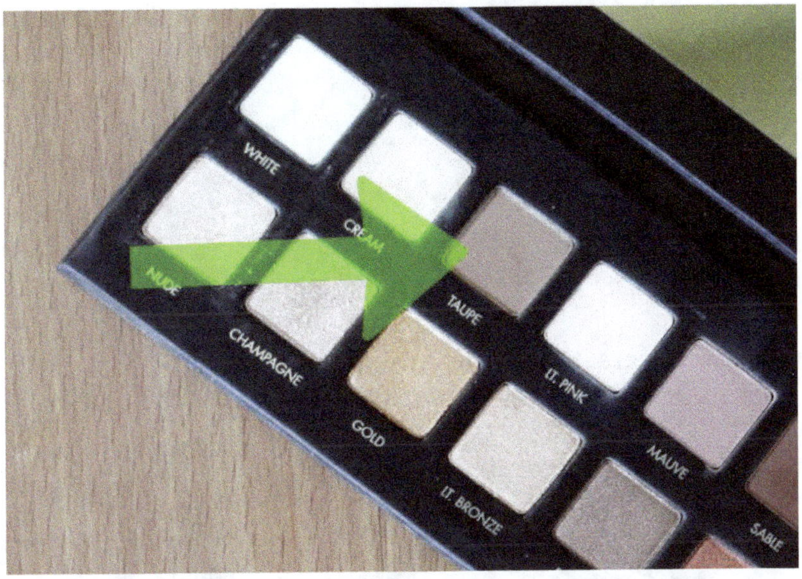

1. Wear neutral browns for a daytime look. Go for reddish browns, such as terracotta, or silvery browns, such as taupe. This is great for school and work.

- If you want to bring out the green a little more, try purple eyeliner or mascara.

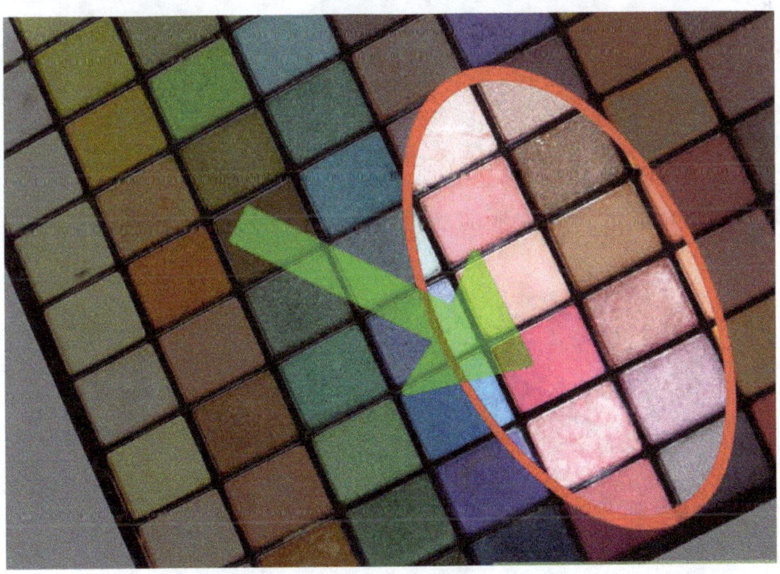

2. Try pinks, purples, and reds to bring out the green. Use warmer, darker, or deeper pinks instead of lighter, cooler pinks. These will help bring out the green in your eyes. For purples, try: eggplant, lavender, lilac, plum, or violet.

- If you don't like to wear red, try a reddish brown instead. It will look more natural while still bringing out the green.

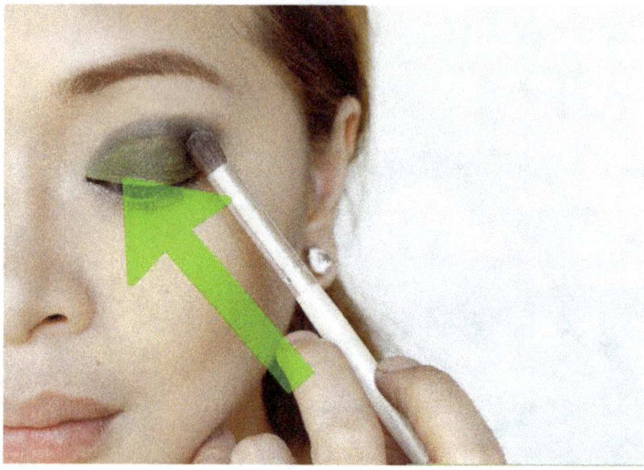

3. Use green eyeshadow with care. Green eyeshadow can help make green eyes sparkle, but it can also make them appear more dull. The trick is to use a darker shade of green, and sparingly.

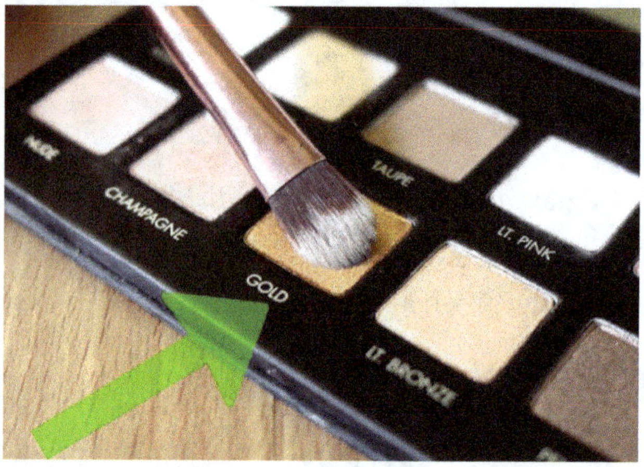

4. Try bronze, copper, or gold. They will help bring out the gold flecks in your eyes. They will also make your eyes appear brighter. Brown or green eyeshadow with gold shimmer are also great choices.

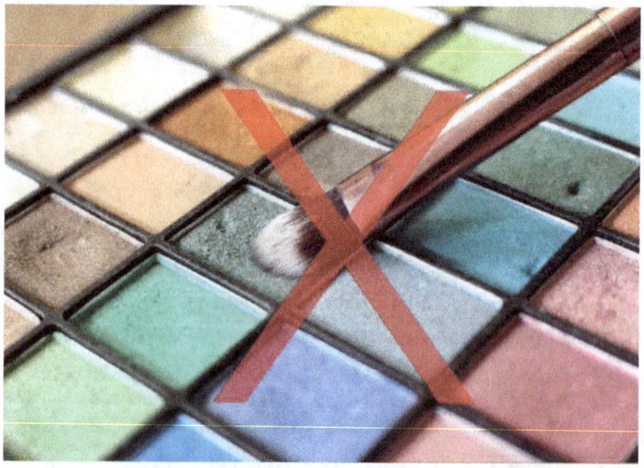

5. Avoid eyeshadow with blue undertones. This includes all shades of blue and blue-ish purples.

Green has too many blue undertones to begin with, so anything blue-tinted will make your eyes appear more dull. This same rule goes for eyeliner and mascara.

- Reddish or pinkish purples are fine.

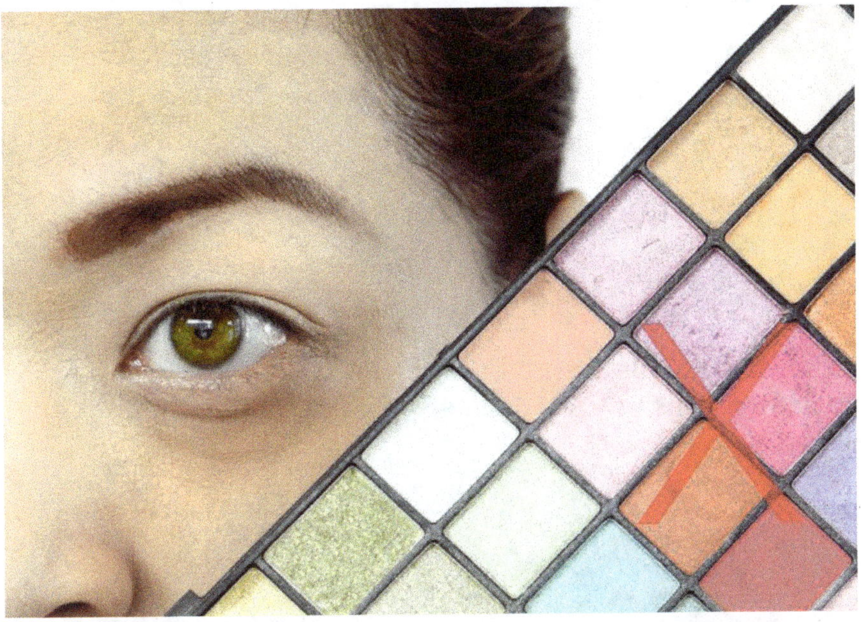

6. Avoid red and purple undertones if you have redness around your eyes. This will bring out the redness even more and make you look tired.

Method 2

Choosing Eyeliner, Mascara, Lipstick, and Blush

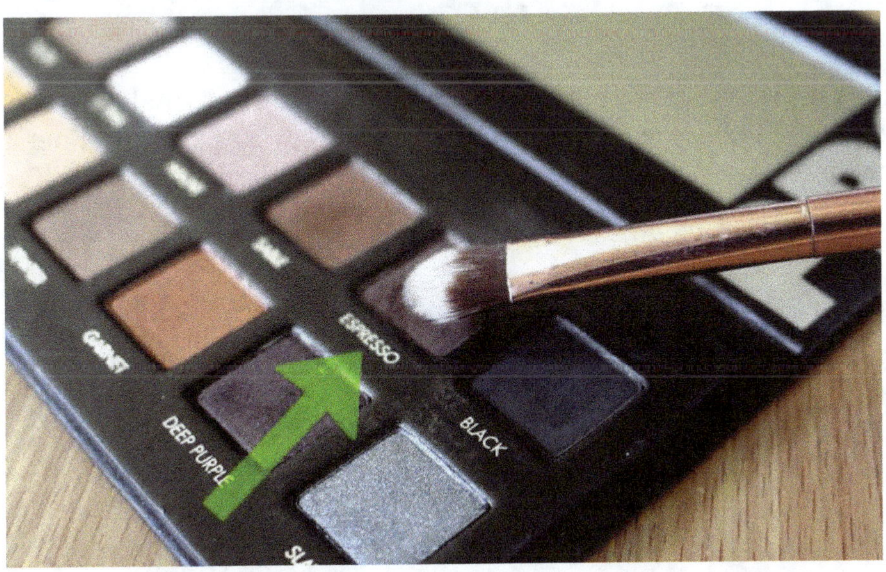

1. Try dark brown or espresso eyeliner. It is dark enough to enhance your eyes, but light enough so that it doesn't close them in. If it is a special night out, you can even try gold.

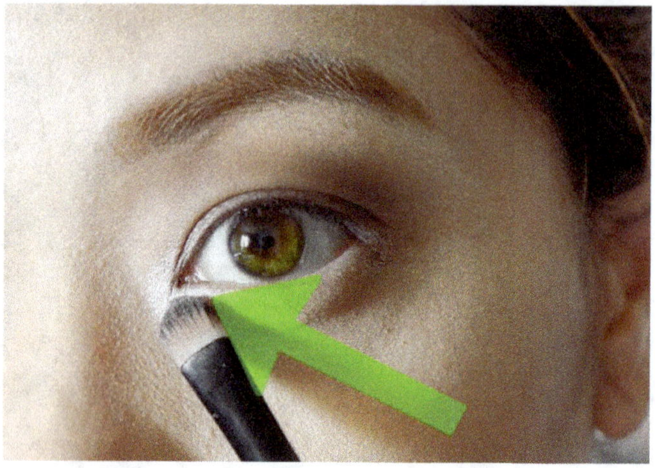

2. Try adding white eyeliner to the inner corner of your eye. Be sure to blend the eye shadow in to make it look more natural. This will help open up your eyes.

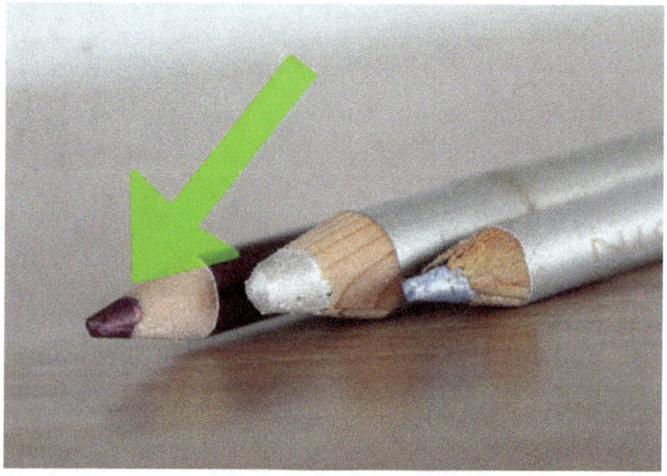

3. Consider using purple eyeliner or mascara. They are a great way to make your eyes look brighter while wearing brown or green eyeshadow. You don't have to wear purple eyeliner and purple mascara at the same time, however. Try pairing charcoal eyeliner and purple mascara.

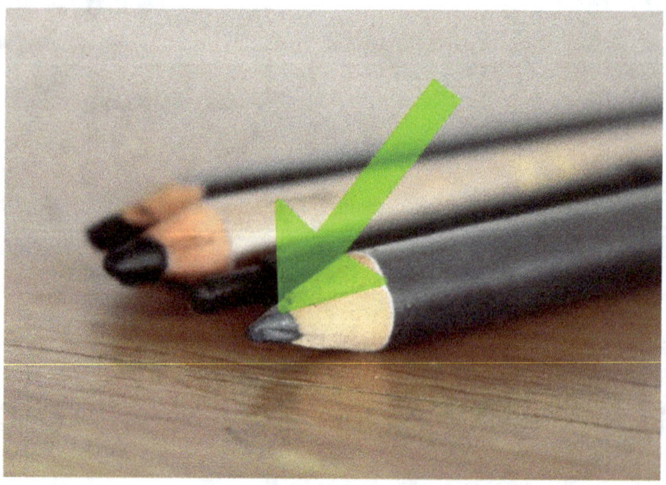

4. Don't be afraid to use black mascara, but avoid using black eyeliner. Instead, go for charcoal, dark gray, or slate gray eyeliner. Black eyeliner is too harsh for green eyes. Black mascara, however, can help define your eyes.

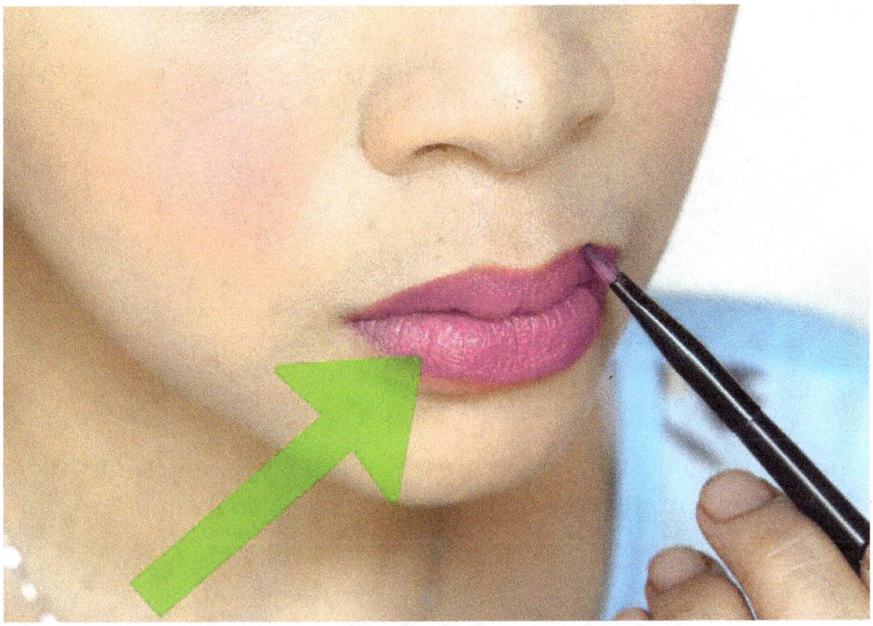

5. Try red, pink, or violet-tinted lipstick. This will give your eyes some nice contrast. To make your lipstick last longer, apply a lip liner all over your lip first. Be sure that you are using a matching shade. Apply your lipstick over the lip liner, blot it, and apply a second coat. Set your lipstick by placing a thin tissue over your lips, then dusting it lightly with setting powder.

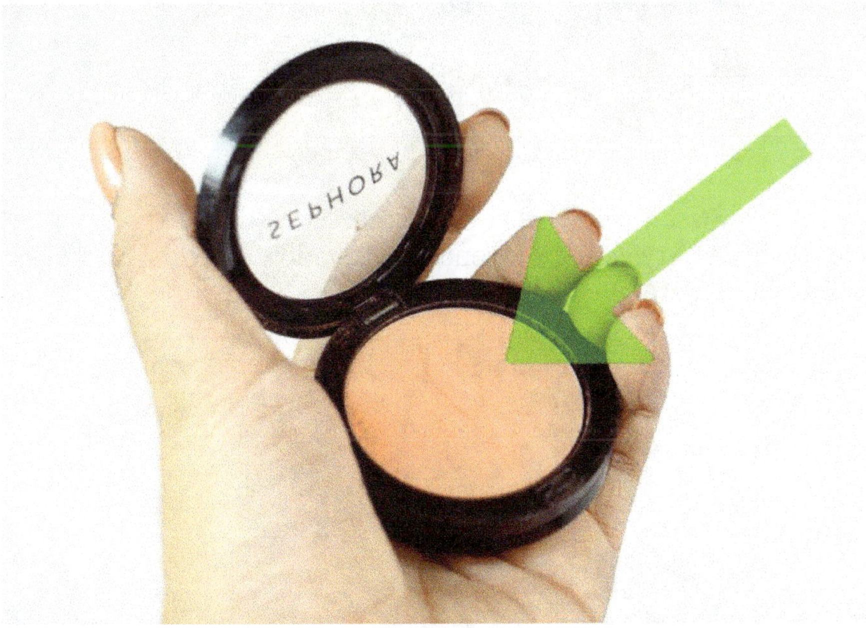

6. Wear a peach-colored blush to compliment green eyes. If you have cool skin, however, you might want to try a pink-tinted blush instead.

Method 3

Getting Color Combination Ideas

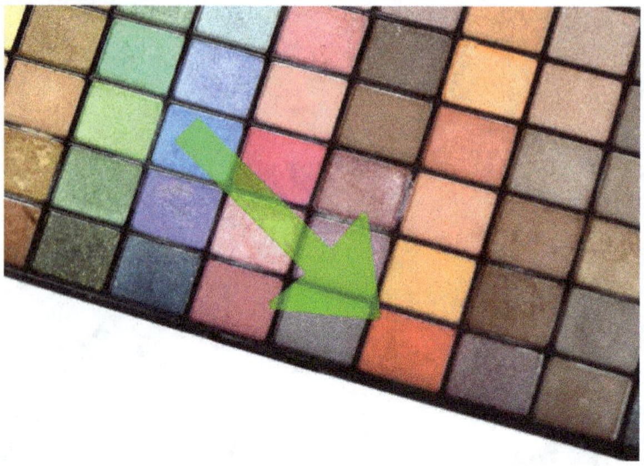

1. Use more red tones if you have true-green eyes. You can also apply some of your blush to your lash line. This will help tie your eye makeup to the rest of your makeup.

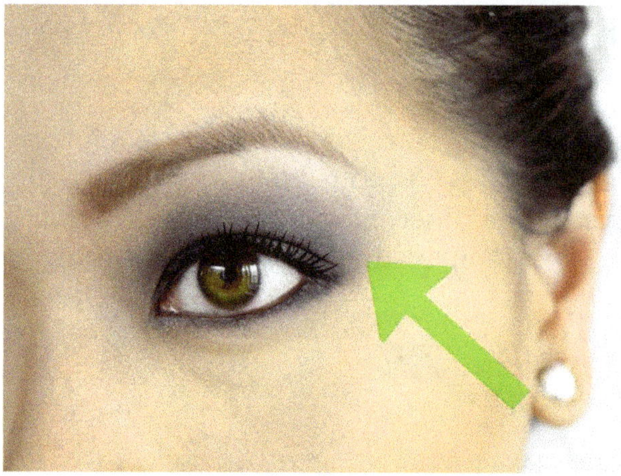

2. Try smokey eyes with a twist if you have golden-green eyes. Instead of using the usual charcoal and silver eyeshadow shades, try wine or lavender eyeshadow instead. Add more definition with some charcoal or dark brown eyeliner.

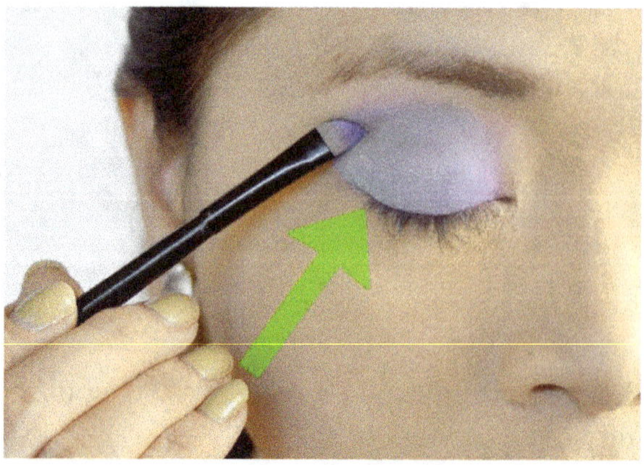

3. Use periwinkle on your lash lines if you have hazel-green eyes. Sweep periwinkle eyeliner on your upper lash line. Dust some periwinkle eyeshadow on your lower lash line. Finish the look with a violet or plum mascara.

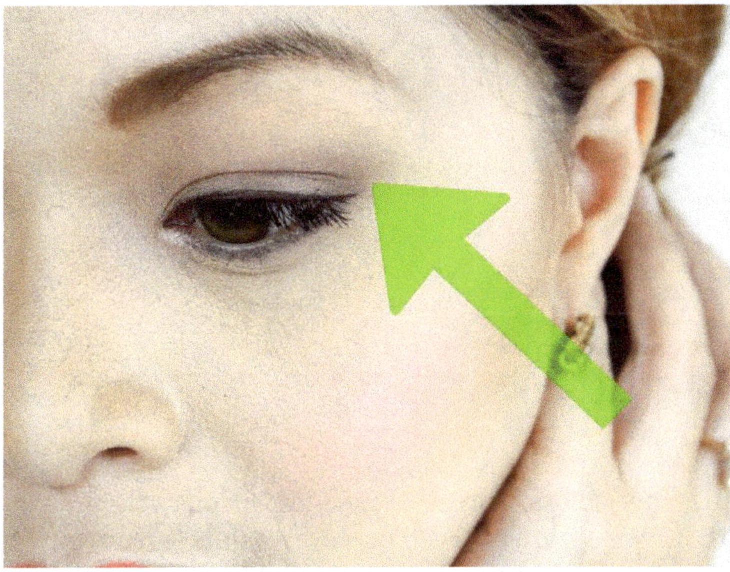

4. Go neutral with browns and golds. Apply gold eyeshadow all over your lid. Then, brush a dark tan shadow to the crease with a crease brush. Tap on some more dark tan eyeshadow to the inner and outer corners of your eyes. Blend everything in, then brush on some dark brown eyeliner and mascara.

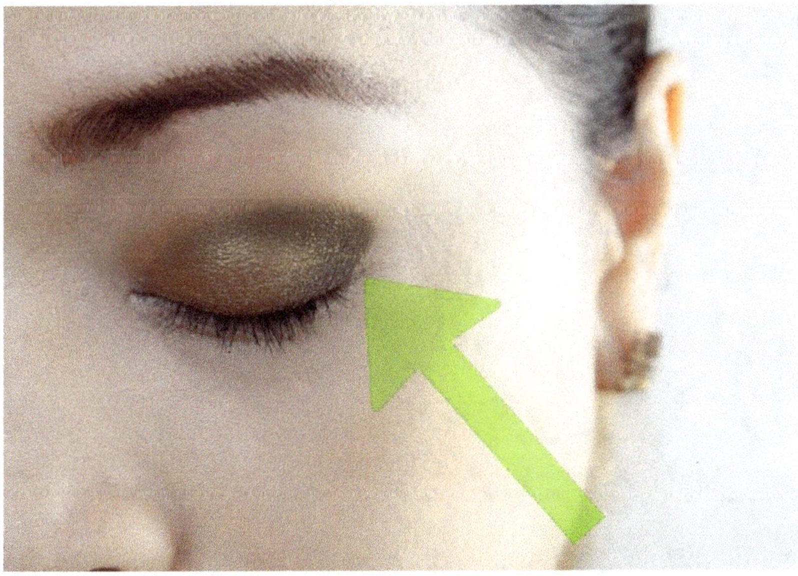

5. Go neutral with peaches and browns. Spread eyeshadow primer all over your eyelid. Brush on a cream color all over your eyelid, from lash line to brow bone. Apply a peach color to your upper lid, from lash line to crease. Dust on some of that same peach color to just below your lower lashes. Apply brown eyeliner to both your upper and lower eyelids. Finish off with brown mascara on both your upper and lower lashes.

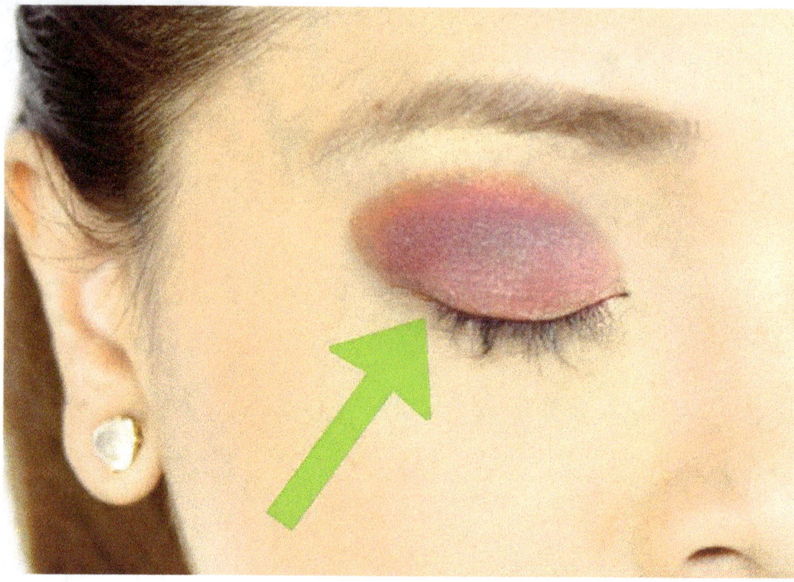

6. Try mixing purple with other colors. Spread eyeshadow primer all over your eyelid. Line your upper and lower lids with brown eyeliner. Brush on a warm purple over your entire lid, from lash line to crease. Apply a strawberry color to the crease. Soften any harsh edges with a blending brush. Dust on some of that same strawberry color to just below your lower lashes. Finish off with some brown mascara on your upper and lower lashes.

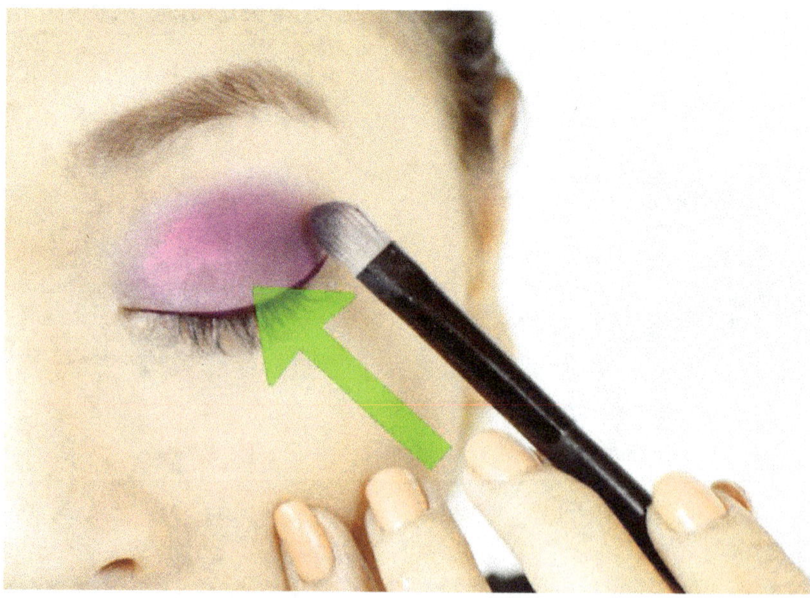

7. Try a monochromatic purple look. Apply some eyeshadow primer. Brush on a medium purple eyeshadow all over your eyelid, from lash line to just past the crease. Apply a lighter purple from just past the crease all the way up to your brow. Finally, brush on a dark purple to your lash line. Blend all three shades to create a smooth, ombre transition. Finish the look off with some charcoal eyeliner and mascara.

- Consider pairing this with clear, glitter lip gloss

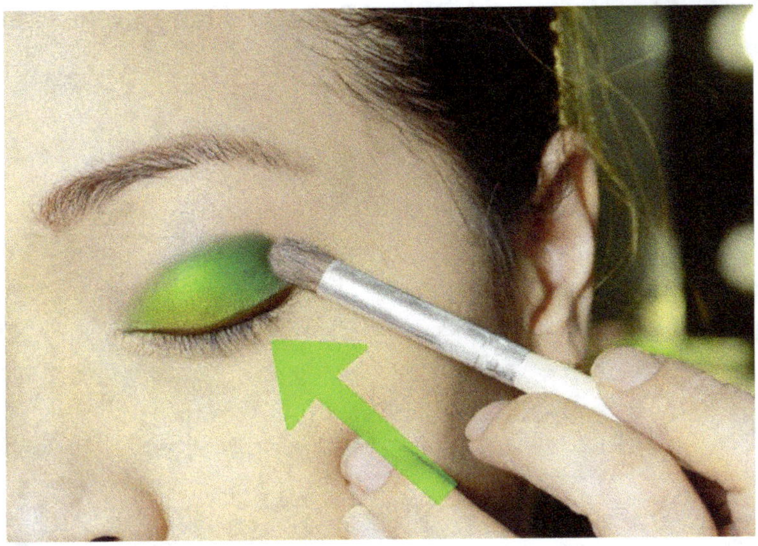

8. Use different shades of green for a monochromatic look. Apply a medium green eyeshadow all over your eyelid, from lash line to crease. Then, apply a lighter green to the inner corner of your eyelid. Finish off with a darker green on the outer corner. Blend the colors together for a smooth, ombre look. If you want, you can add on some eyeliner and mascara as well.

- Apply ivory eyeshadow to your brow bone to give your eye some more definition.
- Try using brown eyeliner or mascara.

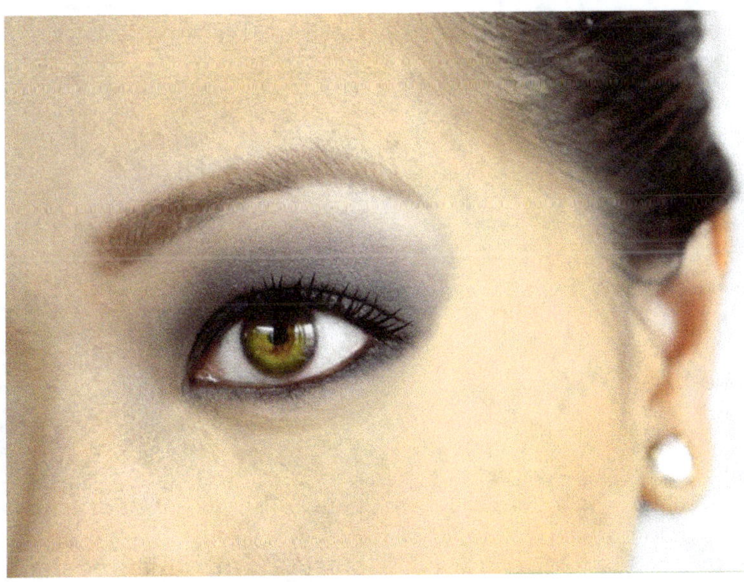

How to Add Rose Gold to your Eyes

A rose gold eye shadow and eye liner can make for a nice, girlish look for a party or social event. To add rose gold, start with a basic foundation using nice, rosy colors. From there, define your eyes with darker eyeshadow and a gold eyeliner. Finnish up by adding eyeliner to your waterline and defining your lashes with a quality mascara.

Part 1

Starting with the Foundation

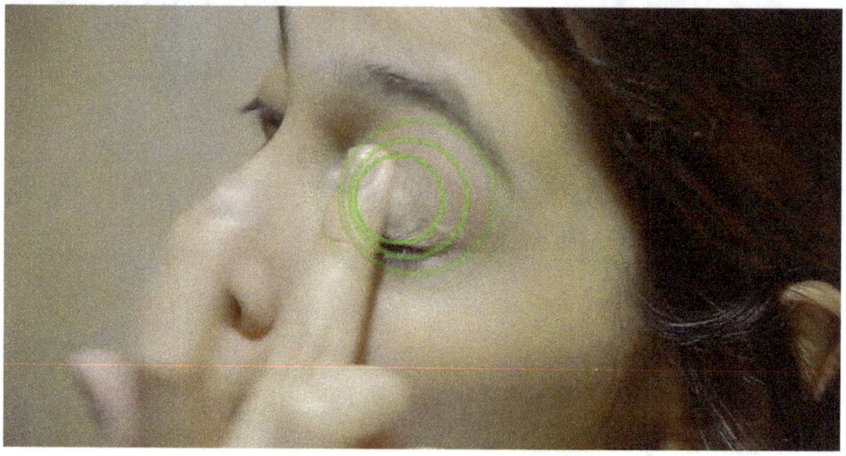

1. Use concealer to form your base. You want your eyeshadow to stand out, as rose gold eyes should really pop. Always start with a concealer to form a nice base on which you'll place your eyeshadow.

- Dab the concealer all over your eyelids and into your brow bone.
- Gently rub the concealer into your eyelids until it's blended into your natural skin tone.

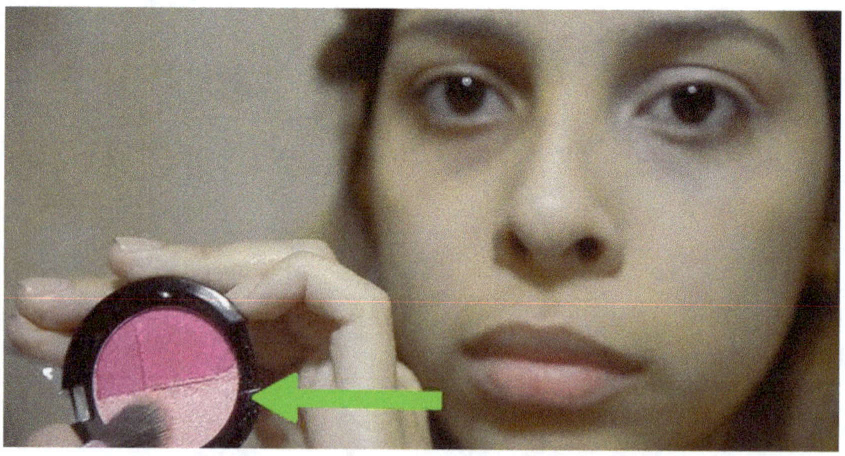

2. Add a lighter shade of eye shadow. You want to start off with a lighter shade of eye shadow. Opt for a shimmery, rosy color to start. To start, use your finger to press the eye shadow onto the outer half of your eye. Then, use your finger to pull the shadow inward to the other corner of your eye. This will create a faded effect. The color should start darker on the outer corner of your eye and lighten as it moves inward.

- Repeat this process on your lash line. Apply a light line of eyeshadow using your fingers that moves from the outer to inner corner of your eye.

- Repeat with the other eye.

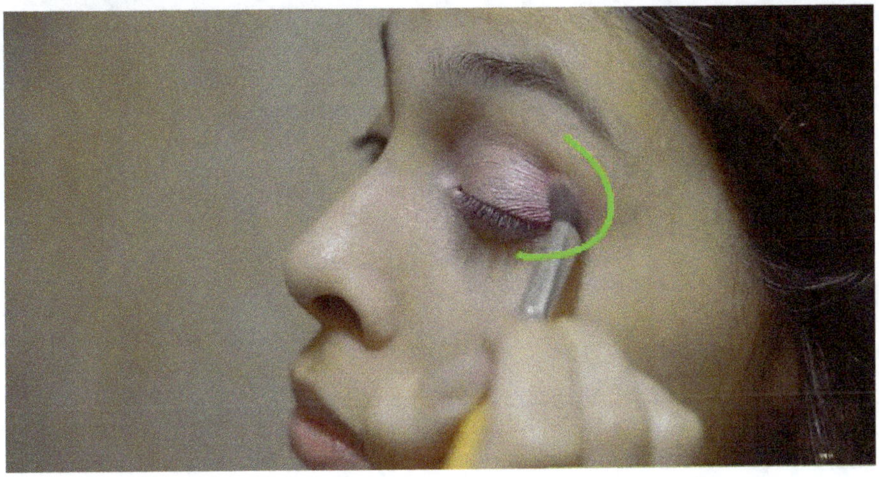

3. Create smokey corners. Once you've added your light layer of eye shadow, create smoky corners using a darker shade of rose-colored eye shadow. Imagine your eyelid is split into three parts: a rectangle in the center and two triangles on either corner.

- Focusing on the outermost corner, fill in this triangle with a darker color of rose colored eye shadow. You can use your fingers or a makeup brush.
- From there, use a shadow brush around the edges of the triangle and into your crease. Use the darker eye shadow to define this corner of your eye.

Part 2

Defining Your Eye

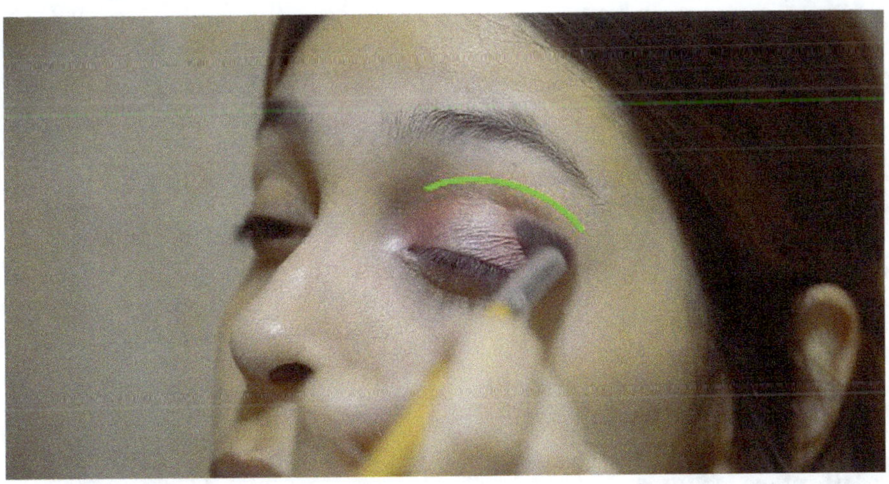

1. Color in your crease. Select a coppery, dark shadow for your crease. Use an angled brush to define your crease by slowly swiping on the eye shadow in back and forth motions. On the inner corner of your eye, draw a horizontal line pointing towards the bridge of your nose with the darker color.

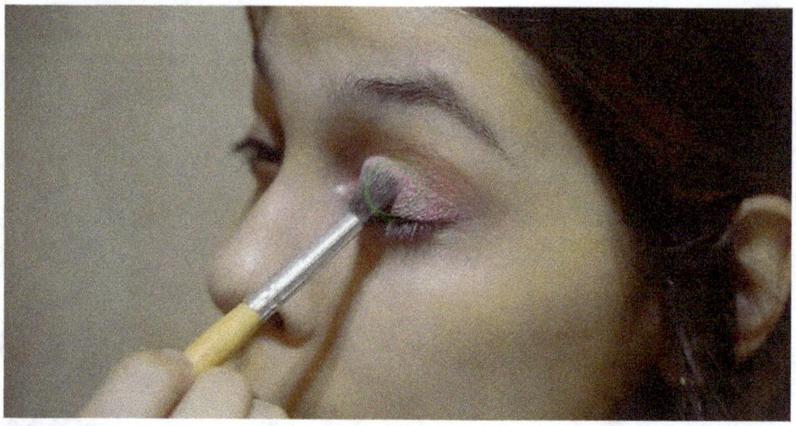

2. Blend your eye shadows together. Take a fluffy blending brush. Use it to blend your eyeshadows together. Use light, circular motions to help all your eye shadow blend together so it looks smooth and even. The horizontal lines should look less defined when you're done.

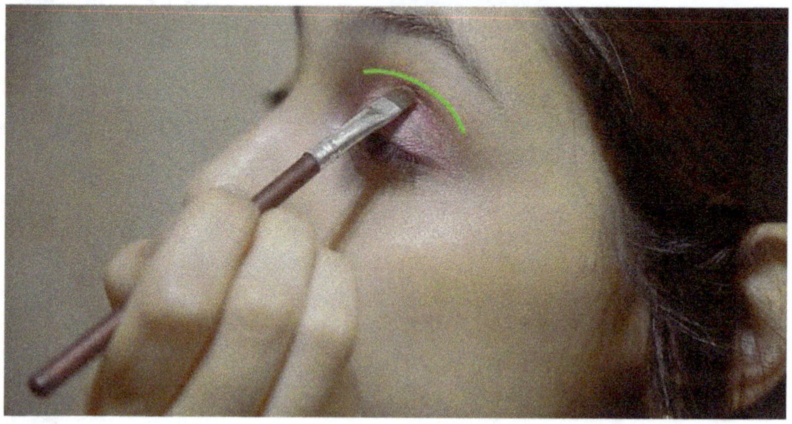

3. Define your crease with a darker eyeshadow. Take another makeup brush. Opt for one that's flatter and skinnier. You will use this to further define your crease with a dark shade of rose colored eye shadow.

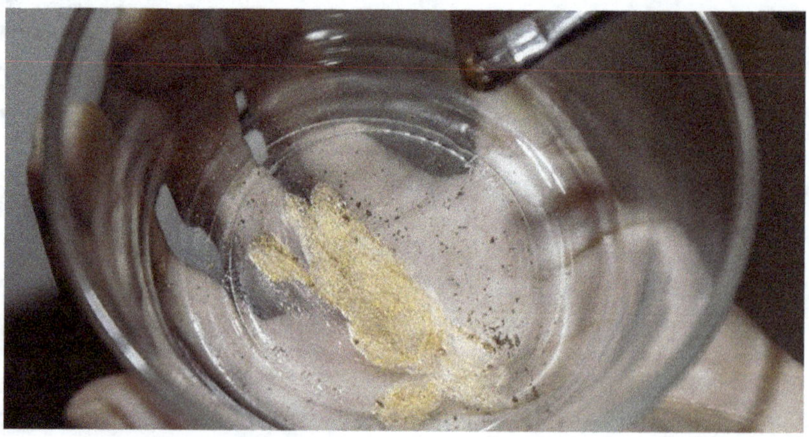

- Starting at the outer corner of each eye, draw a very defined line using a very dark shade of rose colored eye shadow. The line should follow the natural line of your crease.

- When you're done, use a blending brush to blend your crease line slightly into the rest of your makeup.

4. Create your gold liner. Gold eyeliner is important for rose gold eyes. To make gold eyeliner, use glitter and gold pigments and mixing medium.

- On a flat surface, mix your two pigments together.
- From there, add a small drop of your mixing medium. Use a utensil, like a spoon, to mix everything together.

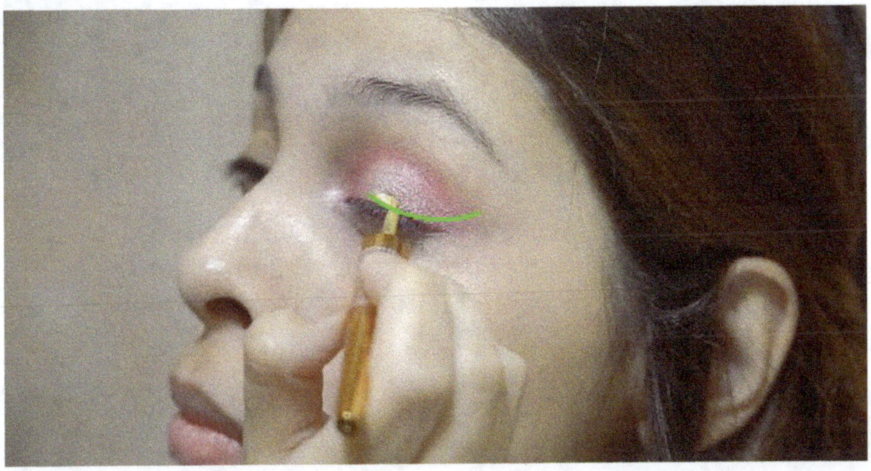

5. Apply your liner to your upper lash line. Use a small pointed make up brush here. Dip it in your gold liner. Draw a thin line running along your lash line. Start at the inner corner of your eye and move outward. The line should get gradually thicker the closer you get to your outer eye.

Part 3

Finishing Up

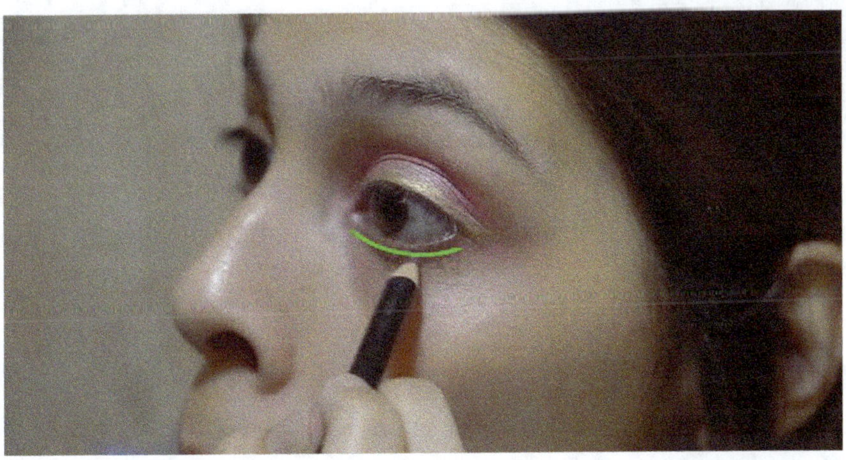

1. Add dark eyeliner to your waterline. You can use brown or black eyeliner to define your water line. Simply add a line of black eyeliner on the water lines of both of your eyes. This should make your eyes stand out more, as they will be dramatically outlined.

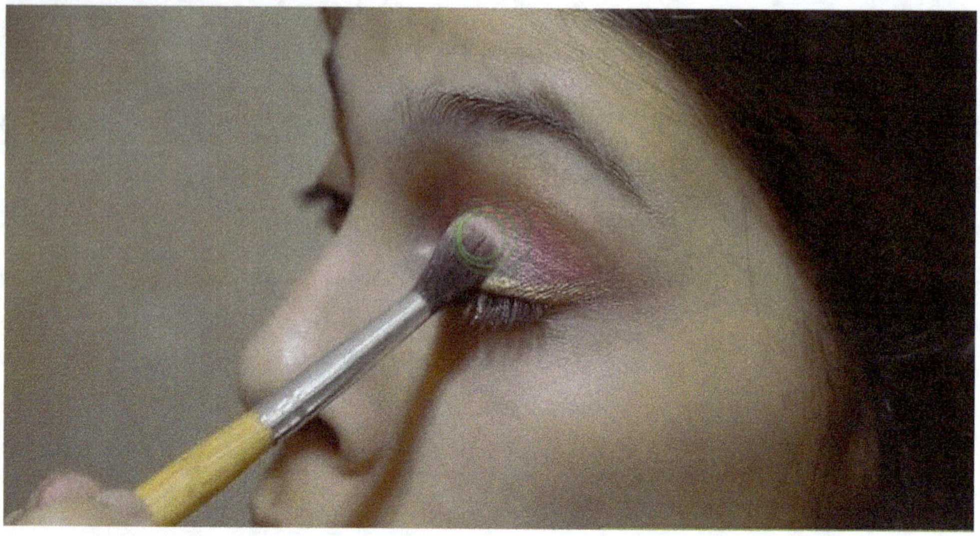

2. Brighten up your eyes slightly if necessary. If your eyes are too dark, you can add some lighter eyeshadow to the center of your eyes. Dab the eyeshadow near the center of your eyelid. From there, you can use a blending brush to blend the eye shadow outward to create a lighter effect.

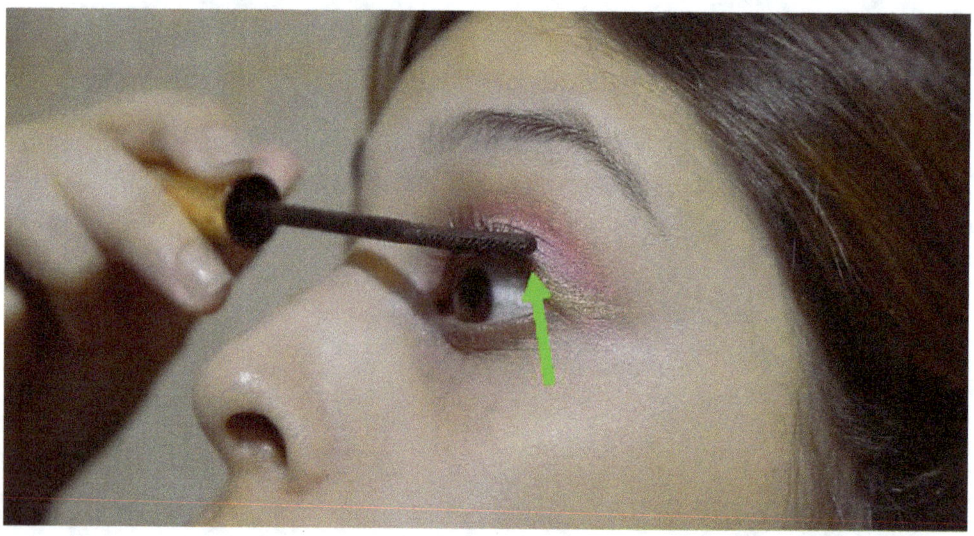

3. Finnish with a quality mascara. Opt for a volumizing mascara, as this will make your eyelashes standout. To apply, use the mascara brush starting at the root. Then, wiggle the brush outward to the end of your eyelashes.

How to Apply Dark Eye Makeup

Want to add extra oomph to your evening look? Dark, smokey eyes are beautiful and glamorous, but they can be tricky to do. This article will show you step-by-step how to apply dark eye makeup, perfect for any night out.

Part 1

Applying Dark Eye Makeup

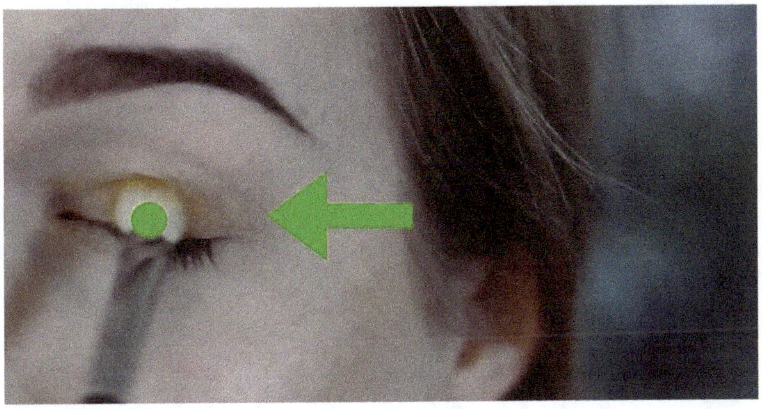

1. Apply a matte, light brown eyeshadow to the crease of your eyelid. Use a soft, fluffy eyeshadow brush with longer bristles to do this. This will give you that nice, soft base color.

- If you have a darker skin tone, a light brown might be too light for you; opt for a shade that is 2 to 3 shades darker than your skin tone instead.

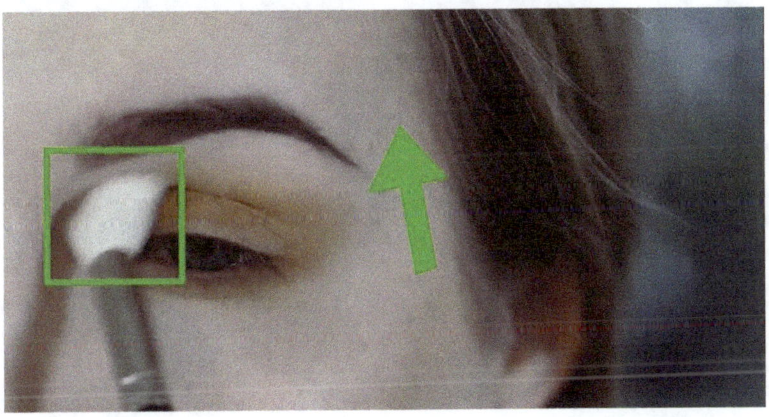

2. Blend the eyeshadow upwards towards your eyebrow. The eyeshadow should be darkest along the crease, and faded to almost nothing as it goes towards your eyebrow.

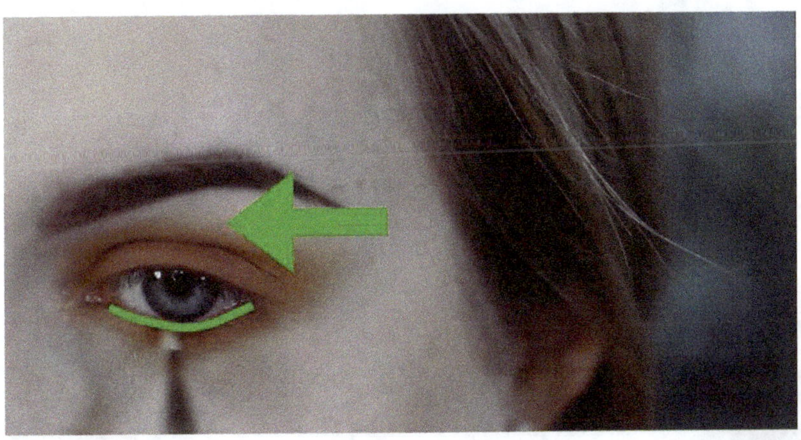

3. Apply a darker brown eyeshadow to the crease. Use a smaller brush with slightly shorter and stiffer bristles to do this. Focus the shadow inside the crease, as well as just above and below it. For this, you can use a somewhat sparkly eyeshadow.

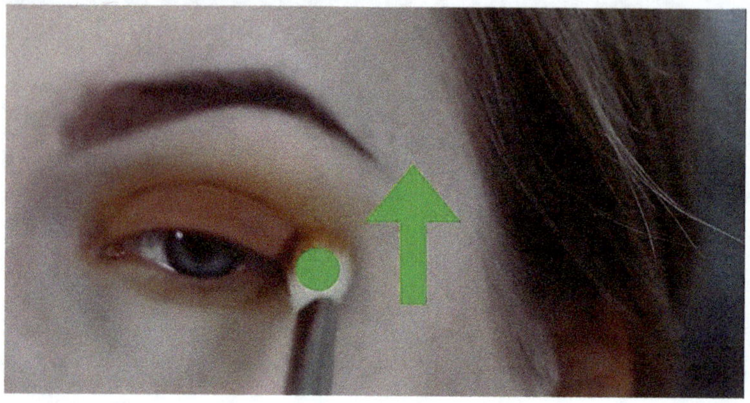

4. Blend the darker brown shade in. Start by blending most it downwards towards your lash line. Finish off by blending it upwards towards your eyebrow, just a little bit past the crease. Don't worry so much about getting the blending on the eyelid perfect, as you will be covering it up.

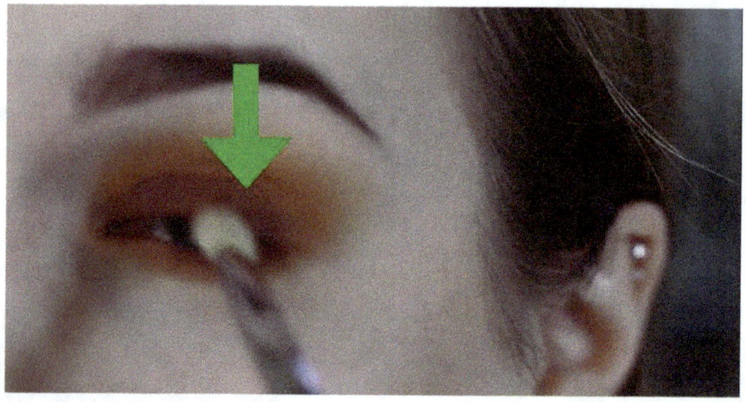

5. Apply a black, gel eyeliner to your eyelid using a brush with short, stubby bristles. Start applying the eyeliner to the center of your eyelid, right along the lash line. Work your way to the corners, making the line thinner as you go. When you are done, you should have a half-circle shape halfway up your eyelid.

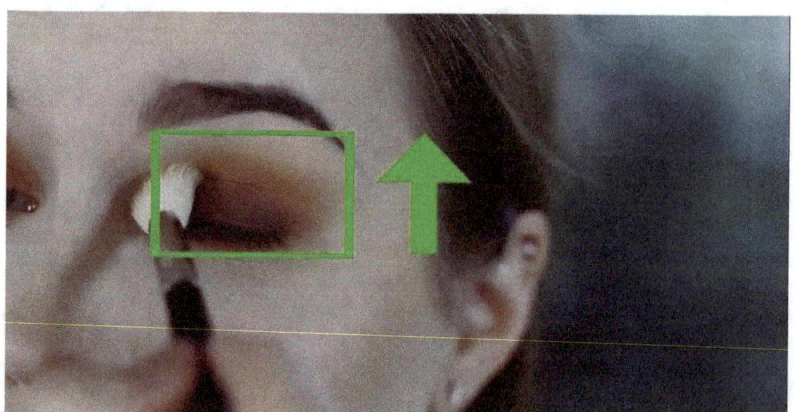

- You can also use black eyeshadow, black kohl, or a black eyeliner pencil.
- If you are having difficulties applying the makeup to your lash line, take a little mirror and hold it below your eyes, in the palm of your hand. Look down into the mirror, and carefully outline your upper lash line.

6. Blend the black eyeliner up towards the crease using short, downward strokes. Do not blend it up too high, however. The black eyeliner will simply act as a base, so that you can get the darkest black possible.

- Finish off your blending by running your brush along your eyelid, just below the crease. This will help soften any harsh edges.

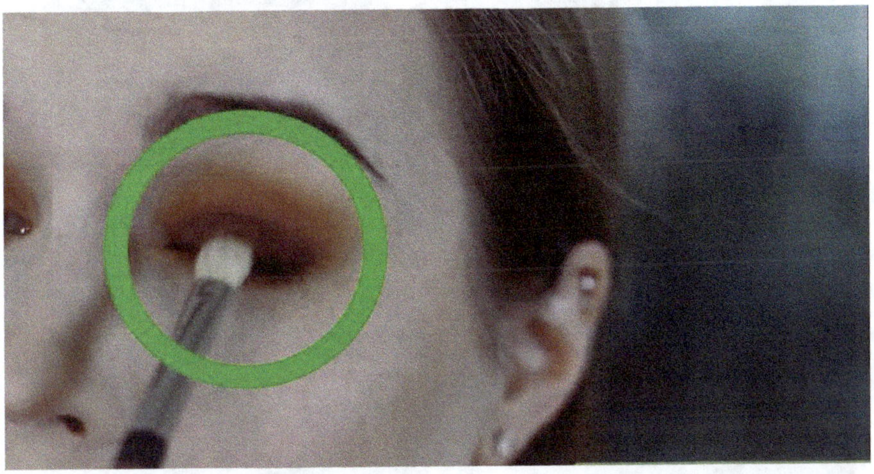

7. Dust black eyeshadow over the black eye makeup using your short, stubby brush. This will help set it, and prevent it from smudging. It will also help take away any shine. If you want, you can use a black eyeshadow with some shimmer in it.

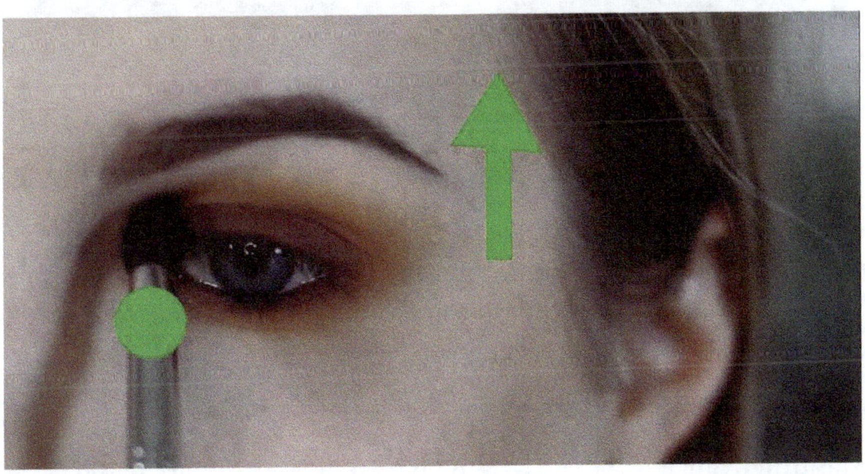

8. Go over the crease again with your darker brown eyeshadow. Use the same brush you used to apply it originally—the one with the stiffer bristles. Be sure to blend it up towards the brow bone. When you are done, you should have a sort of ombre effect on your eyelid, that starts black, and gradates to a lighter brown towards your brow bone.

Part 2

Adding Finishing Touches

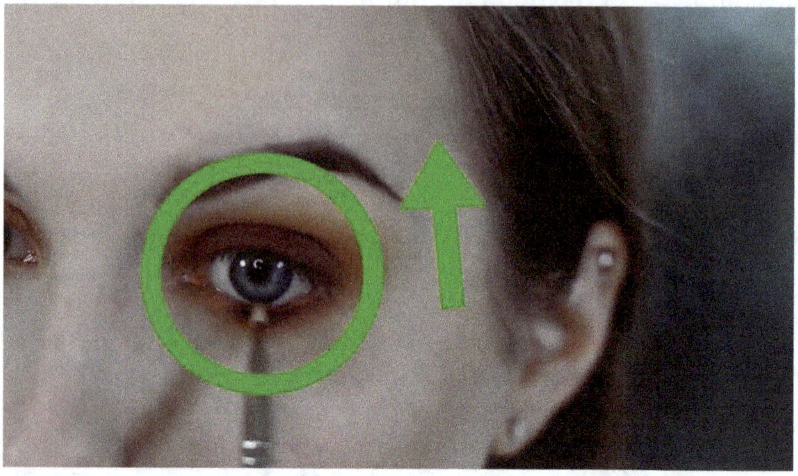

1. Consider tightlining your upper lashes. Use a black eyeliner with a felt tip or brush applicator to fill in the gap between your upper lashes and eyelid. This will help create a smoother transition, and blend everything together.

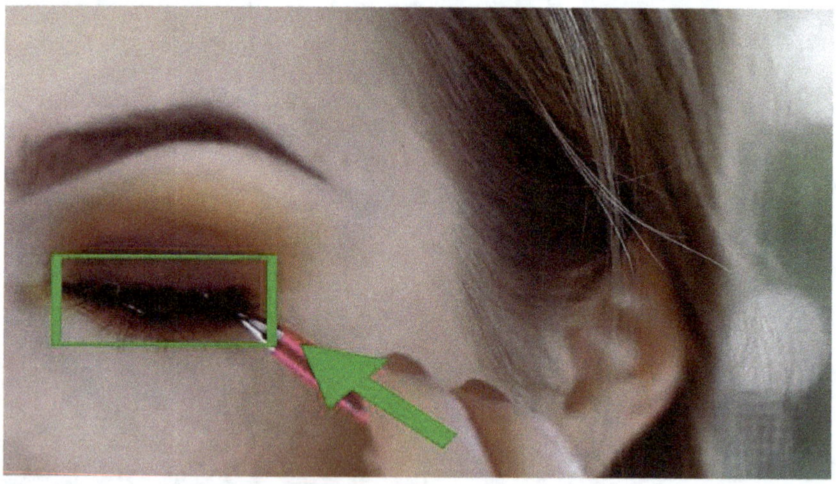

2. Apply some false lashes for a touch of glamour. If you have not already, trim your false lashes down until they fit your eyelid. Apply a thin line of eyelash glue to the back strip of your falsies, and wait until the glue starts to turn tacky. Carefully apply the eyelash, and lower your eyes until it dries.

- Most white glues will start to turn clear when they get tacky.
- Consider holding your falsie in a U-shape between your fingers while you wait for the glue to turn tacky. This will give it a nice curved shape, and help it mold better against your eyelid.
- Learning how to put on false lashes takes practice. Some people use special applicators or tweezers to put them on.

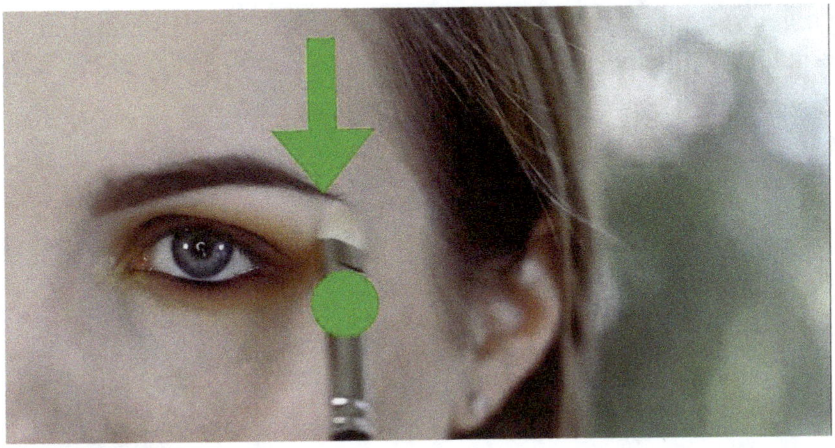

3. Dust on some white eyeshadow to your brow bones and to the inner corners of your eyes. Use a brush with shorter, slightly stiffer bristles to do this. This will help open up your eyes, and make them appear wider, brighter, and more awake.

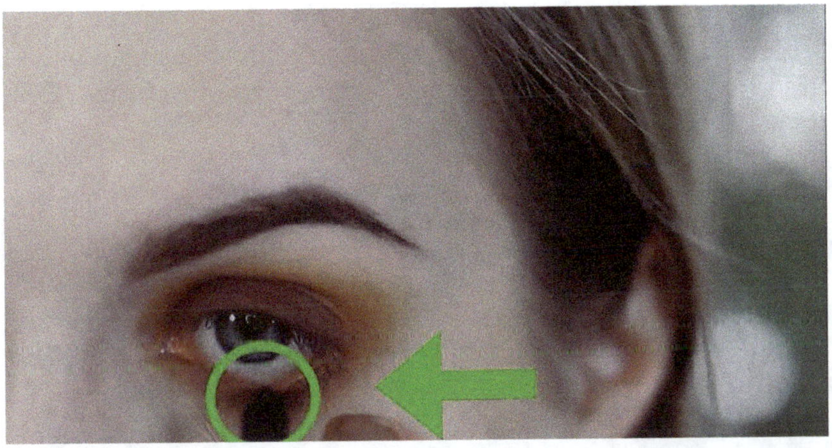

4. Apply some eyeliner and eyeshadow to your lower lashes. This will give your eyes that darker, smokier effect. Begin by lining your lower eyelid with black liner. Dust on some dark brown eyeshadow using a brush with short, stubby bristles. Be sure to follow the outline of your lower eyelid. Blend everything together using a thin, crease brush.

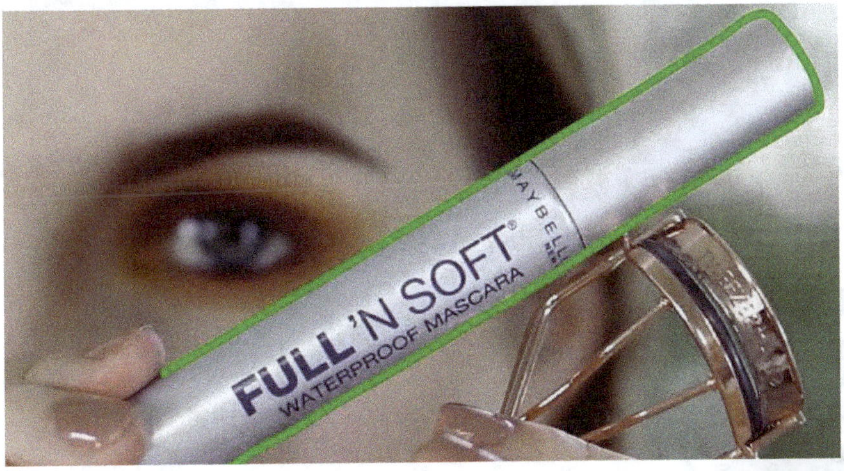

5. Consider applying some mascara to your bottom lashes. This will help balance your eyes out, and make them look less top heavy—especially if you are wearing very heavy false lashes.

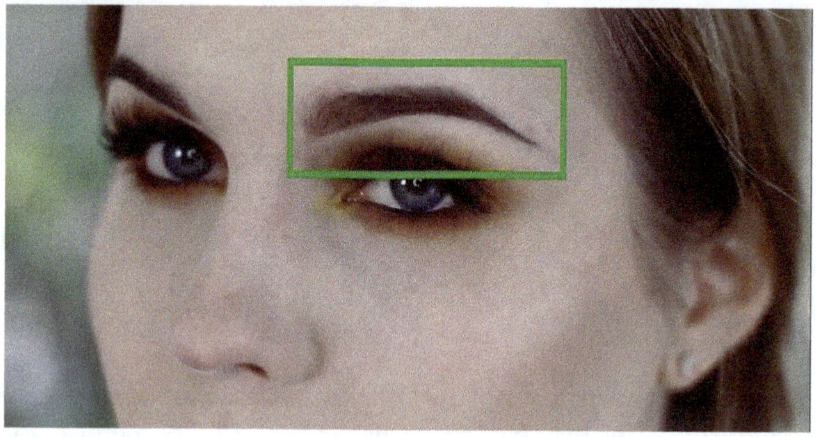

6. Groom and shade your eyebrows. This will give your eyes that nice, clean look. Begin by combing your brows upwards with a "spoolie" brush. Fill in any gaps and sparse areas with an eyebrow pencil; use as light a touch as you can. Next, fill in your eyebrows using a pressed powder and an angled brush; use a softer touch towards the inner corners of your eyebrows. Finish off by combing through your brows with the spoolie brush.

- A spoolie brush looks a little bit like a mascara brush.
- Use colors that closely match your eyebrows. If you have blond or very pale eyebrows, however, go a few shades darker. If you have black eyebrows, use a very dark brown or charcoal.
- To set the look, comb some eyebrow gel over your eyebrows. You can also dust on some translucent setting powder instead.

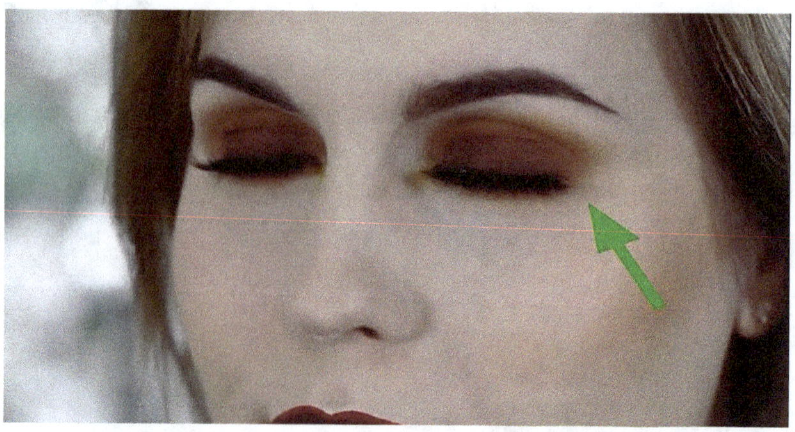

How to Apply Glitter Eye Makeup

Do you want to make your eyes sparkle? Wearing eye makeup that contains glitter is a great way to increase your glam factor. Glitter is a fun way to dress up your everyday look. You can choose to make the look subtle, or use it as the focal point of your whole makeup scheme. Take care to learn to properly apply glitter eye makeup.

Method 1

Creating a Smoky Eye

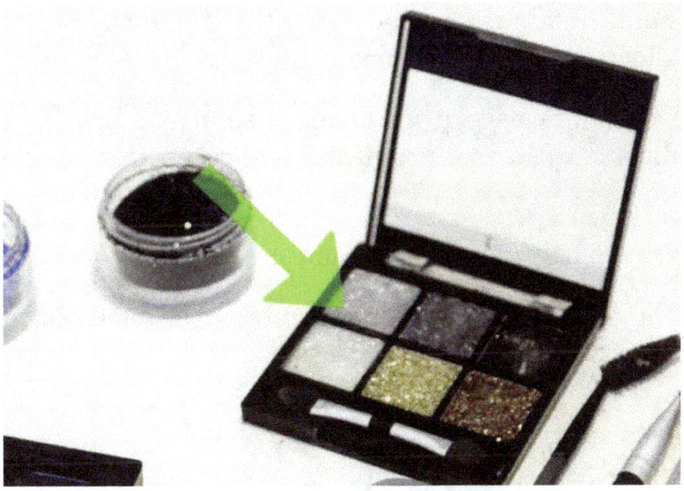

1. Choose the right product. Creating a smoky eye using glitter shadow is a great way to create a sultry, dramatic look. There is a wide array of glittery eye-shadows from which you can choose. One of the most important things to consider is which color of shadow you want. For example, if you are trying to create a more subtle look, try a shadow that closely matches your natural skin tone. This method will make your eyes appear to sparkle.

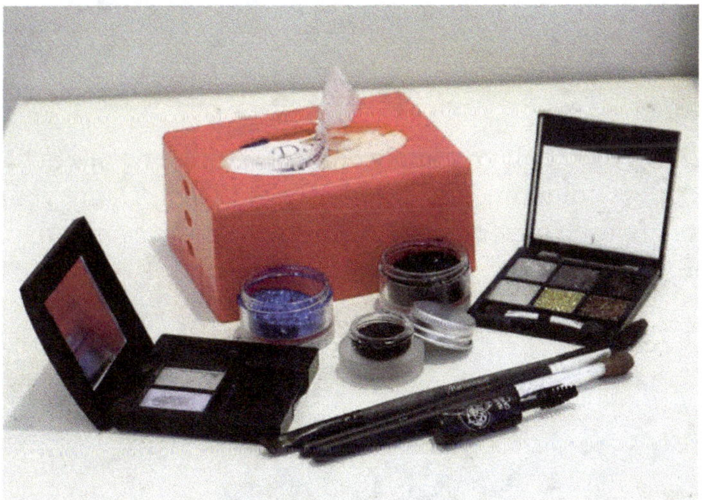

- If you want to highlight your eye color, glitter eye-shadow can help you do that. To make brown eyes pop, use a cream shade. To make green eyes glow, try a shadow with a reddish tint.
- Any of these color palettes can be used to create a smoky eye. Gray is also great for smoky eyes, and works on all skin tones.

- Glitter eye makeup comes in many different forms. You can buy eyeshadow pencils, powders, or gels.
- If this is your first time using glitter, try purchasing an eyeshadow palette. This will let you experiment with multiple shades.

2. Gather your supplies. Once you have chosen the right glitter shadow, it is time to achieve the look you want. Take a couple of minutes to make sure that you have everything you need. To start with, you'll need the shadow and a tool to help you apply it.

- You can apply eye shadow using your finger, a sponge, a brush, or a Q-tip. Many people prefer using a silicone brush as it is sturdier and can better handle the weight of a glitter shadow.
- Have tissues nearby to help you clean up any stray glitter.
- Make sure that you have a gentle eye-makeup remover handy in case you need to remove the shadow and start over.

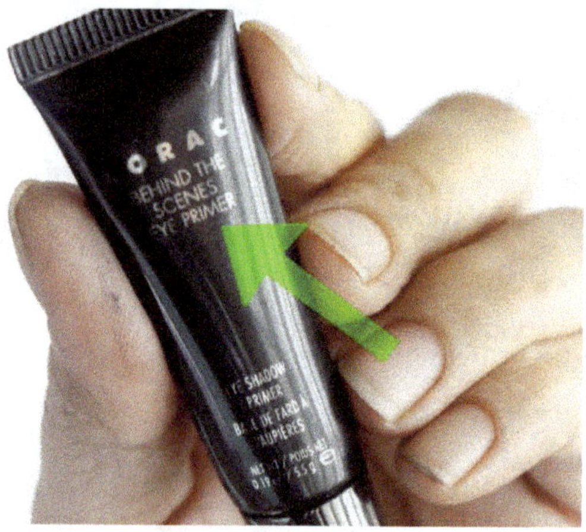

3. Use primer. A primer is a base that you apply before putting on your actual makeup. It will typically be a clear liquid, but is sometimes in powder or gel form. Using your finger, apply a small amount of shadow primer to each of your eyelids. This will create a smooth palette for your shadow and make it last longer.

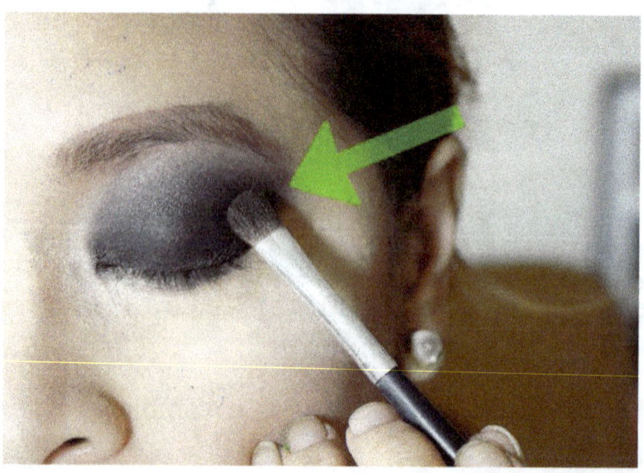

- You can purchase eyeshadow primer at any drugstore or department store. Remember, a little goes a long way.

4. Apply the base shadow. Once your eyes and your tools are ready, it is time to put the glitter shadow on your eyes. Try using several different shades to create a dramatic effect. Begin by applying a charcoal gray shadow. Use a medium brush to cover your lid with shadow.

- Then, use a slightly darker shade to color the inner and outer corner of your eyes. This will help highlight them.

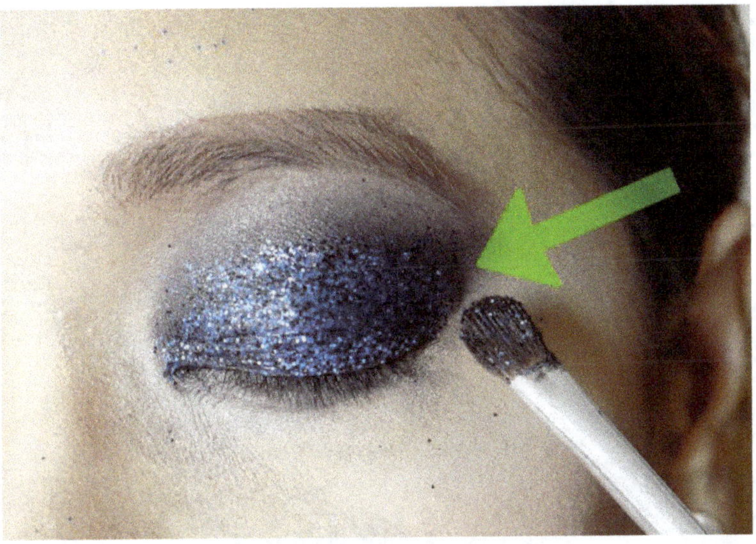

5. Use multiple colors of glitter shadow. Different shades are what create the smoky look. Next, you want to apply the darkest of your shadows. Using a brush, apply a thin line of dark shadow across the crease of your eyelid. This will help create the smoky effect.

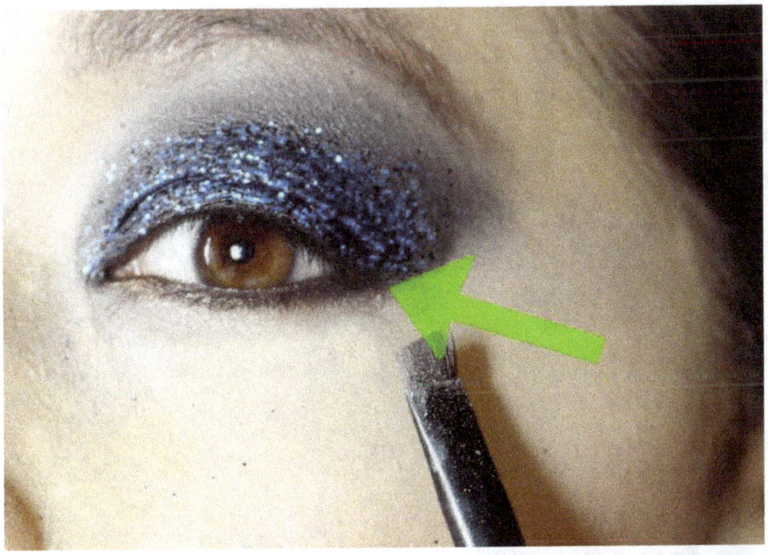

- Remember, it is easier to add more shadow than to take it away. Start with less than you think you might need. You can always apply more.

- Blend the colors. Blending the complimentary colors will help create a softer, yet still dramatic, look. For this step, you can use either your finger or a brush. Lightly smudge each of the colors together so that they are no longer sharply defined.

6. Color the bottom lid. To create a true smoky eye, you need to focus on your lower lid, too. Use a gunmetal shade for this step. Use a small, firm brush and press shadow along your lower lid line.

- To keep the look from being too severe, use a light silver shadow to lighten the overall effect. Place a small amount in the inner corner of each of your eyes.

Method 2

Making a Glittery Cat Eye

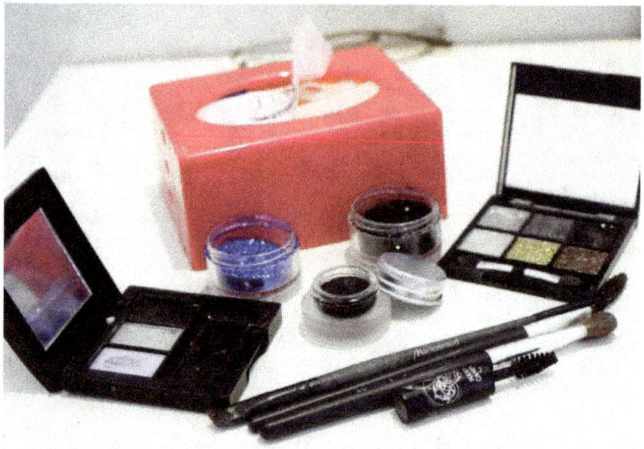

1. Get the right supplies. A cat eye can add an extra wow factor to your look. To make the cat eye pop even more, use eyeliners with glitter in them. To create the perfect cat eye, you will need two different kinds of liner.

- You will need a gel eyeliner pot. You will also need an eyeliner brush.
- Additionally, you will need a felt-tipped liquid liner. One or both of these liners can be glittery.

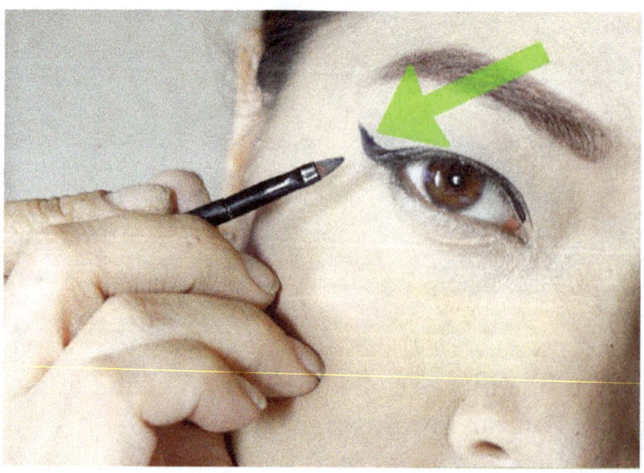

2. Create your outline. Start with the gel liner and the eyebrow brush. Dip the brush in the pot of liner. Draw a line with the brush from the outer corner of your eye towards your temple. Try drawing a line approximately 1/8 of an inch long. You can make it longer if you want.

- This is the "tail" of your cat eye.
- Using the same gel liner, create a series of dots along your upper lash line. Start the dots about 1/4 of the way in from the inner corner of your eye.

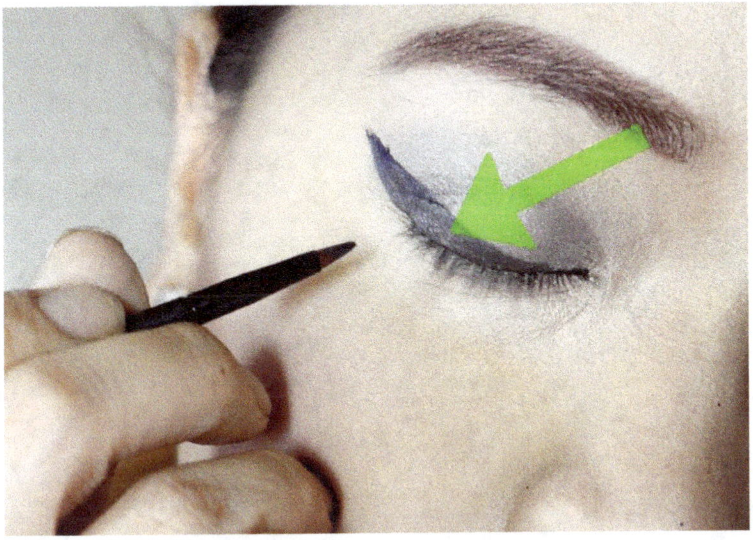

3. Fill in the lines. Now you are ready to fill in the outline that you have begun. Using the gel liner again, draw dashes between the dots. This creates a solid line of eyeliner across your lid.

- Now it is time to connect the tail and the line. Using the gel liner, return to the tail. Draw a small triangle that connects to the line of dots and dashes. This should be a diagonal line that comes off of the tail and angles towards the line across your lid.
- Fill in the triangle shape using the felt-tipped liquid liner.

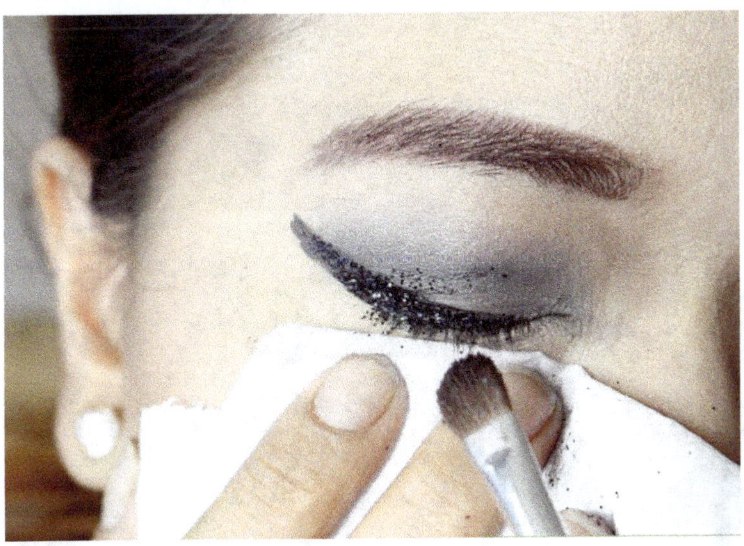

4. Prevent a mess. You don't want to end up with glitter on the rest of your face. Your look will look best if the glitter stays on your eyes. Take steps to keep the glitter from drifting down onto the rest of your face.

- As you are applying the eyeshadow with one hand, hold a tissue beneath your eye with the other hand. This will catch any fallout that occurs.
- Do your eye makeup first. That way, if you make a mistake, you can start over without having to reapply your foundation, blush, or lipstick.

Method 3

Using Multiple Glittery Products

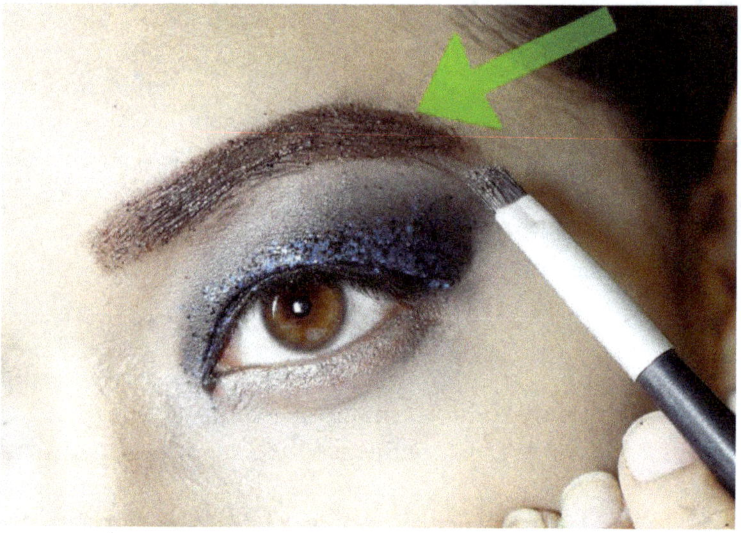

1. Put glitter on your eyebrows. Glittery eyebrows are a major fashion trend right now. You can accomplish the look as long as you have a few specific tools. You will need an eyebrow brush, eyeshadow brush, a glitter base (or lash glue) and make-up grade glitter. Do not use glitter that is intended for crafts or other uses.

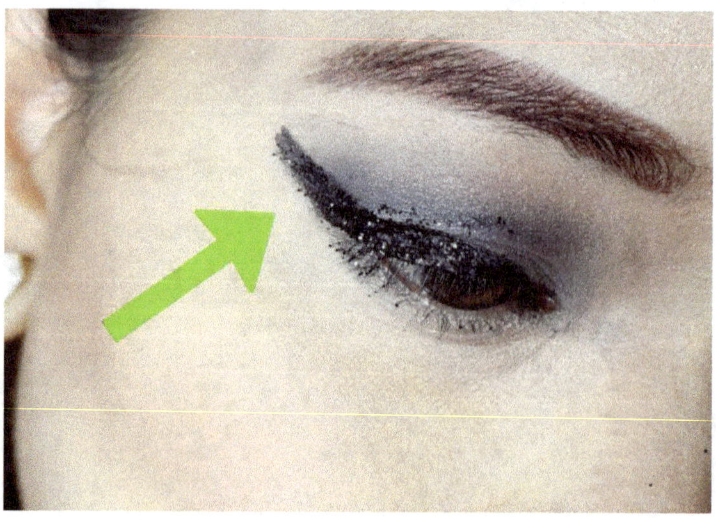

- Brush your brows into place with the brow brush. Next, use the shadow brush to completely cover your brows.
- Dip the shadow brush into the glitter and press onto your eyebrow. Cover your brows with glitter.
- Use the brow brush to comb through the glitter, making sure your entire brow is covered.

2. Wear a glittery liner. Once you have a perfectly shadowed eye, it is time to apply the rest of your makeup. For extra pop, consider using an eyeliner with a glittery shimmer. This will enhance your look, even if you are not doing a cat eye or smoky eye.

- Use a lighter liner if you want to make the glitter eyeshadow the focal point. Use a dramatic black liner if you are going for more of a sultry look.
- Using a glitter liner is a great way to experiment without committing to a full glittery eye.

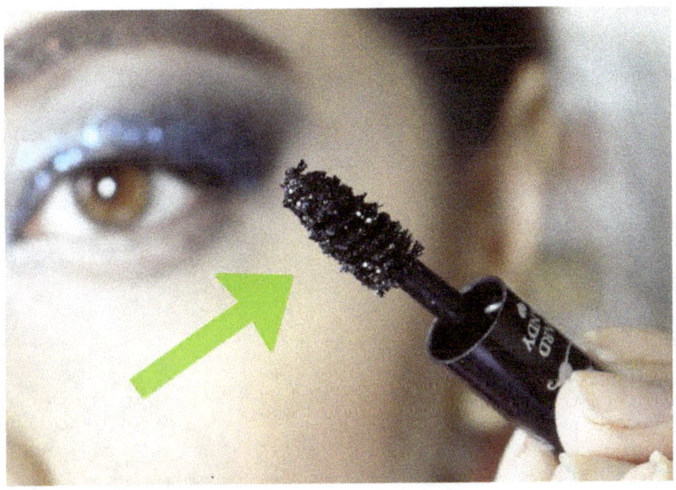

3. Make your eyelashes glitter. Your eyelashes are a great way to get creative with glitter. You can try a mascara that contains a little bit of sparkle. These products come in different colors, and have different amounts of glitter. Try swiping a coat on your lashes for some extra sparkle.

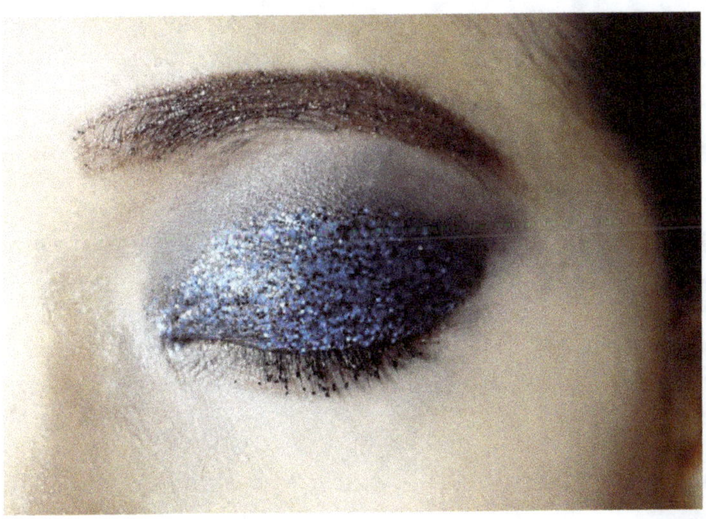

- If you want to ease into using glitter, apply one coat of your normal mascara. After allowing it to dry for 10 seconds, follow with a coat of glitter mascara.
- Try pairing the glittery mascara with a sparkly lipstick. Your look will be festive and fun.

How to Create an Elegant Cat Eye Look with a Colorful Lower Lashline

It is good to use a profile photo with red lips, or with neutral lips. This is a neutral look that is used with a bit of purple eyeshadow on the lower lash line and natural, but long-looking false lashes. If you feel like any of these colors or products don't suit you, you can use other colors or products. If you want to learn how to do the good look on the picture or you want to see the actual look, please keep reading.

Part 1

Starting Off

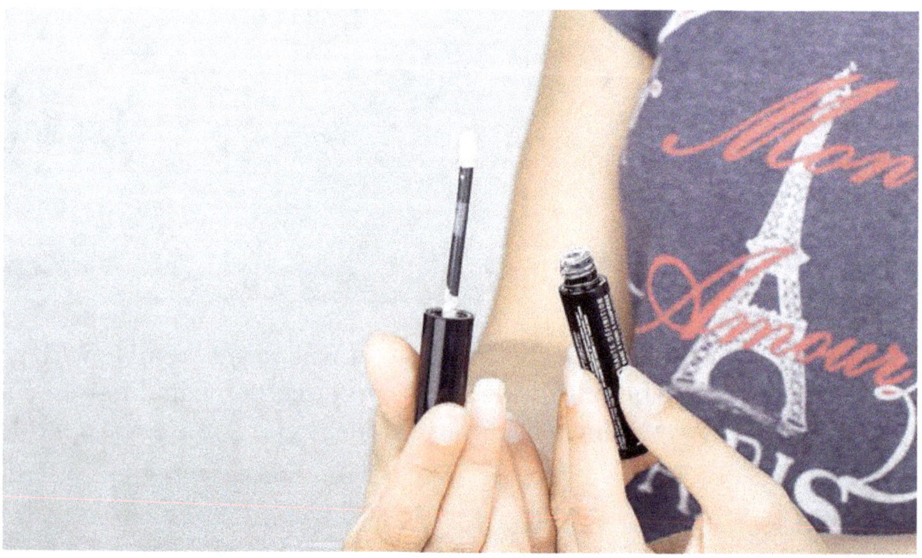

1. Add the base. There are two to three things you have to do before you start the look. The first thing you want to do is apply a primer.

- Apply something like the Mac Paint Pot in Soft Ochre or just a concealer and set it with powder.
- Wait for that to set in and then apply a "Base Shadow." This is an eyeshadow that matches your skin tone and that is matte. You can apply these two things with a flat shader brush, or with your finger.
- Make sure to also apply the primer on your lower lash line.

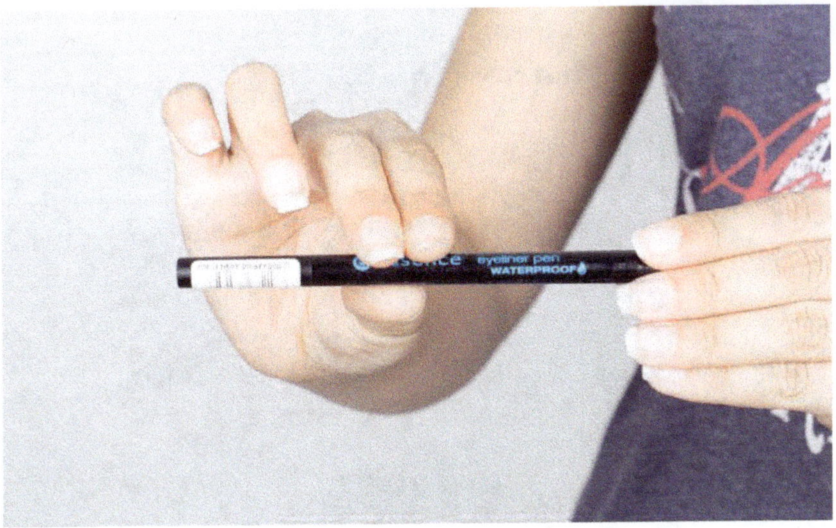

2. Make your lashes look a bit thicker, and fuller. To help the look build up, grab your favorite black, waterproof eyeliner. Make sure its not something like gel liner or liquid eyeliner, pencil is the best.

- Apply this to the tight line, which is also know as the upper water line. If you are not sure what that is, you can look it up on Google, or go up to a Mac store or any other makeup store and they will help you if you have a question.

Part 2

Adding Some Color and Shape

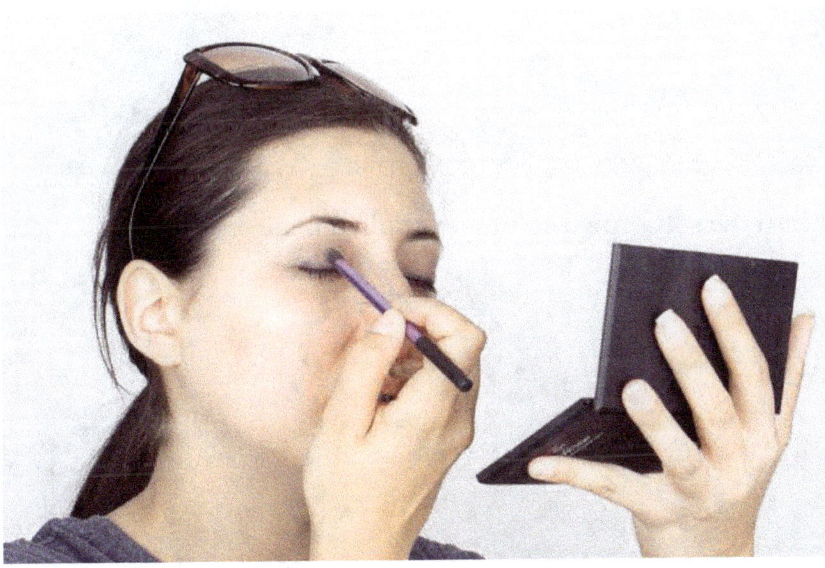

1. Add depth to your eye. Now take a soft brown, matte color on a Mac 217 brush, or any other blending brush you have, and apply that color to your crease. Add some to your "Outer V" and blend that color outwards, but not too far.

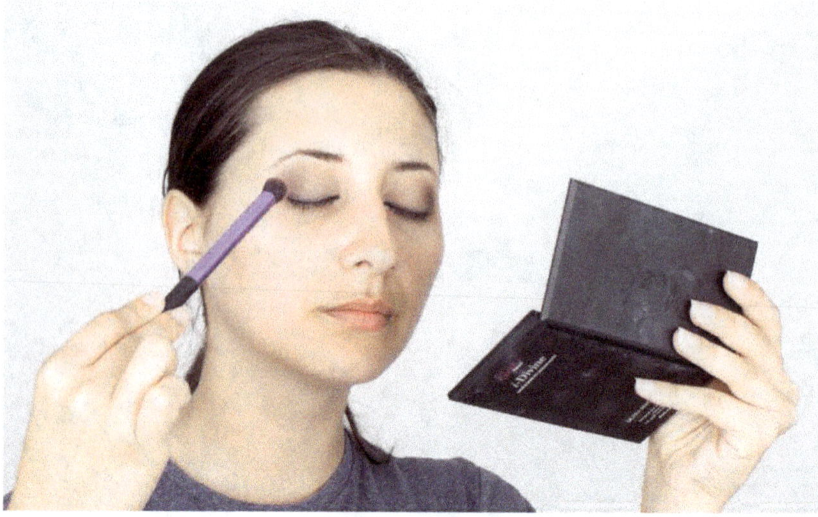

2. Add a bit more color to your eye. Take a gold color on the same blending brush, apply that to your crease and "Outer V" making sure that these colors stay matte all the time.

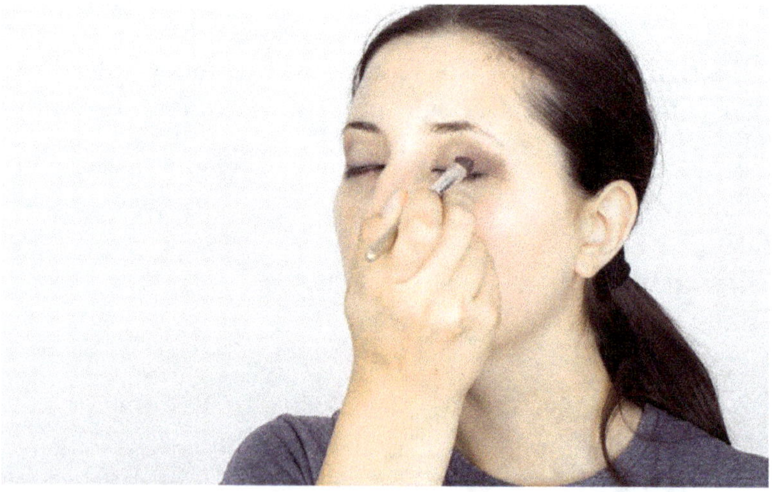

3. Blend this color into the soft brown color you applied before.

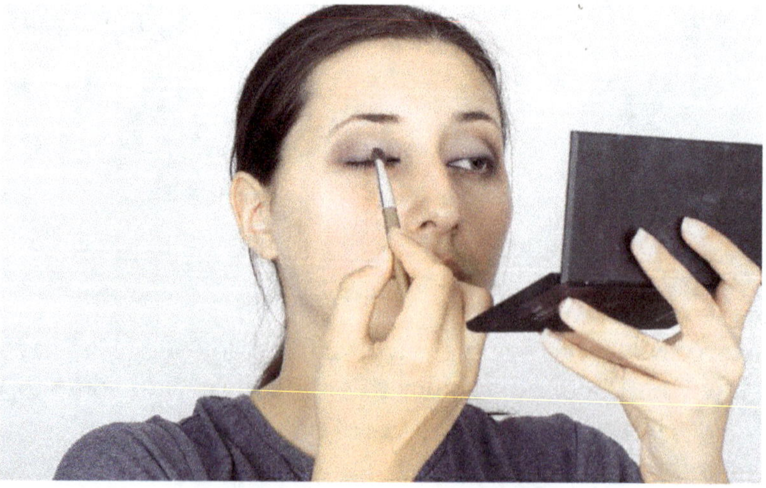

4. Add some color to your lid. Use a lighter color, that's matte, and apply that to your lid with a flat shader brush.

- You can go in with another metallic color and apply that to the middle of your eye to add so more definition and to make your eyes look brighter.
- Since you've added your lid color, the color on your crease has faded out a bit. Well, no worries. Just go back in with that brownish gold color, just a little, on the same blending brush and blend that color out, just enough so that it has a natural transitioning thing going on instead of having harsh lines.

Part 3

Doing the Eyeliner and Lash Part

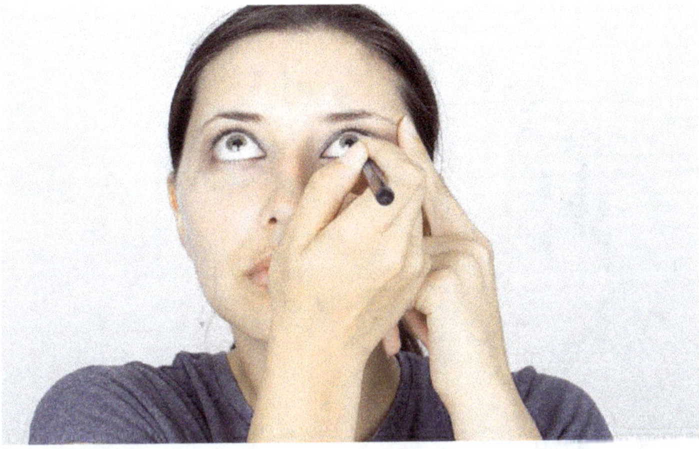

1. Do eyeliner on the inner rim. Now taking your favorite black pencil liner, maybe the same one that you used for the tight line, apply some to the inner rim of your eye, and feel free to retouch the upper water line part.

- Make sure that you go all the way to your inner corner, and then go back up to your tight line. Be careful though, make sure you are applying this eyeliner to the water line and not the lash line. They are the two different things.

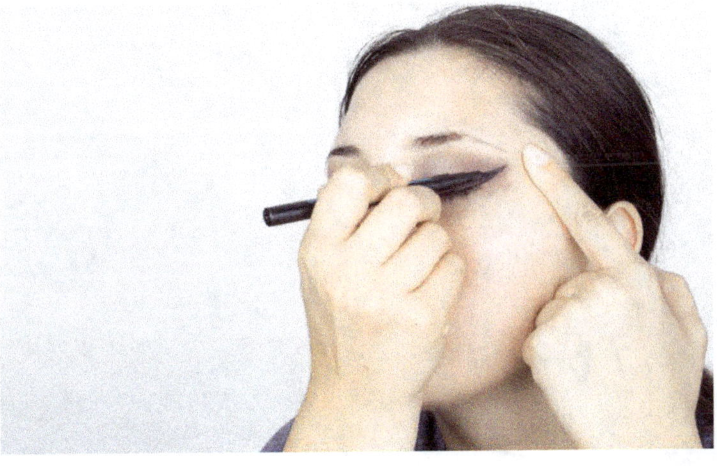

2. Do the cat eye.

- Take your favorite gel liner and an eyeliner brush, and line very close to the upper lash line, starting at the inner corner and towards the edge, almost as if you were using a regular pencil liner.
- Take that same brush, or an angled brush if you'd feel more comfortable, and start the wing. To do the wing, you have to start at the edge of your eye and go out, making sure the line is on a slant and not straight up.
- Connect the two lines that you created, and fill that triangle in.
- Draw a little curved line connecting these two parts and fill that little space in so no one would tell the starting or ending point. If you feel self-conscious or didn't understand anything written here, make sure to watch tutorials about winged liners.

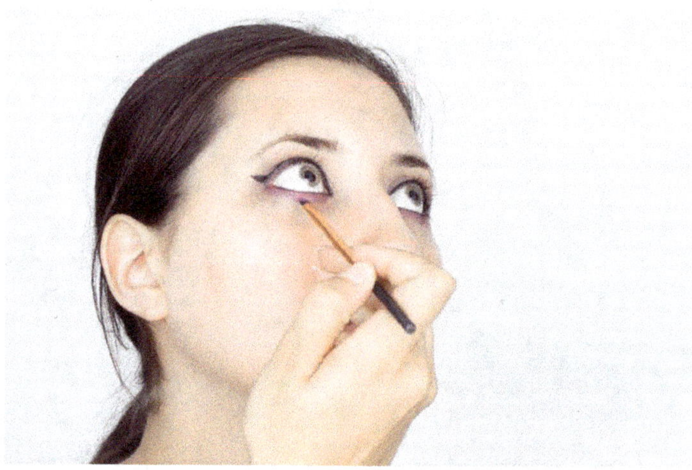

3. Add the purple.

- Take a flat shader brush, or an angled brush, and apply some purple to your lower lash line.
- Start at the outer edge of your eye and stop at the middle portion of your eye.

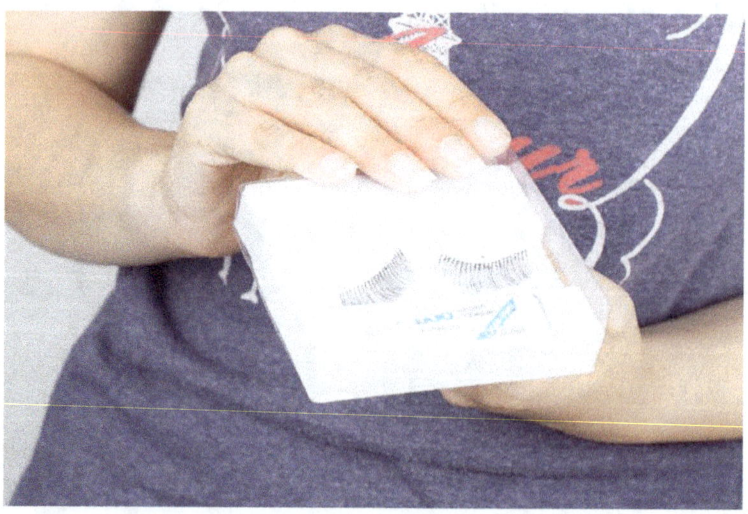

- Take a clean blending brush and blend that out, then re-apply that purple again.
- Repeat this step about three times.

4. Use false lashes. Now, take a set of lashes that looks natural and apply that to both your top and bottom lashes. Finish off with lengthening mascara, or eyelash booster, and you are done.

Part 4

The Finished Look

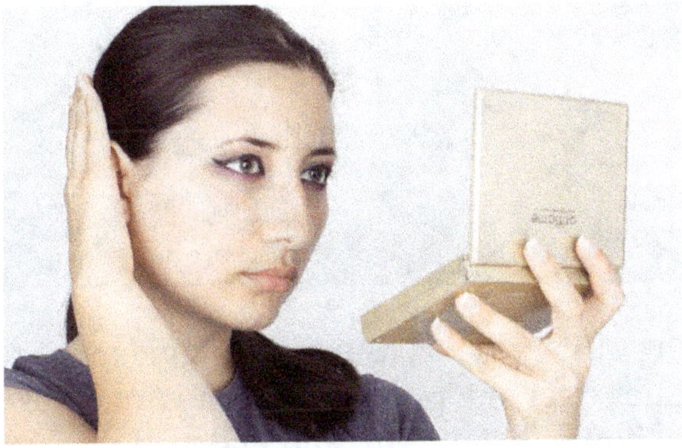

1. Once you are done with the look, it should look like

How to do a Cat Eye on Round Eyes

If you have round eyes (or even if you don't), doing the cat-eye can seem intimidating, especially if you're not very familiar with makeup. If you don't know what the cat-eye is, it's pretty self explanatory, and you've probably seen it done before. It's basically extending the outer corner of the makeup upwards, making your eye appear much like a feline's eye. If you have round cyes, it can seem even more intimidating to do this look. However, round-eyes actually pull off this look perfectly! Read on to learn how to achieve this cool cat look.

Steps

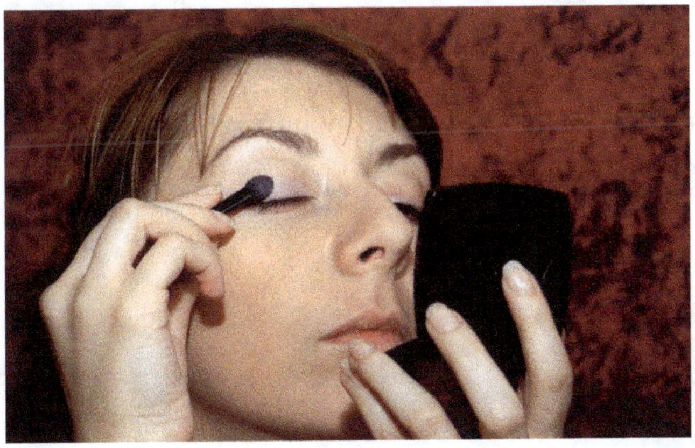

1. Apply your shadow (if desired). This step isn't exactly "necessary", depending on the look you're going for. If you do want shadow, apply it now before your eyeliner. I find that doing this beforehand is easier, but whatever works for you is fine.

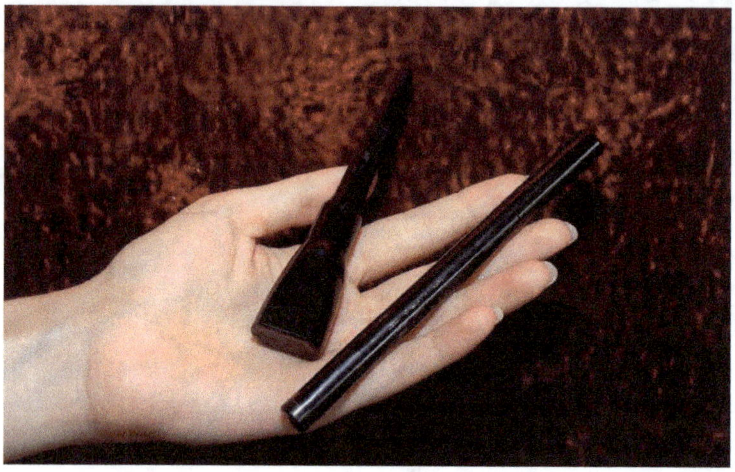

2. Select an eyeliner. For doing a cat-eye look, use a gel or liquid liner. This comes down to personal preference, however, a gel-liner offers more control. There are a huge amount of affordable and awesome liners, both gel and liquid that are $10 and under. If you aren't sure which to use, go to your local drugstore and peruse the makeup section. Or go to Sephora or the makeup section at Macy's. Ask the pros what they would recommend!

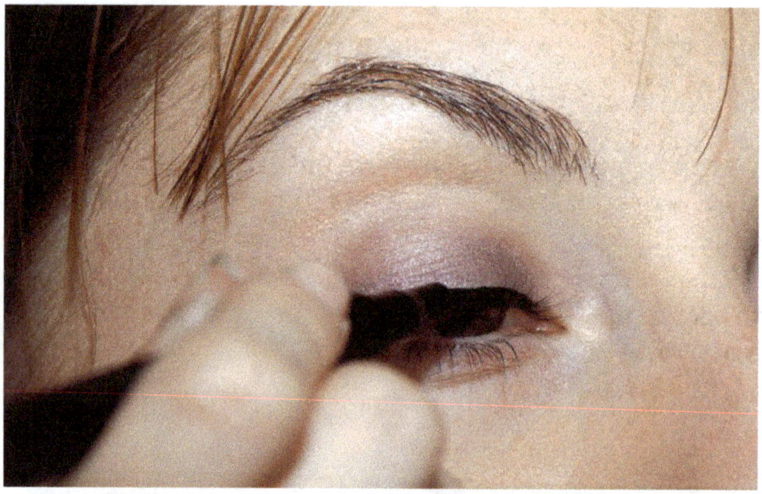

3. Be sure you have the correct tools. This is not necessary if you are using a liquid liner. Most gel-liners come with a small brush. If it did not include a brush, or if the brush is of low-quality, invest in a good liner brush. Sonia Kashuk created a line of makeup brushes that are sold at Target. They're inexpensive and are of great quality. Remember, if you use low-quality products/tools, your makeup will reflect this fact.

- For gel-liner
    - If you chose to go with the gel-liner, take your eyeliner brush and dip it into your gel-liner.

- Evenly coat the tip of the brush. Steady your hand on something. Either sitting down in front of a mirror & resting your elbow on a firm surface, or resting your pinky on your cheek to steady your hand.
- Since the goal of this is to not cause your eye to appear more round, begin applying the eyeliner just after the round peak of your eye.
- Drag the brush close to your lash line, using small, firm strokes. If necessary, re-apply the liner to your brush.
- Create the line to be thicker at the outer corners. Not only is this essential to creating the desired look, it is also vital in reducing the roundness of your eyeball.

- For liquid-liner: Liquid liner is, in a way, easier to apply than gel-liner. It is thinner & easier to create a wing spontaneously with just a small flick. Also, it does not require you to purchase an additional brush or wash the said-brush. It's all-inclusive!
    - Use the same technique as the gel-liner, applying on the outer portion of your eye & using the same wing-technique.
    - However, be careful not to let the liquid liner get on your upper eyelid. Make sure it's dry!

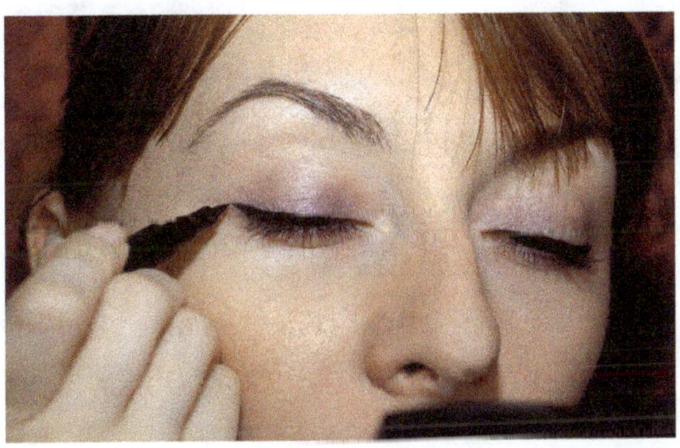

4. Wing it, wing it out, girl. After the outer corner has been thickened, you have reached the defining moment of this makeup look: the wing. Take your brush, and make a small flick up toward the end of your eyebrow. Depending on your personal preference, you can make this as short or as long as you like. It's just important to A) make sure it is even on both eyes and B) make sure it is connected properly to the rest of the eyeliner. Make sure it is free of gaps!

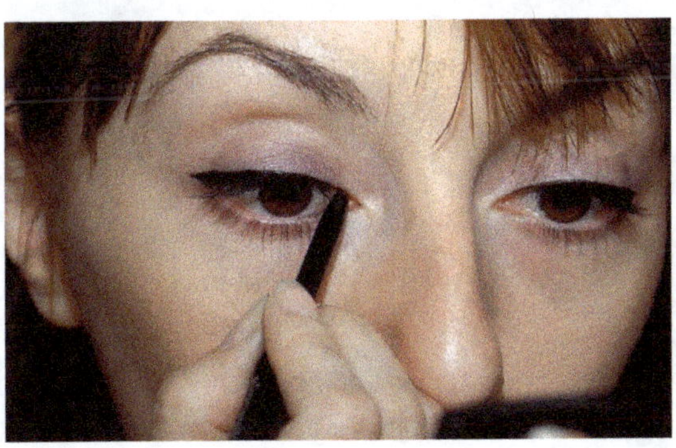

5. Optional; Apply eyeliner to the inner corner. If you have wide-set eyes, I find that this is a good way to reduce that effect. Take your eyeliner (gel, liquid, or pencil-style) and apply it to the upper inside corner of your eye. I wouldn't necessarily apply it to the bottom inside corner, but whatever floats your boat!

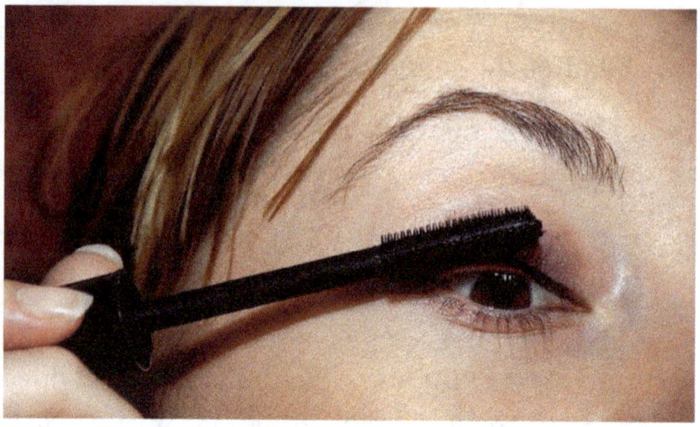

6. Wear Mascara/false-lashes. It just brings an extra level of drama. If you do falsies, cut 'em in half evenly & apply to the outer corner with lash-glue. This gives it an even more feline look by accentuating the outer half of your eye. If you don't want falsies, suit yourself. It still looks cool either way.

How to do a Colorful Smoky Eye Look

A smoky eye is the perfect sultry, attractive look for an evening out. But if you're tired of the usual black, gray, and even brown smoky looks, it may be time to add a little color. Creating a colorful smoky eye is just as simple as creating a neutral one; you just have to choose a bold, fun color to substitute for the black. You can create a traditional smoky eye with your colorful shades or go for a striking halo smoky eye where dark colors sandwich a light shade on the center of your lid. If you're ready to try a bolder eye look, a colorful smoky eye may be for you.

Part 1

Choosing a Color for Your Smoky Eye

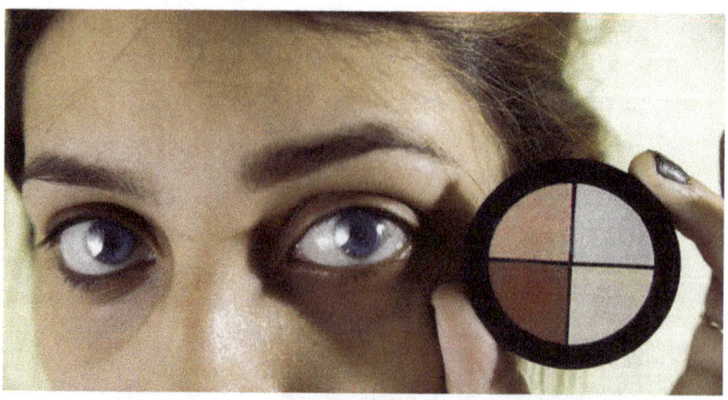

1. Use warm orange shades for blue eyes. When it comes to choosing colored shadows for a smoky look on blue eyes, warm orange shades are usually the most flattering option. Orange is opposite

blue on the color wheel, so orange toned shadows create a bold contrast with blue eyes that really make them pop.

- Some orange tones to consider include burnt orange, copper, coral, amber, rust, pumpkin, and tangerine.

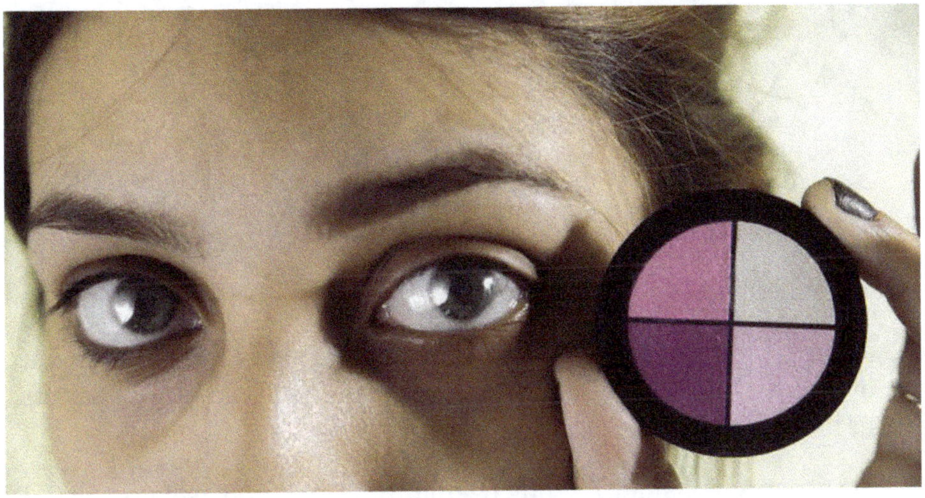

2. Select red and pink shades for green and hazel eyes. For green and hazel eyes, you'll get the most flattering colorful smoky eye if you use cranberry and pink shadows. Red is opposite green on the color wheel so it creates the most striking contrast for eyes that are green or have green flecks.

- Some red and pink tones to consider include cranberry, maroon, wine, brick, dusty rose, mauve, and magenta.

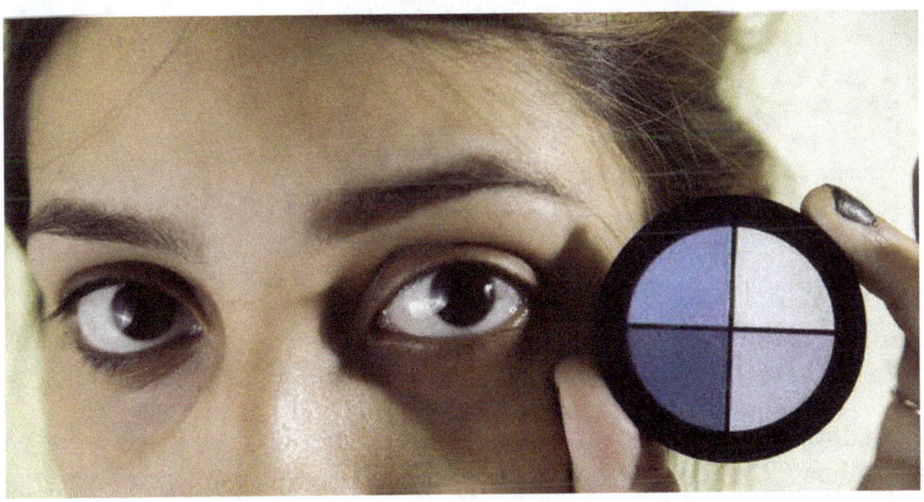

3. Grab blue or green shades for brown eyes. Brown eyes typically feature orange and red undertones, so blue and green shades typically offer the best smoky eye look. That's because orange is opposite blue and red is opposite green on the color wheel.

- Some blue tones to consider include cobalt, navy, teal, violet, and midnight blue.
- Some green tones to consider include olive, forest green, emerald, and moss.

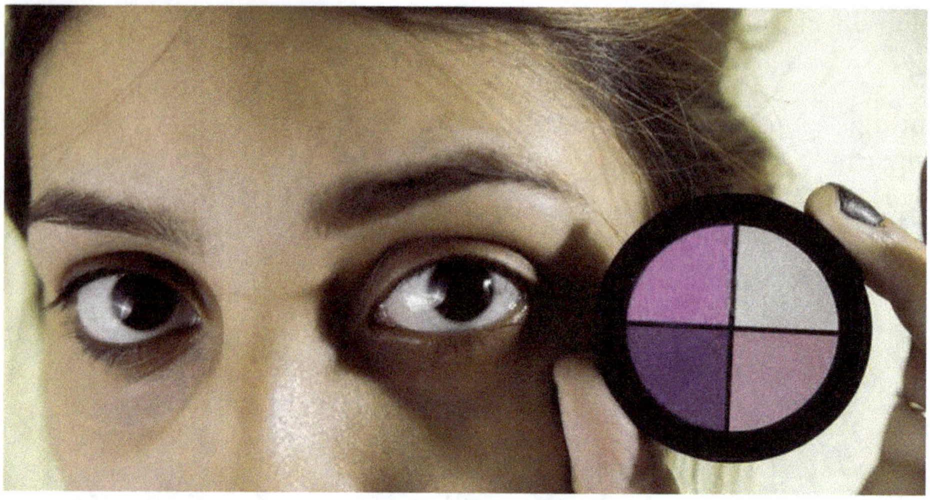

4. Opt for purple shades no matter what your eye color. Purple is the most universally flattering shade of eyeshadow, so it typically works well for everyone. It is especially beautiful with brown and green eyes, but blue-eyed people can wear it too.

- Some purple tones to consider include eggplant, plum, and royal purple.

Part 2

Applying a Traditional Colorful Smoky Eye

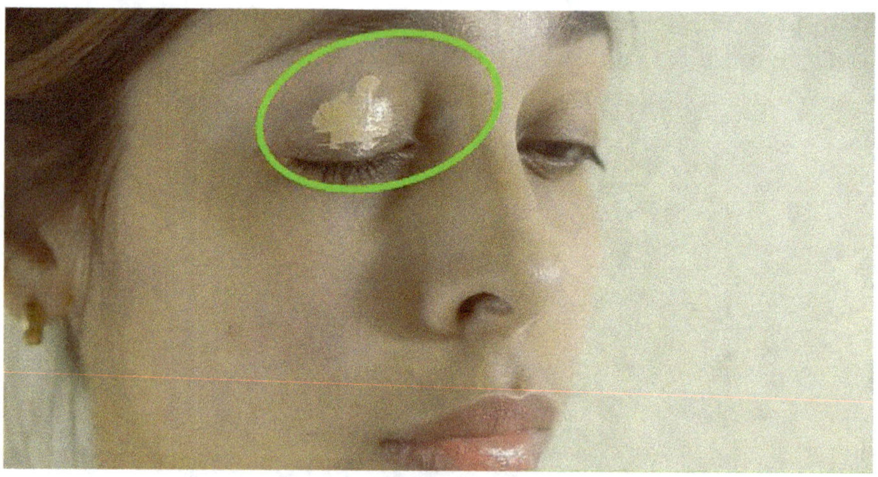

1. Apply an eyeshadow primer or base. An eyeshadow primer provides a base for your shadow to stick to so it lasts all day. Use a clean finger to spread the primer from your lash line to your brow.

- If you don't have an eyeshadow primer, you can substitute concealer. Smooth it over your eyelid just as you would with primer.
- If you have dark skin or just want to make sure that your colorful smoky eye is as vibrant as possible, it helps to use a white base as your primer. Blend a white cream eyeshadow over your eyelid so the colors that you place on top of it really pop.

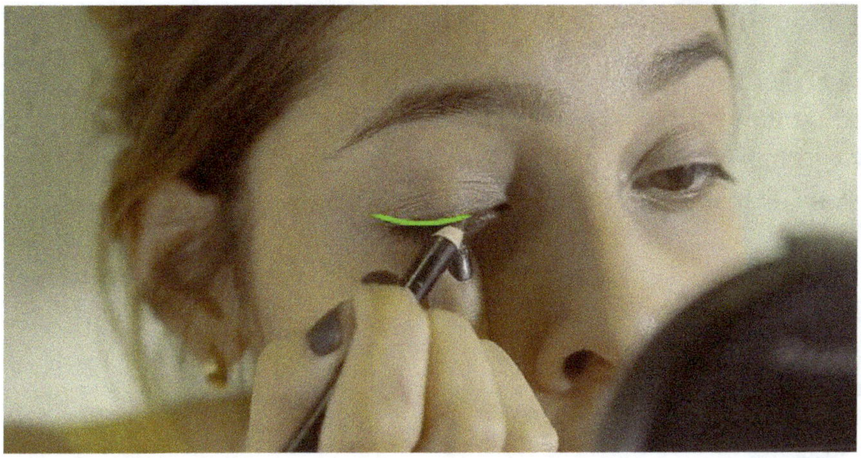

2. Smudge dark eyeliner along your upper and lower lash lines. To get the classic smoky look, you need to li your upper and lower lash lines with a creamy eyeliner pencil. After you've applied the liner, use a pencil brush or cotton swab to softly smudge it. Black liner is traditionally used for a smoky eye, but you can also use a dark liner that coordinates with your shadows.

- If you're doing a blue smoky eye, you can substitute a navy eyeliner.
- If you're doing a green smoky eye, you can substitute a forest green eyeliner.
- If you're doing a orange smoky eye, you can substitute a bronze or warm brown eyeliner.
- If you're doing a purple smoky eye, you can substitute a plum eyeliner.
- If you're doing a red or pink smoky eye, you can substitute a reddish brown eyeliner.
- Like black, a charcoal gray eyeliner can also work with any colorful smoky eye.

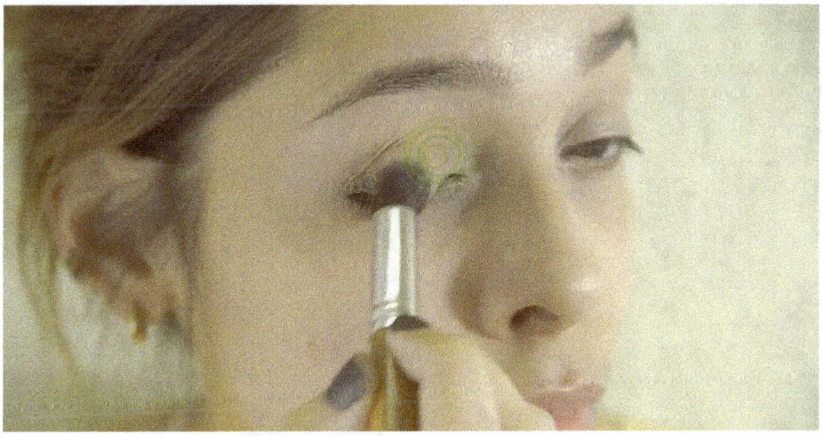

3. Sweep a neutral shadow through the crease. To help the colorful shadows you use in your smoky blend more easily, you want to use a subtle transition color in the crease. Use a fluffy crease brush to softly blend a neutral eyeshadow that's two or three shades deeper than your skin tone through your crease.

- The crease of your eye is the area above the lid where your eye naturally folds.

- A brown or tan shade is usually the best option for a transition shade.
- If you're worried about your smoky eye looking too stark, you may want to use a transition shade with some warmth. Your bronzer can do double-duty as your transition shade if that's the case.

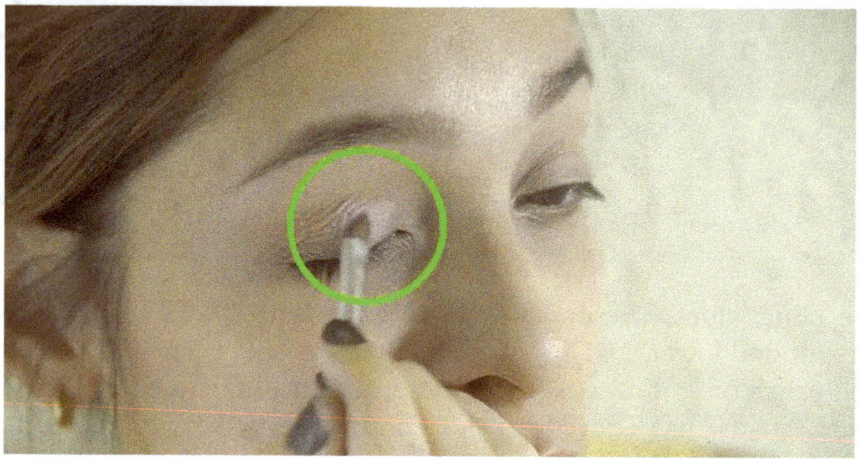

4. Press a mid-tone colorful shadow onto the lid. After you've added the transition shade to your crease, use a flat eyeshadow brush to apply a mid-tone shadow in your choice of color to your lid. Use a pressing motion to apply the shadow to avoid fallout, and be sure to smooth the shadow over the eyeliner that you've applied.

- A mid-tone shade basically means a shadow that falls between light and dark shades on the color spectrum. You don't want to use the darkest colorful shade that you have on the lid, but the shadow should be darker than your usual lid colors.
- Use a clean fluffy brush to blend the edge of your lid color into the transition shade for a seamless look.

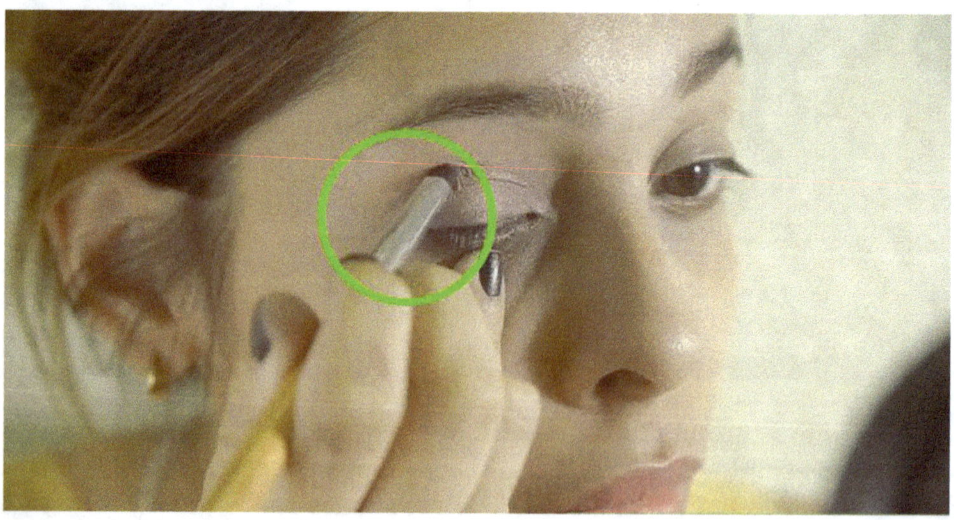

5. Deepen the outer corner of the eye with a dark colorful shadow. To add depth to your smoky eye, use a pencil brush to apply a dark colored eyeshadow that coordinates with your lid color to the

outer corner of your eye. Make a sideways "V" shape so one line is angled down toward the lash line and one line is angled up toward the outside of the crease.

- Make sure to blend out the shadow that you add to the outer corner with a clean, fluffy brush so there aren't any harsh lines.
- When it comes to choosing a dark shade to use in the outer corner, opt for the same color family as your lid shade. For example, if you've used a emerald green on the lid, you might use a forest green in the outer corner.
- If you don't have a dark shadow that coordinates with the color that you've chosen for your smoky eye, you can substitute black.

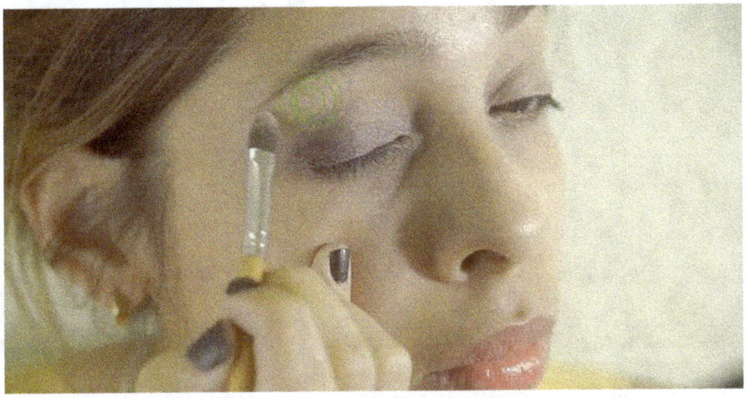

6. Highlight your brow bone and inner corner. To keep your smoky eye from looking too dark, it's important to use a light shadow to highlight your brown bone and inner corner. Sweep a light shade, such as ivory, cream, beige, or tan, beneath your brow with a small, fluffy brush, blending it into the transition. Use a small detail brush to dab a small amount of the same shadow to the inner corner around the tear duct.

- You can use a matte or shimmery shadow to highlight your brow bone and inner corner. However, with a smoky eye, it's especially flattering to use a shimmery shade for the inner corner because it will reflect the light so your eyes appear brighter.

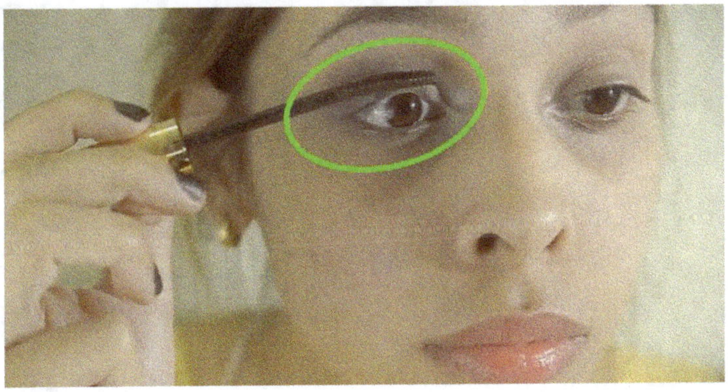

7. Coat your lashes with mascara. With dark shadow on your eyes, it's easy for your lashes to get lost. Finish off your look with one to three coats of your favorite mascara to help them stand out against the colorful smoky shadow.

- To really open up your eyes with smoky shadow, it's a good idea to use an eyelash curler to curl your lashes before you apply the mascara.
- Make sure to apply some mascara to your lower lashes too. They'll have trouble standing out against the dark liner that you've smudged there.

Part 3

Creating a Colorful Halo Smoky Eye

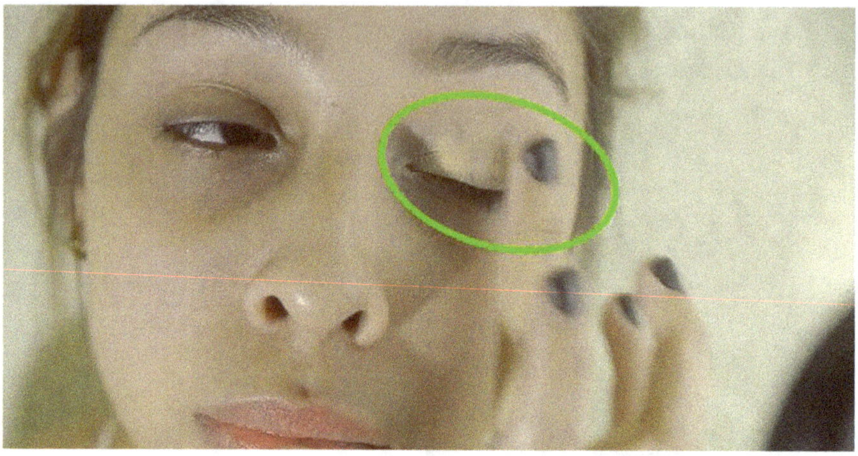

1. Smooth on an eyeshadow primer. To keep your colorful smoky shadows in place all day, you must start with an eyeshadow primer. Dab a small amount of primer onto each eyelid, and blend it up through the crease.

- It's a good idea to rub whatever primer is left on your finger along your lower lash line, so the colors that you apply there will stay in place.

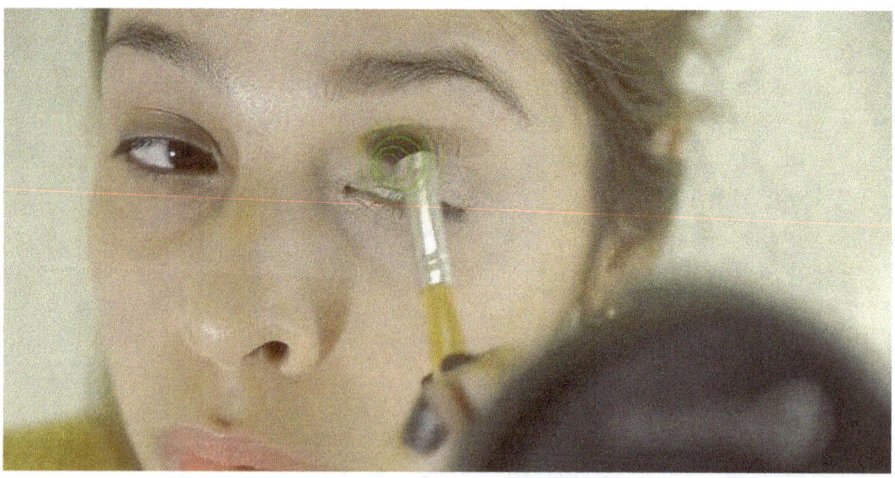

2. Blend a neutral transition shadow through the crease. Just as with a classic smoky eye, you want to apply a transition shade to the crease to make it easier to blend the colors out. However, because you want all the attention on the colors on your lid, choose a light neutral shadow that's only a shade or two darker than your skin tone. Sweep it through the crease with a fluffy crease brush.

- Make sure to blend the transition shade well after you apply it so it has a soft look.

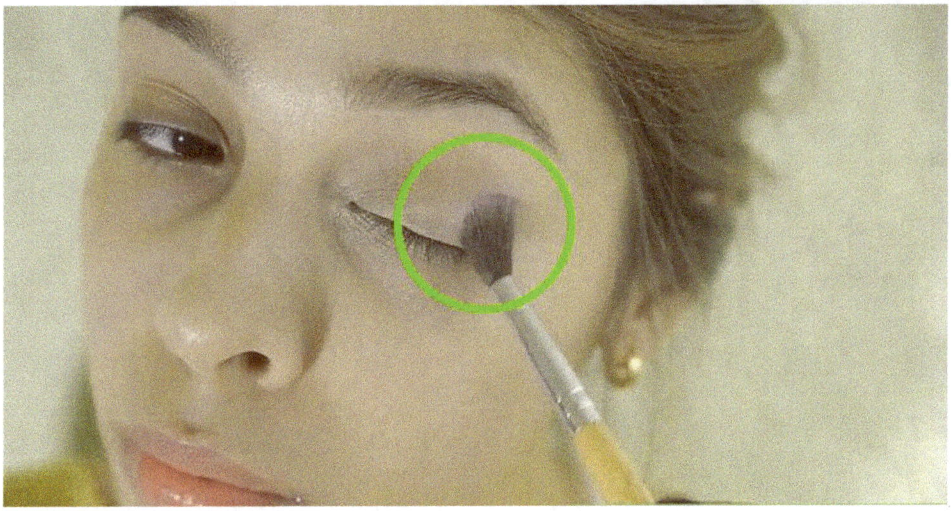

3. Apply a mid-tone colorful shadow to the inner and outer corners. With your transition shade in place, use a small fluffy shadow brush to apply a mid-tone shadow in the color family that you've chosen to the inner third and the outer third of your lid. Blend the shadow slightly into the crease above the respective areas.

- Be sure to leave the center of your lid and crease free of eyeshadow.

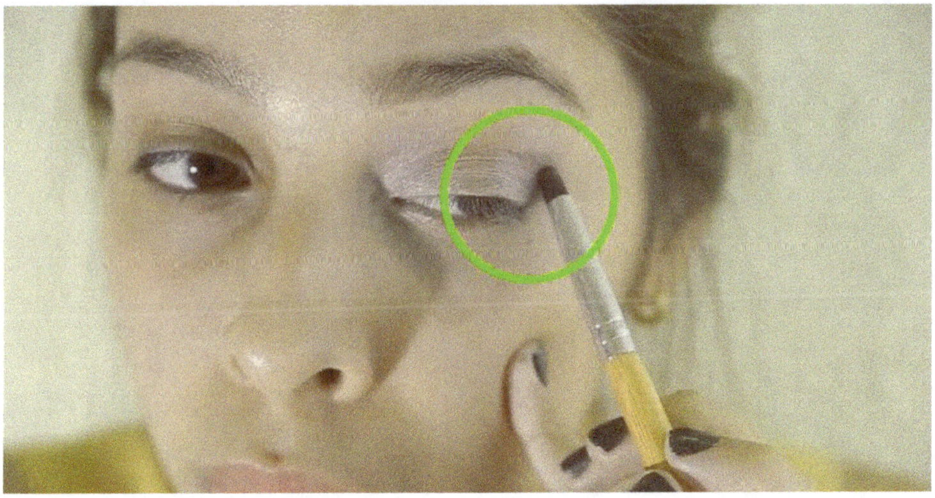

4. Darken the inner and outer corners with black shadow. With a small, tapered blending brush, apply a small amount of black shadow over the colored shadow in the inner and outer corners of your lid and crease. You shouldn't cover the colorful shadow completely; concentrate the black in outer edges of both areas.

- You don't necessarily have to use black shadow for darkening up your eyes. Instead, use a dark shadow from the same color family as the colored shadow you've used. For example, if you've used a royal blue in the inner and outer corners, darken them up with a navy blue shadow.

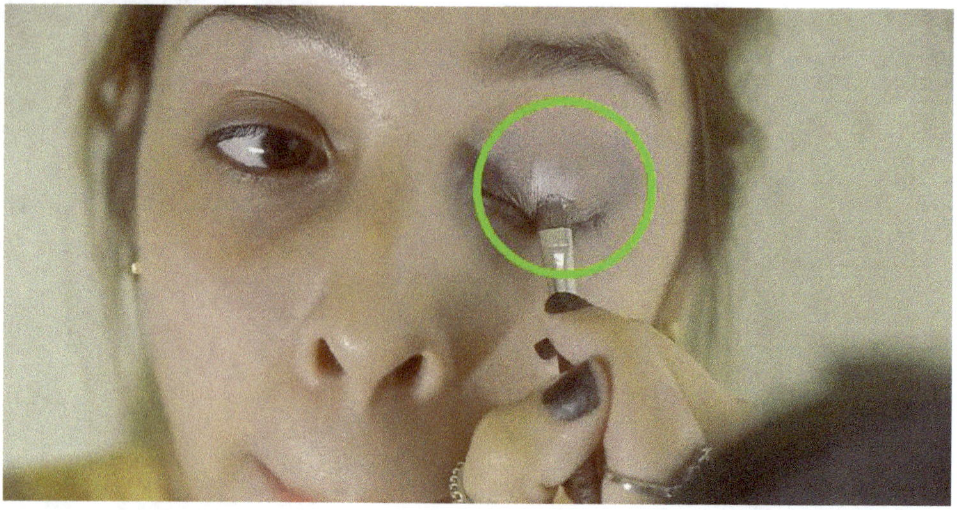

5. Press a light colored shadow to the center of the lid. After you've darkened up the inner and outer corners, use a flat shadow brush to apply light shade from your chosen color family to the center of the lid. A shimmery or metallic shadow is the best option because it will stand out even more.

- If you want to be sure that the lighter shadow really stands out, you can dab a small amount of a white cream shadow over the center of your lid before applying the shadow.
- Use a small fluffy brush to blend the lines between the dark and light colors so the shadow looks soft and smoky.

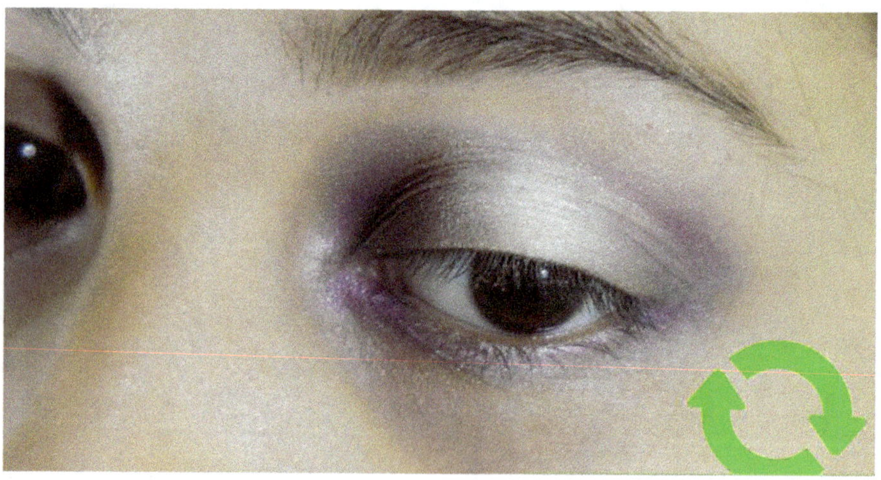

6. Repeat the steps on your bottom lashline. With the shadow done on your lid, apply shadow to your lower lashline in the same manner. Use a pencil brush to apply the mid tone shade to the inner and outer corners, a darker shadow on just the outermost corners, and the light shade in the middle.

- You can repeat the same process on your waterline, the bit of skin on your lower lid above your lashes, by using a light pencil liner in the center and a dark pencil liner on the outer and inner corners. However, you can also use a dark liner across the entire waterline or skip liner there completely.

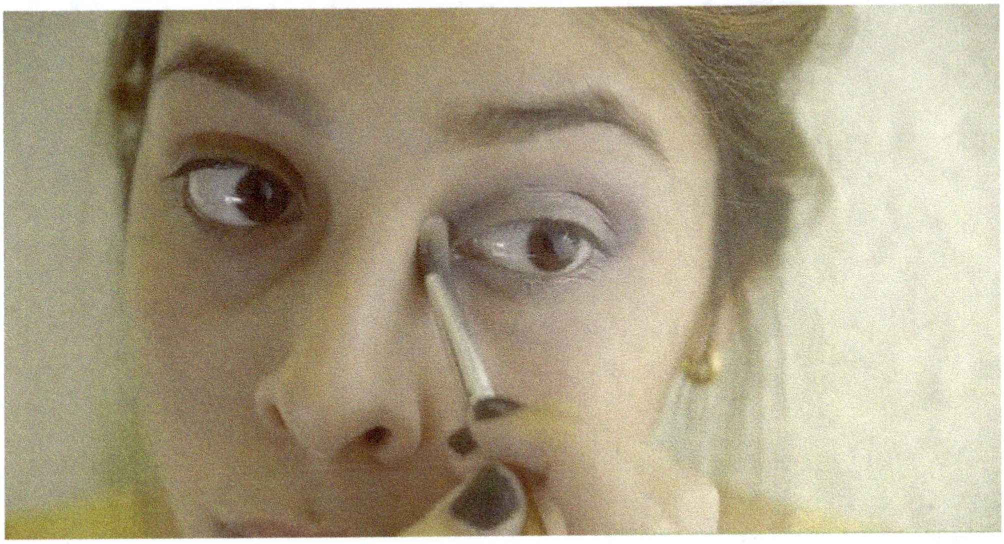

7. Highlight the inner corner. To ensure that your eyes look bright even with a dark color on your inner corners, it's especially important to highlight that area. Use a small detail brush to trace the area around your tear duct with a light, shimmery shadow.

- Depending on how light the shadow you used on the center of your lid is, you may want to use it to highlight the inner corner. Otherwise, use an ivory, cream, beige, or pale gold shadow.

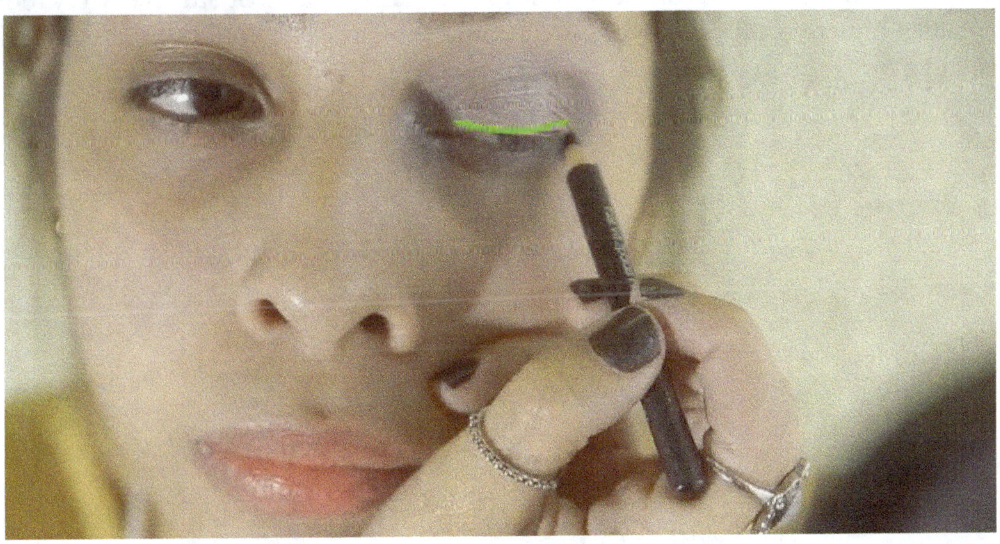

8. Smudge dark liner along your upper lash line. Once your eyeshadow is finished, use a dark eyeliner pencil to line your upper lashline. Smudge the liner with a pencil brush or cotton swab to keep the look smoky.

- You can use a black liner or a dark liner that coordinates with the colorful eyeshadows that you've used.
- The liner is an optional step. You can skip it completely if you prefer.

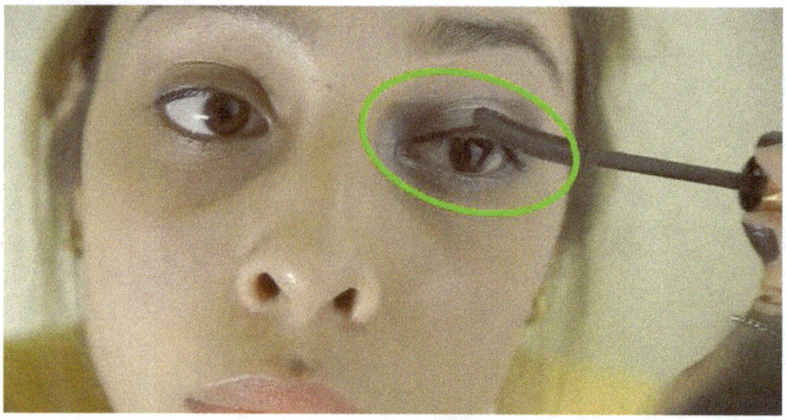

9. Add several coats of mascara to your lashes. To finish off your look, apply two to three coats of your favorite mascara to help your lashes stand out. Brush through your lashes with a lash comb to ensure that they are no clumps.

- If you like, you can also add some false lashes to really make your eyes look fluttery.

How to do Black Eye Makeup

Black eye makeup is timeless, and can be used for nearly any style, from an everyday look to a deep smokey eye. Learn how to easily achieve some popular eye makeup looks, as well as how to create a fake bruised eye for stage makeup!

Method 1

Achieving a Smoky Eye Look

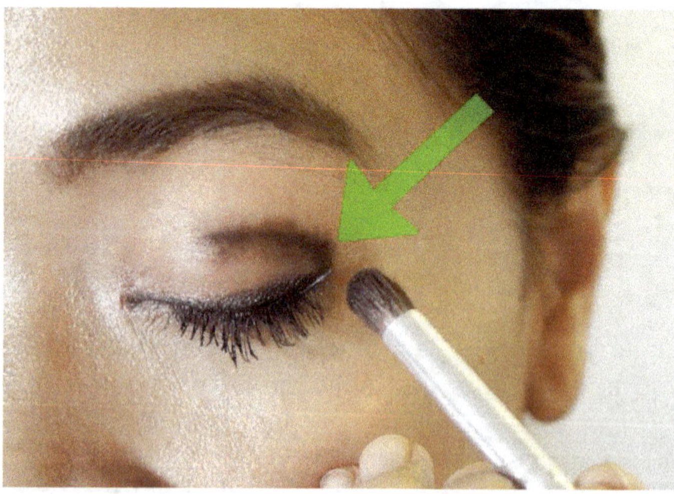

1. Apply your darkest eyeshadow to the outside corner. Take the darkest color eyeshadow you want to use (black or dark gray) and swipe it on in an arch shape just above the crease of your eyelid, from the outside corner to the middle of the eyelid. Then apply it right along the lash line.

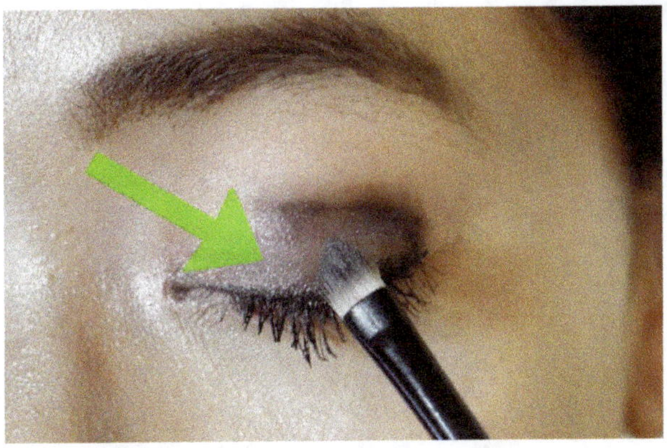

2. Put a lighter shade of eyeshadow in the middle of your eyelid. Apply a slightly lighter gray color to the middle of the eyelid, and blend it in with the darker color in the corner using a small soft brush.

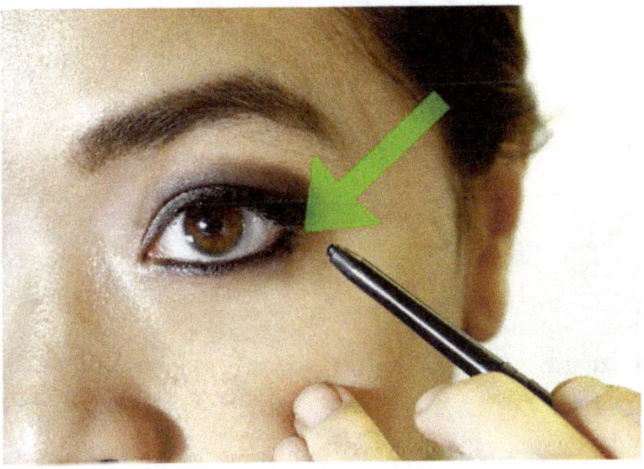

3. Line your top and bottom lashes. Use a black eyeliner pencil to carefully line your top lashes, drawing from the inner corner to a point at the outer corner, staying as close to the lash line as possible. Then do the same to the bottom lash line and your waterline (the side of your bottom lashes closest to your eyeball) by pulling your undereye skin down slightly.

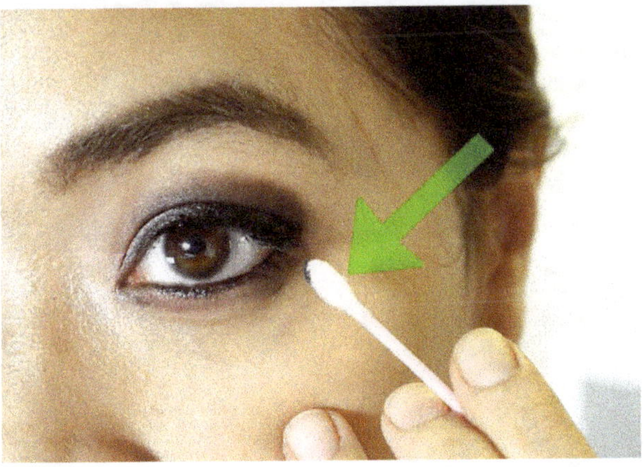

- Use a gel or liquid liner for your upper lash line if you like, but only use pencil on your waterline, because liquid liner will easily transfer to your eyeball from your waterline and irritate your eye.

4. Smudge the bottom liner. Use a smudge brush, q-tip, or your fingertip to gently smudge the liner on your bottom lashes, creating that signature hazy, smokey look. You can smudge the top liner too if you wish.

- If you want more color below your eye, you can also dab on a gray eyeshadow with a firm-bristled brush just below the liner.

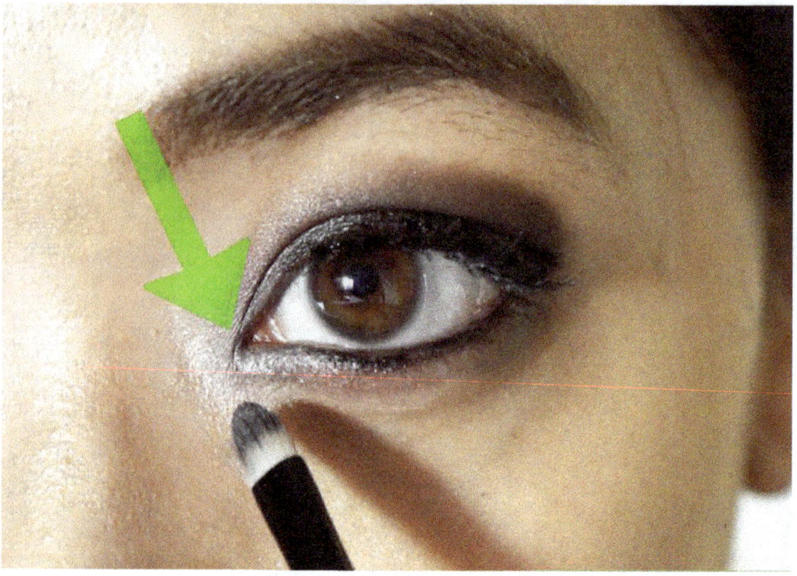

5. Apply a light color to the inner corner. Use a light silver, cream, or shimmery white eyeshadow or a highlighter pencil in the inner corner of your eye. Blend if needed to create an even and gradual change from light to dark across your eyelids.

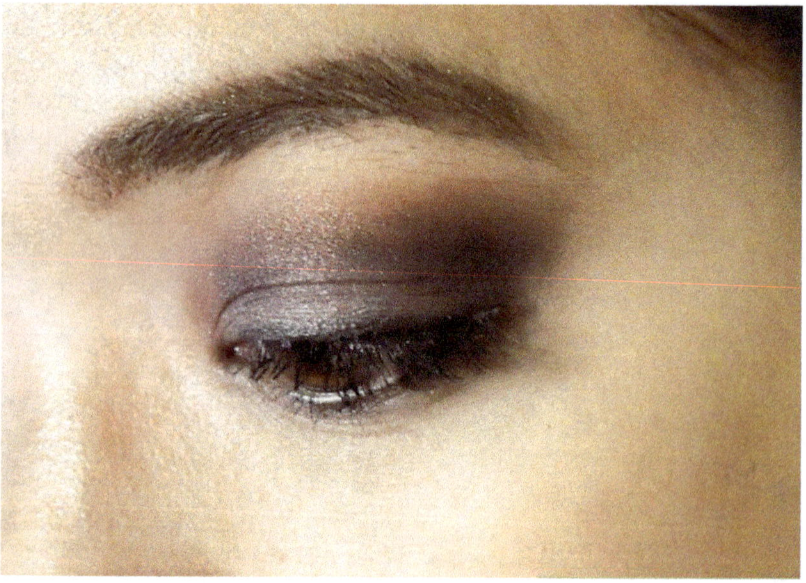

6. Brush on plenty of mascara. Get a black volumizing and lengthening mascara and apply it liberally to your top and bottom lashes, pulling the brush out from base to tip in a repeated motion.

Method 2

Getting the Perfect Cat Eye

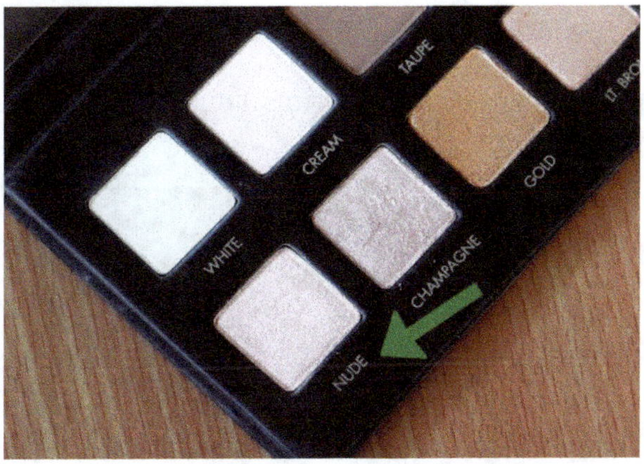

1. Choose a light or nude eyeshadow. Blend a light eyeshadow color across your eyelids to provide contrast for the cat eye. You can use a slightly darker shade to brush into the outside corner and crease if you wish.

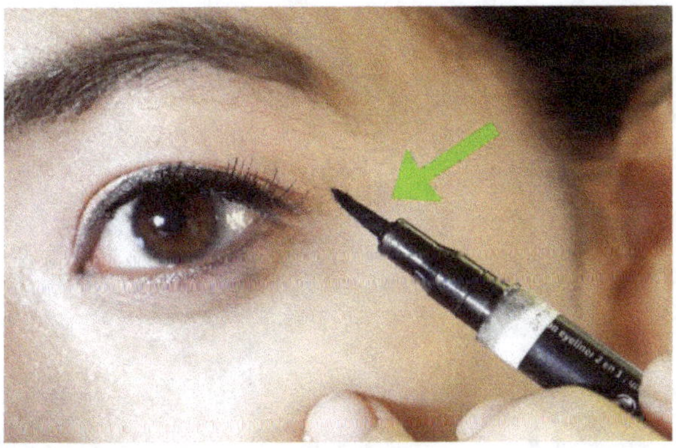

2 Use a black eyeliner for your top lash line. Make small strokes of eyeliner across your top lash line until you have a straight, even line. Start at the inner corner or just outside it, and increase the thickness of the line as you draw further out toward the outside corner.

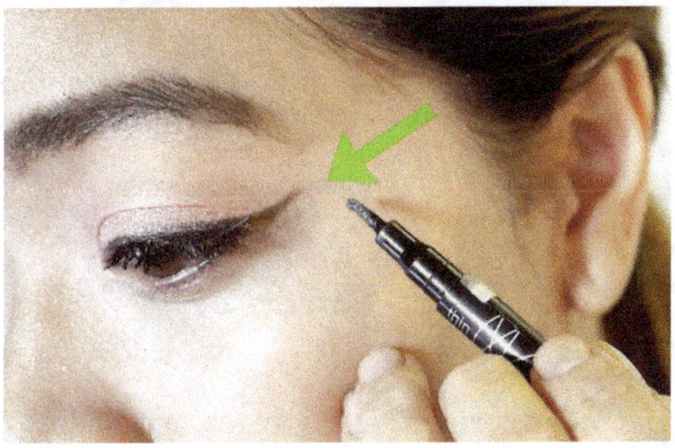

3. Achieve the signature wing tip. Draw a thin line of eyeliner from the outside of your bottom lash

line into a fine point past your eyelid, up and out as far as you like in the direction of the end of your eyebrow. Then draw a line that smoothly connects the liner on your eyelid to this point, creating an unfilled triangle. Fill in this triangle with liner to finish.

- You can use a piece of clear tape or the curve of a spoon to help guide the shape of the wing.
- Liquid or gel eyeliner works best for creating a sharp, clean line, but you can use a pencil eyeliner if if has a sharp point.

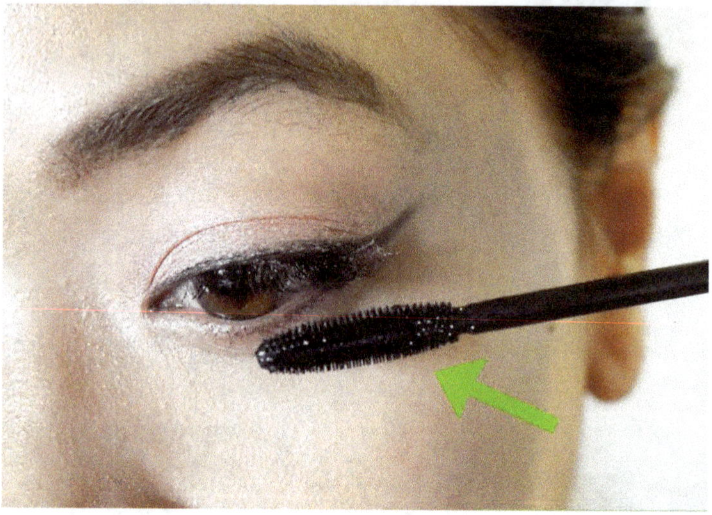

4. Add mascara. Brush on several coats of a black lengthening mascara to complete the look.

Method 3

Pairing Black with Other Colors

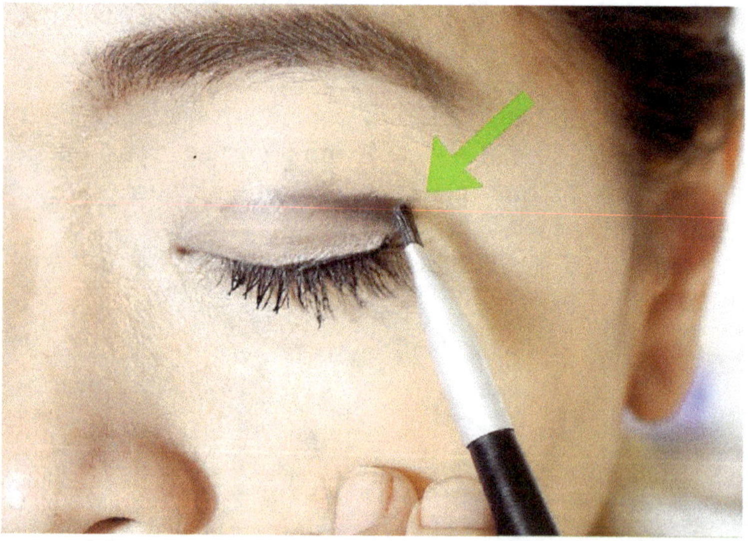

1. Use black eyeshadow in the outer corners. Apply black eyeshadow to the outer corner of your eye, sweeping it up in an arc just above the crease line and down across your lash line.

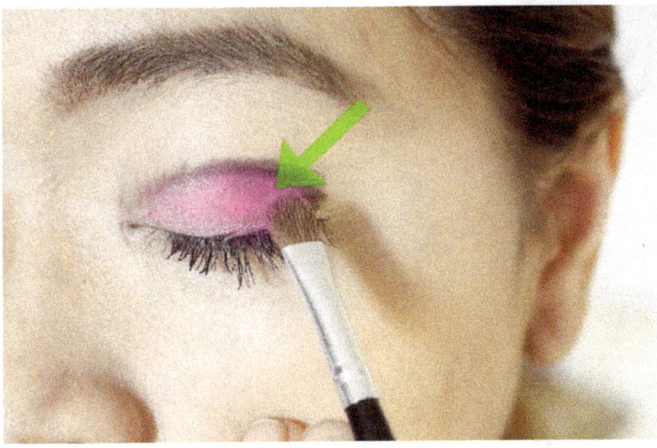

2. Add color to the eyelid. Add a vibrant color of shadow like purple or blue to the eyelid, with a darker shade closer to your black shadow and a lighter shade closer to the inside corner. Then blend the lighter shade, darker shade, and black together with a soft brush to create an even gradient just like a normal smokey eye.

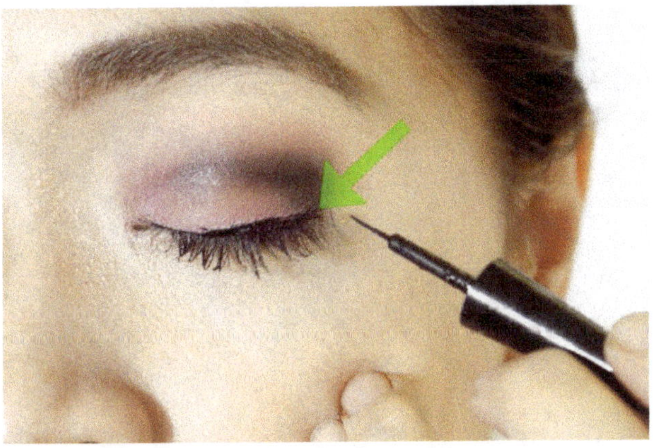

3. Apply black eyeliner. Use a pencil, gel, or liquid black eyeliner to draw an even line across your top lash line, from inside corner to outside corner, staying as close to the lash line as possible. You can line the bottom lash line in the same way if you like.

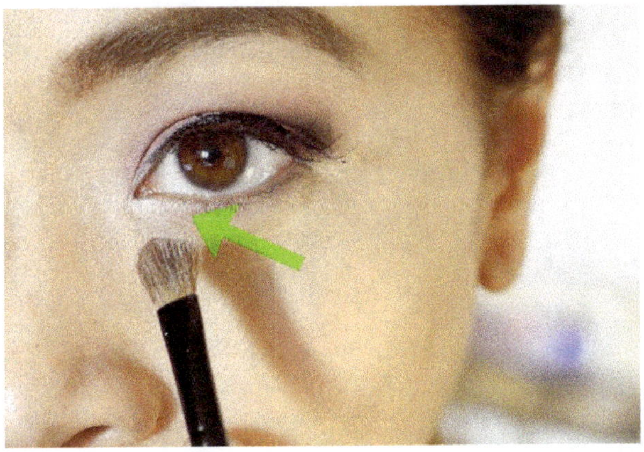

4. Highlight the inside corner. Use a light or white eyeshadow or highlighter in the inner corner of

your eyes to complete the gradient. You can also use the same or a lighter shade of the color you have on your inner lid for the corner.

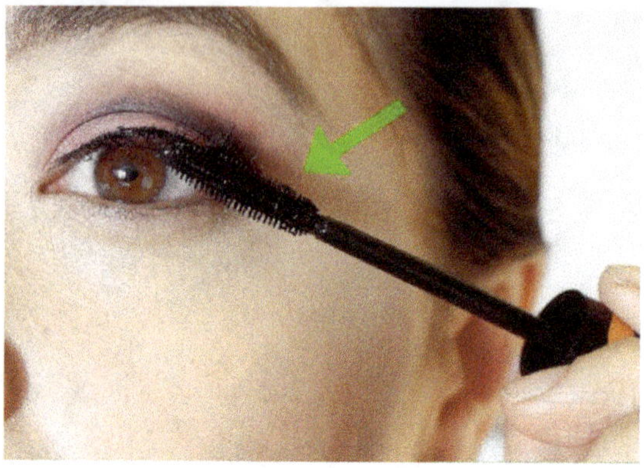

5. Finish with black mascara. Apply mascara by sweeping the brush from roots to tip, repeating several times.

Method 4

Creating a Black (Bruised) Eye

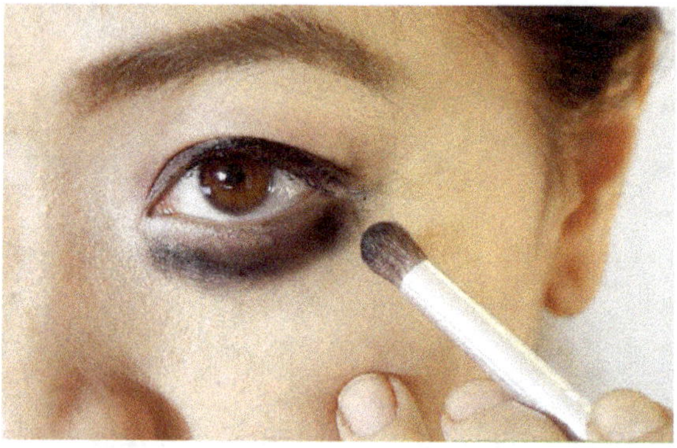

1. Line your eyes with black. Use an eyeliner pencil or black eyeshadow and a brush to create a thick line on the top and bottom of your eye. Smudge it with your finger, a smudge brush, or a q-tip.

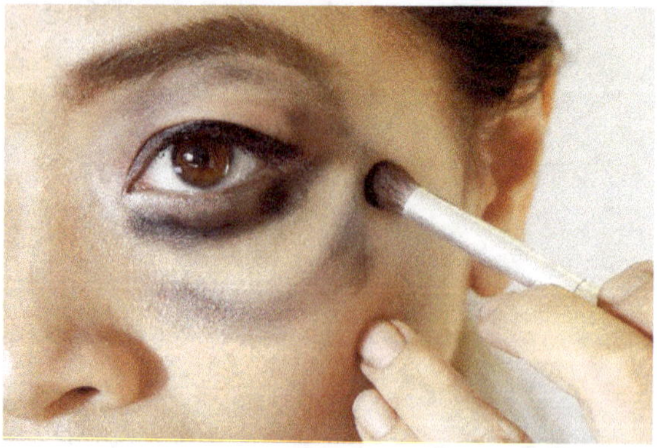

- Don't worry about lining your eyes carefully or smudging evenly. In this case, the messier it looks, the better!

2. Add black to your bottom socket, brow, and nose. Apply the same black eyeliner or eyeshadow from the inner corner of your eye down toward your cheek, following the curve of your eye socket. Smudge it, then use the extra on your finger, smudge brush, or q-tip to add a little smudge to the side of your nose and the outside of your eyebrow.

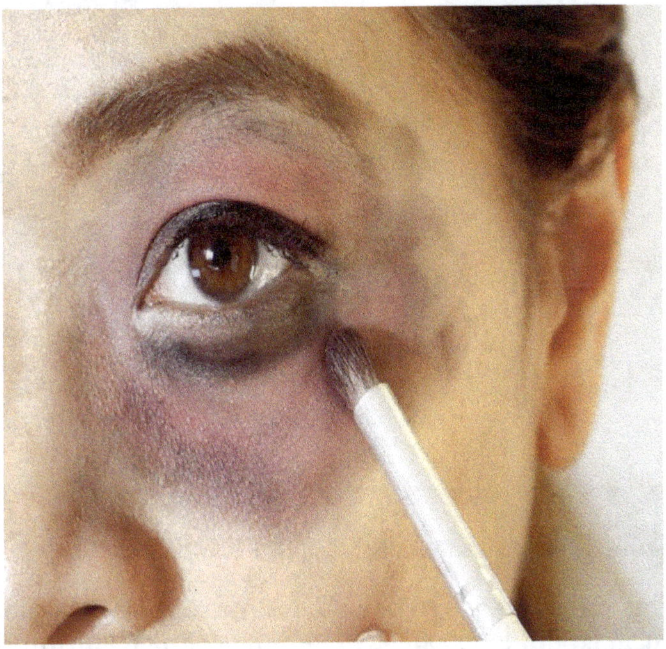

3. Add bruise colors. Use a dark burgundy eyeshadow in an arc just above the eyelid crease and extend it past the outside corner of your eye to your temple. Then use the same burgundy to go over the bottom socket curve that you lined with black before. Use a blood-red eyeshadow along your bottom lashes and blend it downward. Smudge all of the color together to make it look more natural.

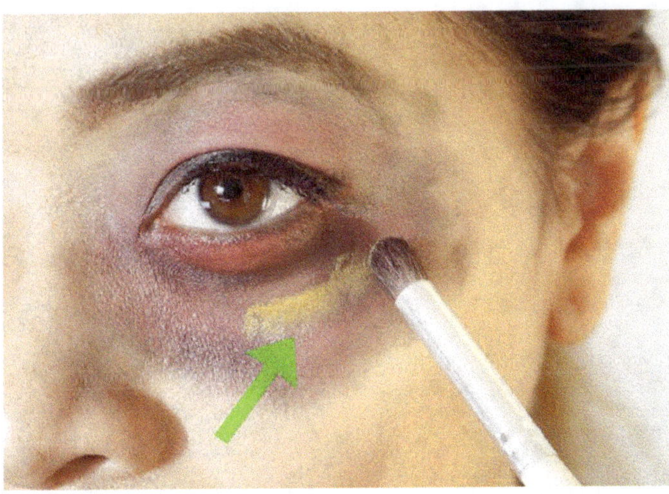

4. Finish with yellow. Add a light yellow eyeshadow wherever you want to create the appearance of swelling, for example: between your lower lash line and your lower socket makeup, above your eyebrow, or below the lower socket on your cheekbone.

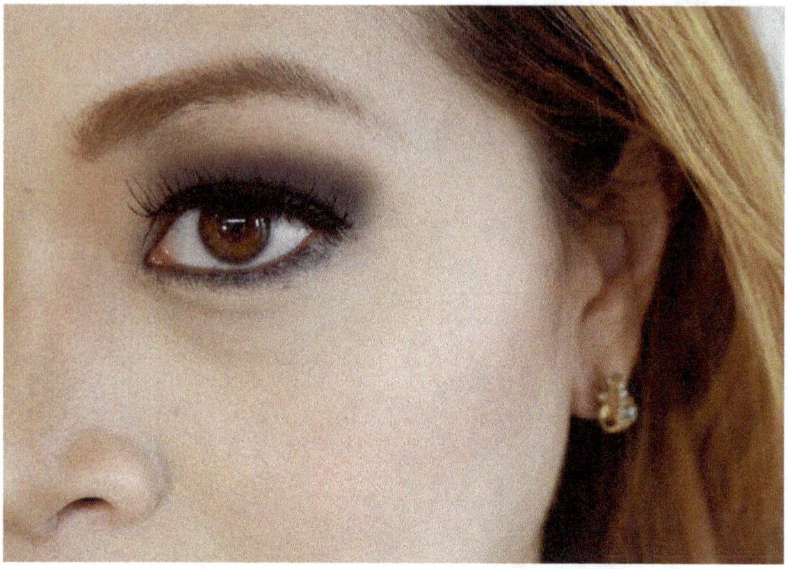

How to do Eye Makeup for Blue Eyes

Blue eyes are tranquilizing and gorgeous to behold, but the wrong makeup can make them appear dull and faded. The right makeup, however, will enhance your beautiful blue eyes, making them appear brighter. Use this article to learn how to bring out the blues in your eyes and make them appear brighter.

Part 1

Using the Right Eyeshadow Color

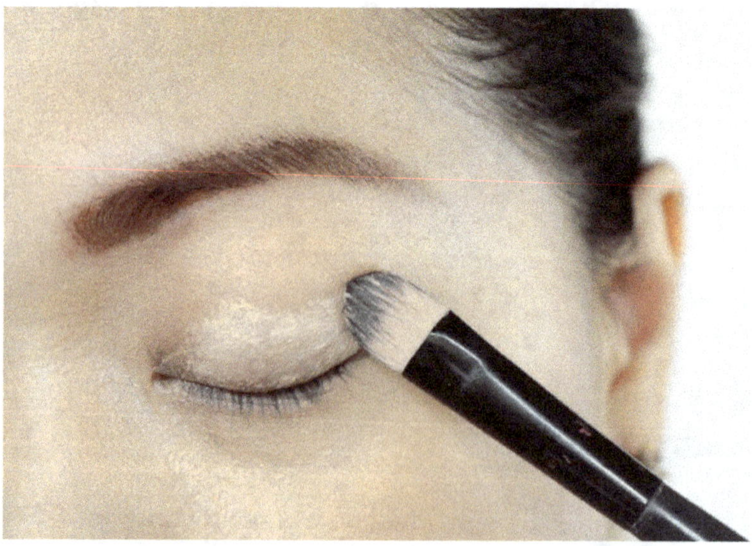

1. Use eyeshadow primer under your eyeshadow. This will help enhance the color of your eyeshadow, making it appear brighter, which in turn will also make your eyes appear brighter.

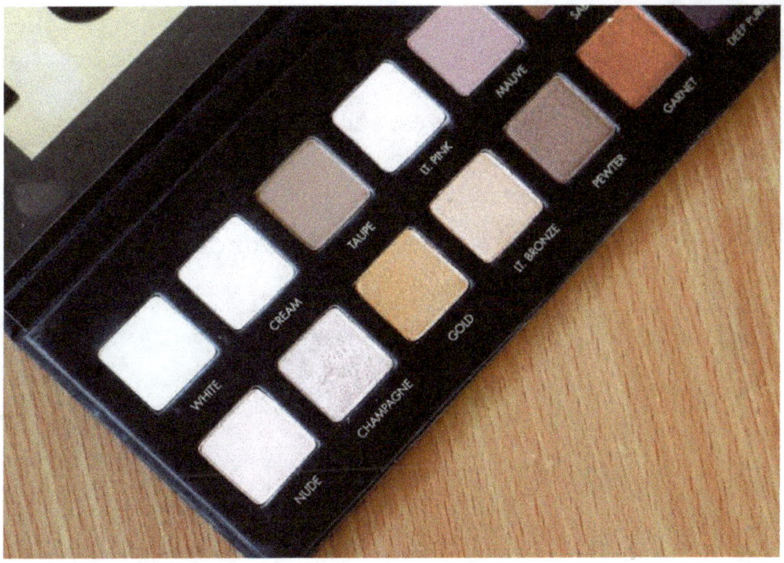

2. Choose eyeshadow with contrasting colors. One of the best ways to bring out the blue in your eyes is to use contrasting colors. This means choosing eyeshadows in neutral and earth tones, warm colors, and colors opposite of blue and green on the color wheel. Here are some suggestions:

- For neutral and earth tones, use beige, camel, sable, sienna, tan, taupe, terracotta, and warm brown.
- For opposite colors, use red, orange, gold, copper, and bronze.
- For warm colors, use pastel orange, rose, and light pink. You can also use a warm purple with red undertones, such as plum.

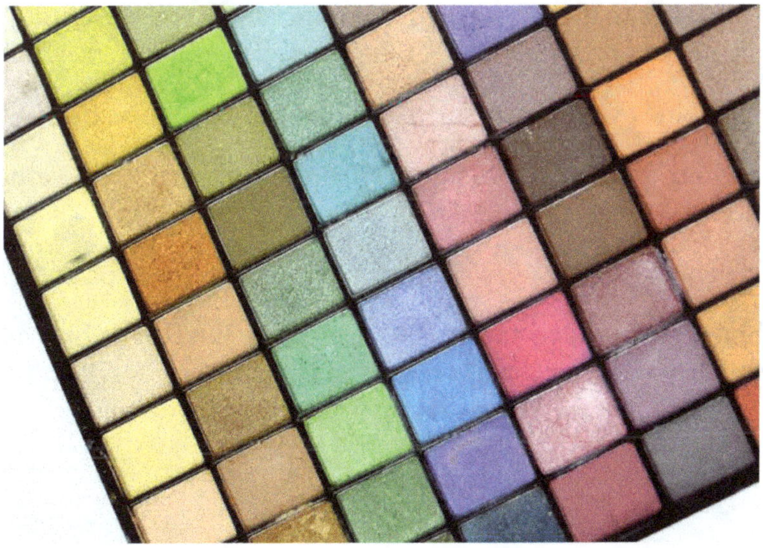

3. Consider using cool colors. You can also use cool-colored eyeshadow, such as blues, greens, and purples. Purple eyes shadow pairs great with blue eyes, while blue should be used with care. If you have flecks of green in your eyes, you can use green eyeshadow to bring those flecks out. Here are some suggestions:

- You can get away with wearing blue-colored eyeshadow, so long as the blue is darker than your eye color, such as navy or midnight blue. Be sure not to overdo the blue eyeshadow.
- Wear greens to bring out blue-green eyes, such as turquoise.
- Wear purples, such as dark purple, heather, lavender, lilac, or plum.
- You can also wear ash, black, charcoal, silver, slate, or dark grey.

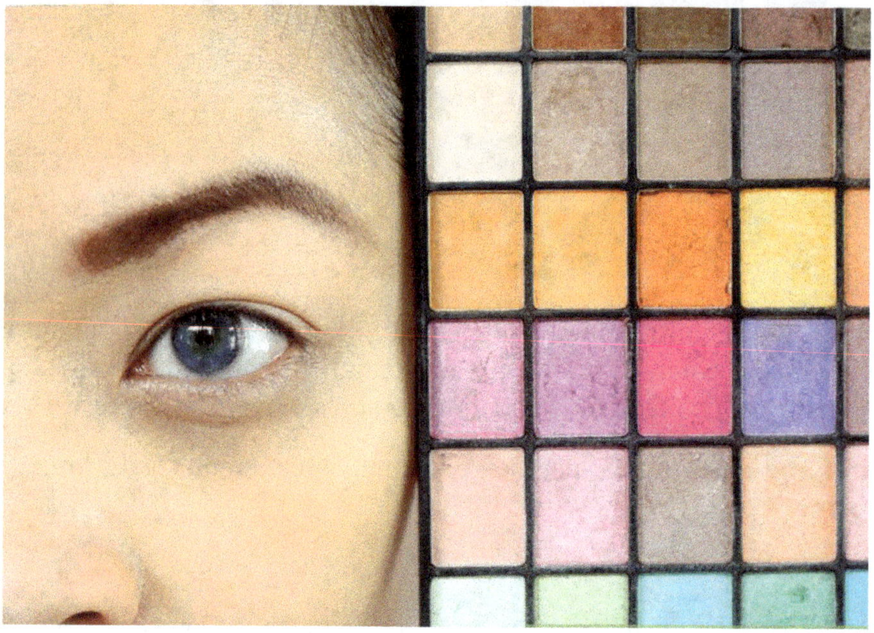

4. Know what color eyeshadow works suits light, medium, and dark blue eyes. There are different shades of blue when it comes to eyes, ranging from dark blue to blue green to blue-grey. Here are some color suggestions, based on the shade of blue your eyes might be:

- If you have light-blue eyes, wear neutral browns and orange or bronze tones.
- If you have medium-blue eyes, consider going for blacks, browns, camel, charcoal, copper, heather, or moss.
- If you have dark or deep blue eyes, use light, nude browns, or pastel oranges
- If you have blue-gray eyes, go for warmer tones, such orangey browns, copper, coral and khaki. You can also wear darker blues, such as teal and midnight blue, and grays, such as charcoal and silver. Lilac will also work well with blue-gray eyes.
- If you have blue-green eyes, use warm colors, such as bronzes, oranges, reds, terracotta, and sienna.
- If you have bright blue eyes, use lighter colors, such as ash, camel, gold, gray, sable, or taupe.
- Purple works well for all types of blue eyes.

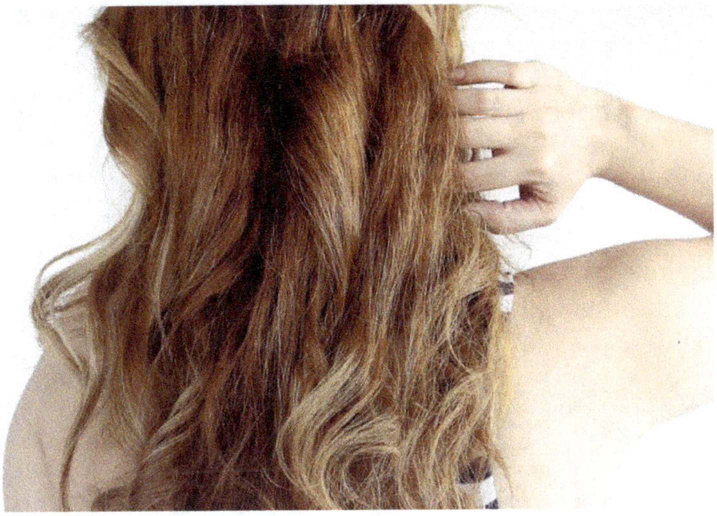

5. Match the eyeshadow color to your hair color and skin tone. Certain colors look better against certain skin tones and hair colors. If you are having difficulties choosing an eyeshadow color, then try to work with your skin tone and hair color instead. Here are some suggestions based on skin tone and hair color:

- If you have fair skin and blonde hair:, consider wearing rich browns, warm pinks, or plums. Pair your eyeshadow with some brown eyeliner and lots of mascara.
- If you have fair skin and dark hair, go for golds and brighter pinks. Pair your eyeshadow with a darker eyeliner and some lengthening mascara.
- If you have red hair, consider wearing dark rust and copper shades with a bit of sage green. Pair this with brown eyeliner and mascara.
- If you have tan skin and dark or brunette hair, try a deep peach or plum. Pair this with brown or black eyeliner and mascara.

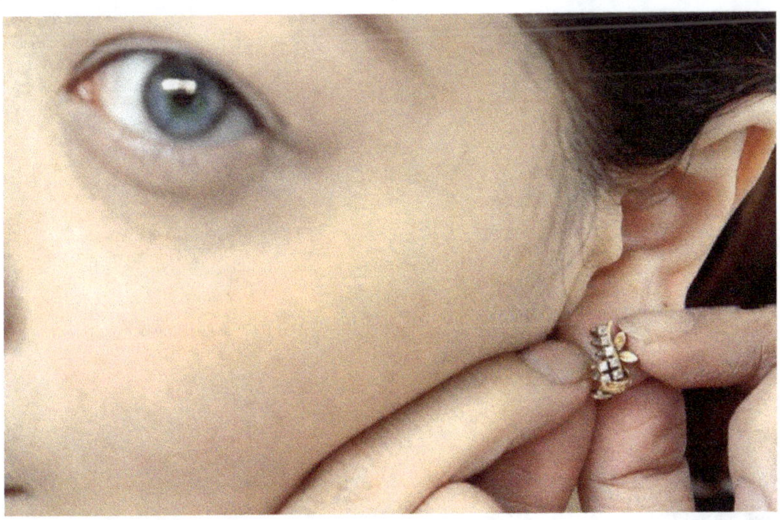

6. Choose an eyeshadow color to match the occasion. If you have difficulties from choosing an

eyeshadow color, you can narrow your choices down by matching the color to the occasion. Here are some examples:

- If you are going to work or school stick with brown, rose, terracotta and neutral shades.
- Lavender and light purples work well for daytime events, while deep plum works best for evening events.
- If you are going out on a date or a fancy dinner, consider using a metallic eyeshadow, such as gold, silver, shimmery pink, and shimmery turquoise.

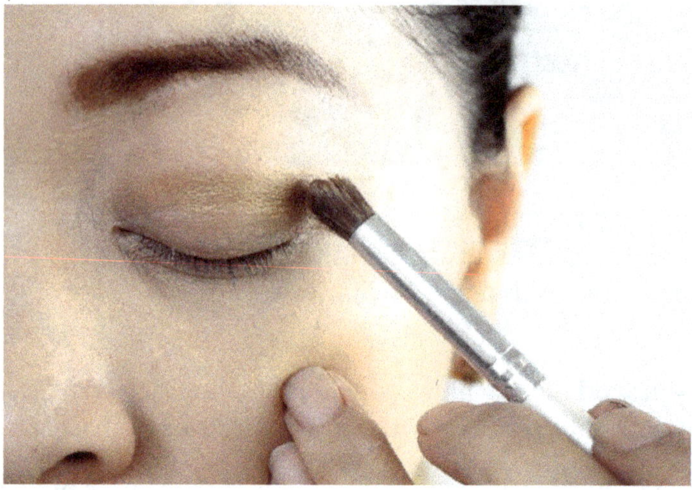

7. Consider using bronzer instead of eyeshadow. For a subtle golden effect, dust a little bit of bronzer in the crease of your eyelid. Using your fingers or a makeup brush, blend it into the rest of your eyeshadow. The light should catch the bronzer just enough to bring out the blue tints in your eyes.

- Use liquid bronzer beneath eyeshadow. If your bronzer isn't in powdered form, use it as eyeshadow primer. Rub a little over your eyelid, then lightly layer your normal eyeshadow on top.

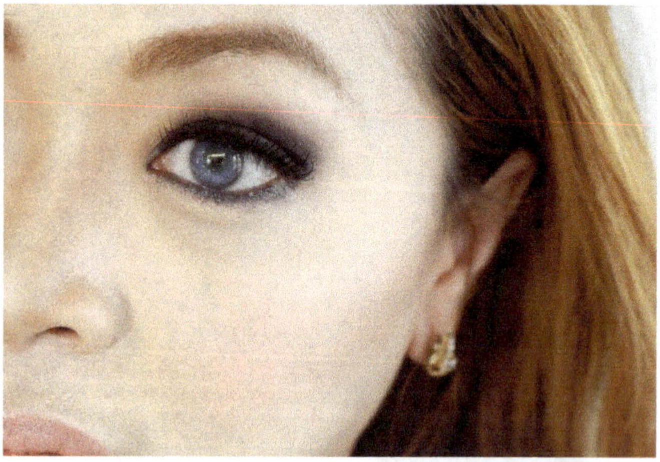

8. Try a modified smoky eye. Instead of using heavy blacks and grays to create a smoky look, try dark brown, gold and dusky pink. The warm tones will showcase your eyes.

Part 2

Using the Right Colors of Eyeliner

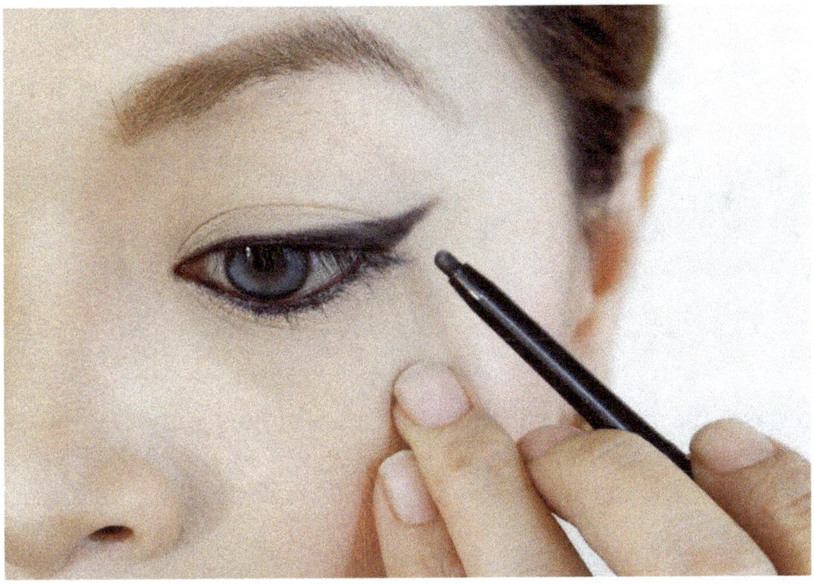

1. Use black eyeliner with care. Black might be too cool and overpowering for blue eyes, especially if you have light-colored hair; however, if used correctly, it can really bring out your eyes. Consider using liquid eyeliner to apply a thin line along your upper lid, and extend it just past the lash line in a wingtip.

- For a less intense look, consider using charcoal or gray instead.

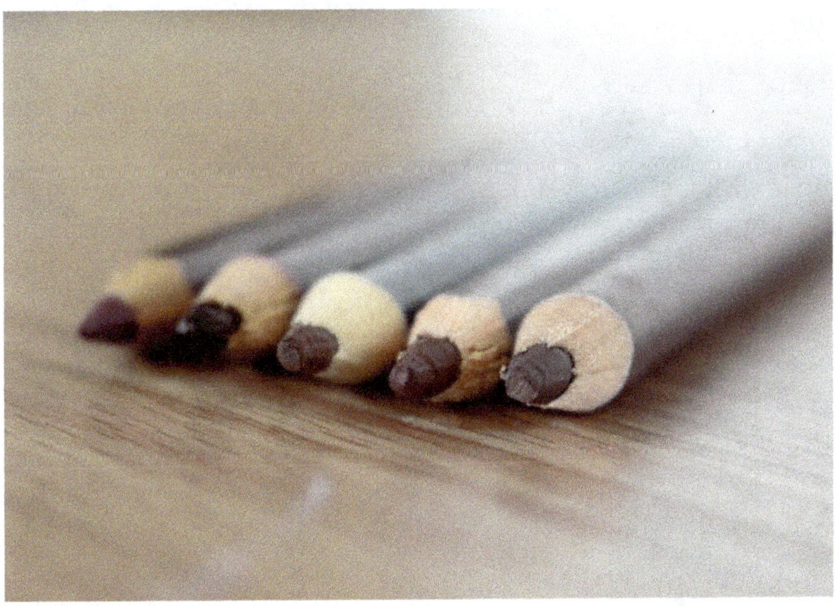

2. Consider using eyeliner in neutral shades. The warm tones found in brown or taupe will contrast with your blue eyes, making them appear brighter. Neutral-toned eyeliner works best for work, school, and daytime events.

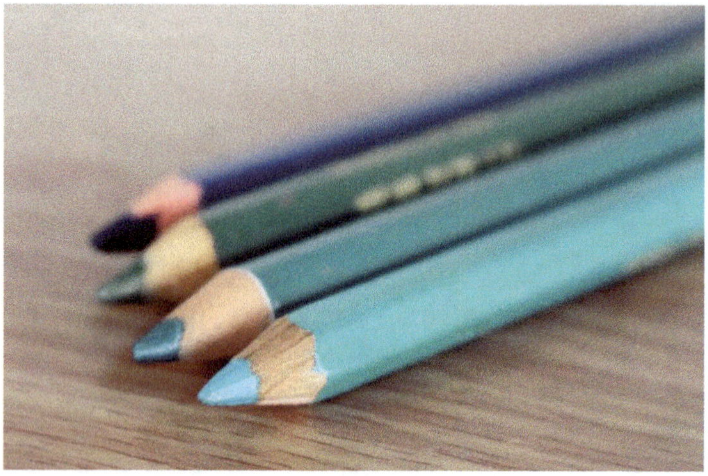

3. Try a cool-colored eyeliner. Colors such as purple, midnight blue, teal, or turquoise will bring out the blue in your eyes, making them appear brighter. Green-toned eyeliner, such as teal or turquoise, works especially well with blue-green eyes, as it will bring out the green flecks.

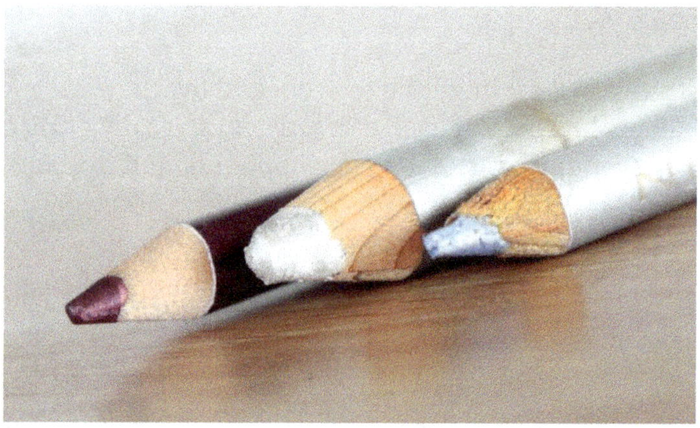

4. Add some shimmer with metallic eyeliner. Colors such as bronze, copper, gold, or silver will not only make your eyes appear brighter, but they will also add some sparkle when you blink.

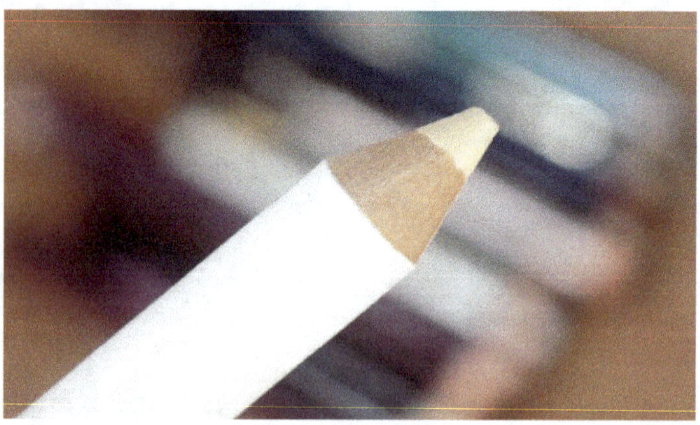

5. Try beige eyeliner on lower lashes. Instead of using a white eyeliner to disguise your waterline

(the pink area between your lashes and your eyes), try beige. It'll blend in with your skin better, and the warmth will draw out the color of your eyes.

Part 3

Using the Right Colors of Mascara

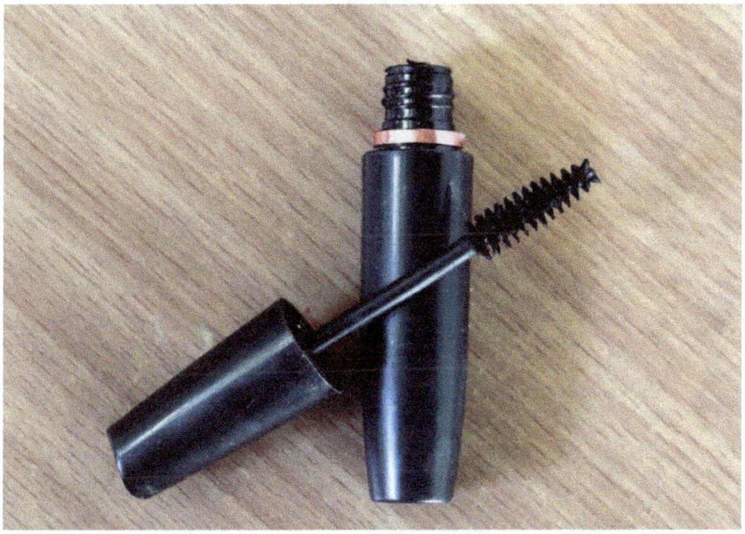

1. Use black mascara freely. Black mascara is classic, and suitable for all eye colors, including blue. Consider using something with lengthening properties. Because of its intensity, however, black mascara works best for evening events. Here are some more suggestions:

- For a less-harsh look, reach for dark brown, dark blue, or charcoal mascara.

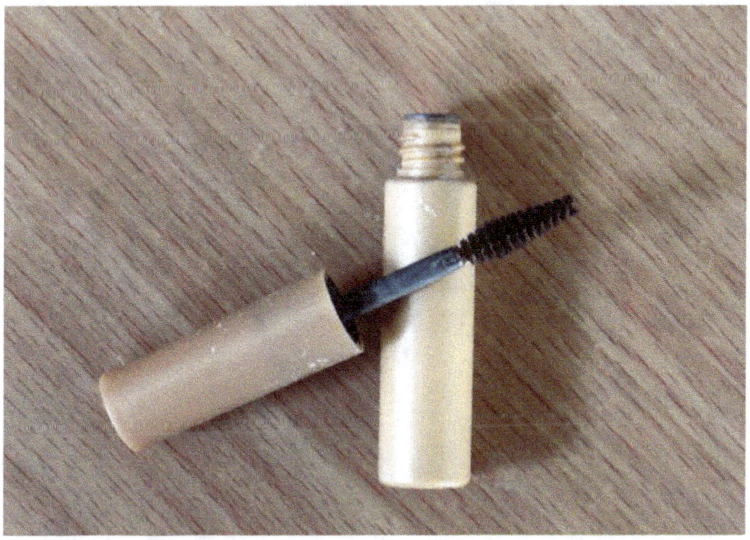

2. Reach for the brown mascara. It will also give you a softer look, that is perfect for work, school, and other daytime events. Brown mascara works especially well for those with blonde, light brown, or lighter red hair; it will give you a more natural but still well-defined look.

- Dark brown mascara will create a subtle contrast with your blue eyes, making them appear brighter.

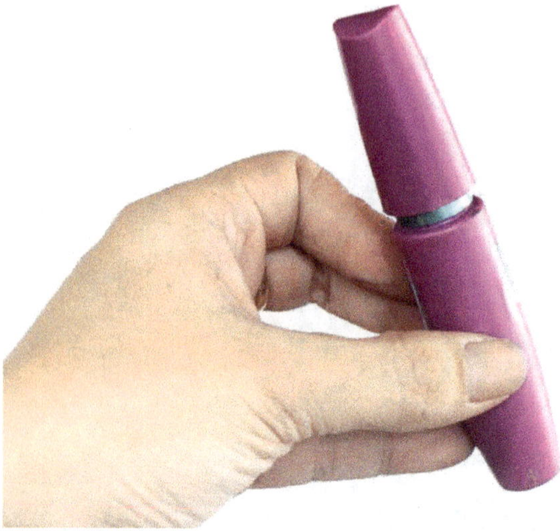

3. Try cool colors. Mascara doesn't have to be black or brown. You can also use some colored mascara. Not all colors will work with blue eyes, however. Here are some suggestions for colored mascara that will help your eyes appear brighter:

- Dark blue mascara can draw attention to your eyes without overpowering them. It will give you a similar look that black mascara gives you, without being as harsh.
- Turquoise mascara is great for those with blue-green eyes. It will help brink out the flecks of green, making your eyes appear brighter.
- Wear purple mascara to bring out the blue in your eyes. If you have a warmer skin undertone, consider using a warmer purple, such as plum. If you have a cooler skin undertone, use a cooler purple, like violet.

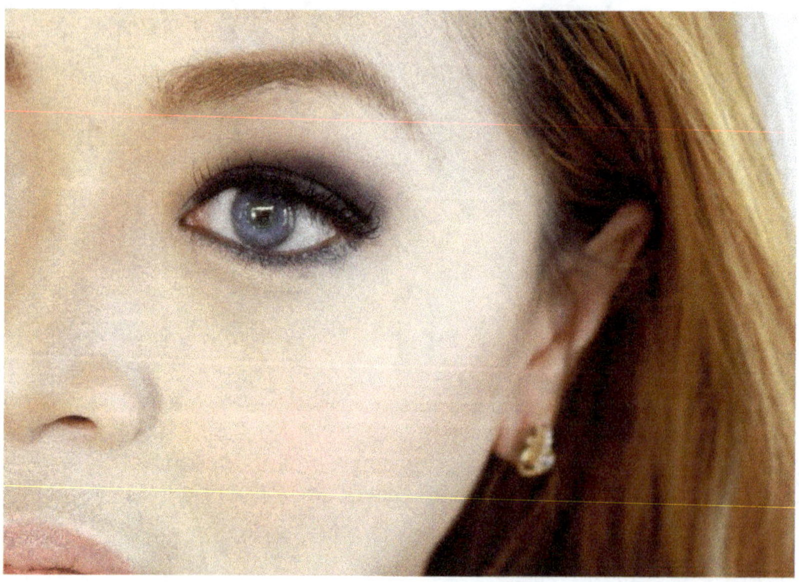

How to Remove Eye Makeup Instantly

Fast removal of eye makeup is important for those nights when you come home late and want to drop into bed as quickly as possible. There is no need to purchase expensive products, however, as you can rely on simple products already in your home: vegetable oils and lotion.

Steps

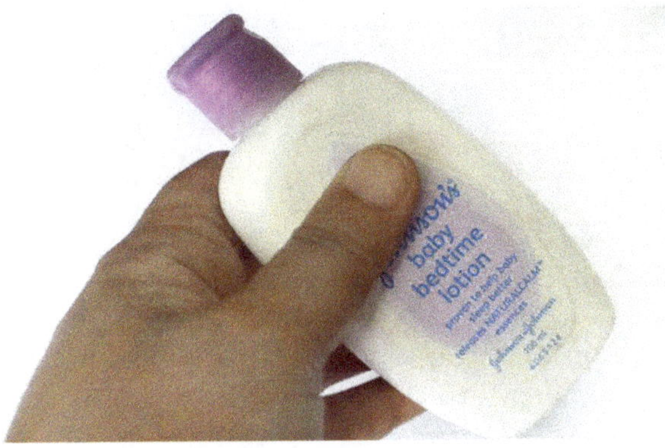

1. Grab a bottle of gentle, unscented lotion (baby lotion works particularly well) or a type of vegetable oil, including olive oil (recommended), coconut oil, sesame oil, jojoba oil, and wheat germ oil. Head to a bathroom sink where you can wash your face.

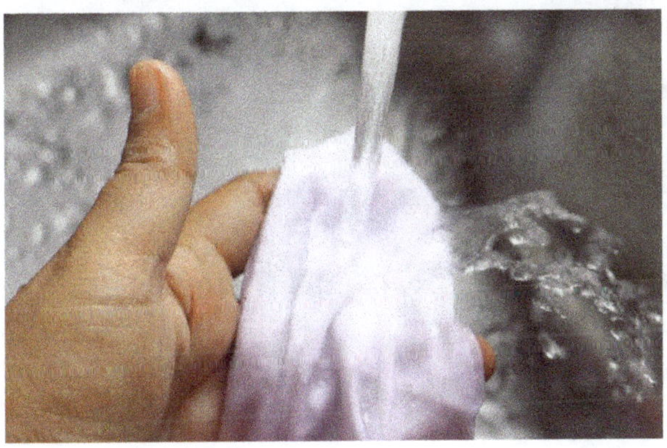

2. Assemble a washcloth or towel. Run it under warm water and wring it out thoroughly so that it is damp.

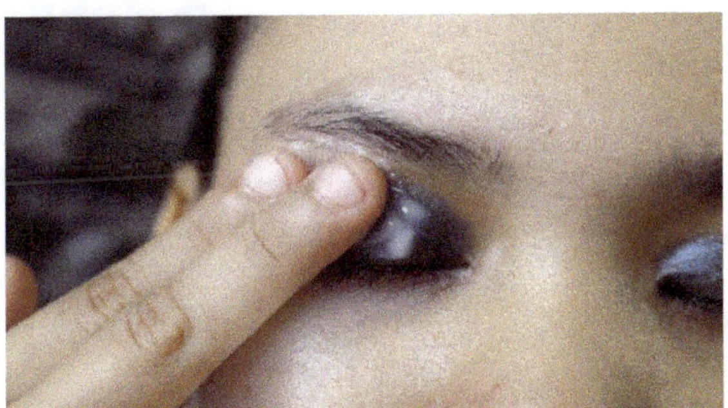

3. Place a dime-sized portion of lotion or vegetable oil on your eyes, rubbing it thoroughly onto

your eyelid. Be careful not to get the product in your eyes, as it will cause your makeup to run into your eye and irritate it. The vegetable oil will break down the formulation of eyeliner and eyeshadows, making them easier to remove.

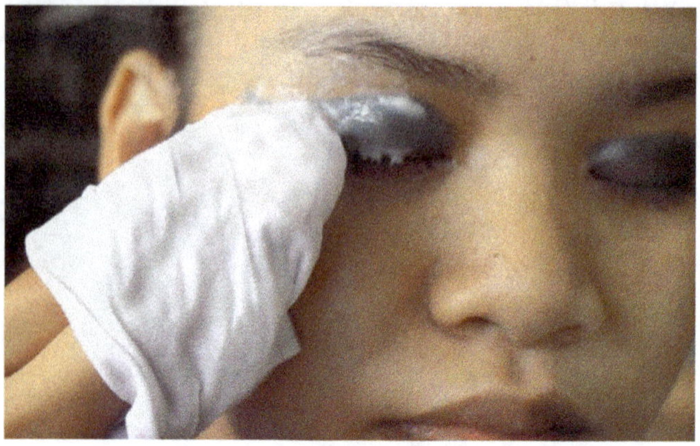

4. Wipe off the lotion or oil with the damp washcloth (or a disposable napkin/tissue). Rinse your eyelids thoroughly -- again, taking care to not let anything get into your eyes. All the eye makeup should come off seamlessly.

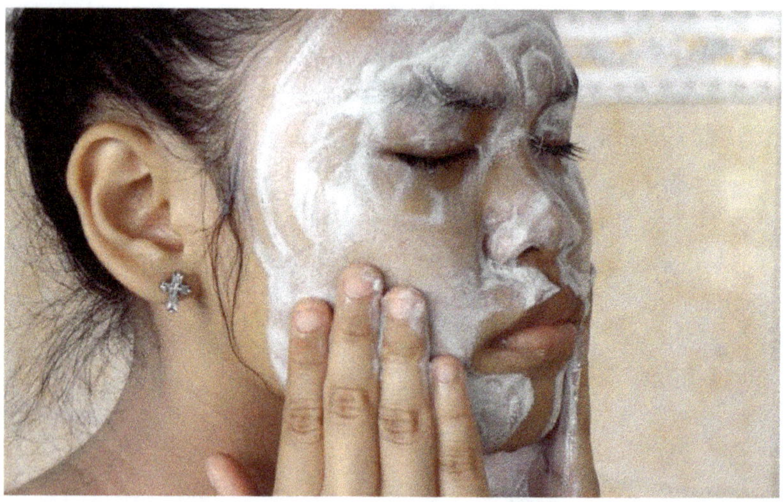

5. If you have the time, follow this procedure by washing your face with a gentle, makeup-removing facial cleanser, such as the First Aid Beauty Face Cleanser or Camaieu Perfuma's Waterless Milk Cleanser. Use something that removes makeup, surface oils and other grime that can collect on your face for the best deep clean.

Permissions

All chapters in this book are published with permission under the Creative Commons Attribution Share Alike License or equivalent. Every chapter published in this book has been scrutinized by our experts. Their significance has been extensively debated. The topics covered herein carry significant information for a comprehensive understanding. They may even be implemented as practical applications or may be referred to as a beginning point for further studies.

We would like to thank the editorial team for lending their expertise to make the book truly unique. They have played a crucial role in the development of this book. Without their invaluable contributions this book wouldn't have been possible. They have made vital efforts to compile up to date information on the varied aspects of this subject to make this book a valuable addition to the collection of many professionals and students.

This book was conceptualized with the vision of imparting up-to-date and integrated information in this field. To ensure the same, a matchless editorial board was set up. Every individual on the board went through rigorous rounds of assessment to prove their worth. After which they invested a large part of their time researching and compiling the most relevant data for our readers.

The editorial board has been involved in producing this book since its inception. They have spent rigorous hours researching and exploring the diverse topics which have resulted in the successful publishing of this book. They have passed on their knowledge of decades through this book. To expedite this challenging task, the publisher supported the team at every step. A small team of assistant editors was also appointed to further simplify the editing procedure and attain best results for the readers.

Apart from the editorial board, the designing team has also invested a significant amount of their time in understanding the subject and creating the most relevant covers. They scrutinized every image to scout for the most suitable representation of the subject and create an appropriate cover for the book.

The publishing team has been an ardent support to the editorial, designing and production team. Their endless efforts to recruit the best for this project, has resulted in the accomplishment of this book. They are a veteran in the field of academics and their pool of knowledge is as vast as their experience in printing. Their expertise and guidance has proved useful at every step. Their uncompromising quality standards have made this book an exceptional effort. Their encouragement from time to time has been an inspiration for everyone.

The publisher and the editorial board hope that this book will prove to be a valuable piece of knowledge for students, practitioners and scholars across the globe.

Index

www.ingramcontent.com/pod-product-compliance
Lightning Source LLC
LaVergne TN
LVHW080924210926
848485LV00004B/718